The Patient's Desk Reference

DISCLAIMER

The authors and publisher of *The Patient's Desk Reference* are not licensed health professionals; consequently, they are not recommending or endorsing any health or medical advice or treatment mentioned in any of the information sources cited herein. This book was written solely for the purpose of helping the reader identify some of the medical and health information sources that are available to the public. No professional evaluation of the medical accuracy or appropriateness of any source is intended. The authors and publisher disclaim liability for any direct or indirect medical or health consequences that may arise from the use of this book or any sources cited in it. The reader should consult with a health care professional before undergoing treatment.

The Patient's Desk Reference

Where to Find Answers to Medical Questions

Melvyn N. Freed, Ph.D.
Karen J. Graves, M.S.L.S.

Macmillan Publishing Company
NEW YORK

Maxwell Macmillan Canada
TORONTO

Maxwell Macmillan International
NEW YORK   OXFORD   SINGAPORE   SYDNEY

Macmillan Publishing Company
866 Third Avenue
New York, NY 10022

Maxwell Macmillan Canada, Inc.
1200 Eglinton Avenue East, Suite 200
Don Mills, Ontario M3C 3N1

Macmillan Publishing Company is part of the Maxwell Communication Group of Companies.

Library of Congress Catalog Card Number: 93-10267

Printed in the United States of America

printing number
1 2 3 4 5 6 7 8 9 10

Library of Congress Cataloging-in-Publication Data

Freed, Melvyn N.
    The patient's desk reference : where to find answers to medical questions / Melvyn N. Freed, Karen J. Graves.
        p.   cm.
    Includes bibliographical references and index.
    ISBN 0–02–897153–1
    1. Medicine, Popular. 2. Medicine—Information services.
3. Medicine—Bibliography. I. Graves, Karen J. II. Title.
RC81.F865 1993
610—dc20   93-10267
                                                      CIP

The paper used in this publication meets the minimum requirements of American National Standard for Information Sciences—Permanence of Paper for Printed Library Materials. ANSI Z39.48-1984.   ∞™

Contents

Preface   *ix*

CHAPTER 1   In Search of Health Information   1

    Diagnosing the Problem   *1*

    The Treatment   *2*

    Choosing the Medicine   *3*

CHAPTER 2   Where Should I Go to Find Health Information
in Printed Sources?   5

    Agencies, Organizations, Associations, Boards, and Companies   *5*

    Aging and the Aged   *13*

    Alternative Medical Care   *14*

    The Body's Structure and Functions   *16*

    Childhood and Adolescent Health   *18*

    Definitions   *31*

    Dental Health   *33*

    The Disabled   *38*

    Diseases and Disorders of Adults   *39*

    Drugs: Use and Abuse   *54*

    First Aid   *61*

    Food Facts   *63*

    Health and Matters of Law   *72*

    Health Care Centers and Services   *73*

    Health Care Equipment and Prosthetics   *82*

    Health Care Professionals   *83*

    Health Information Source Listings   *86*

v

Mental Health	*88*
Occupational Health and Safety	*92*
Physical Fitness and Sports	*92*
Poisons and Non-Toxins	*95*
Rehabilitation	*96*
Sexuality, Reproduction, and Genetics	*97*
Surgery	*102*

CHAPTER 3	Descriptive Profiles of Printed Sources	105
	Abstracts and Indexes	*106*
	Bibliographies	*107*
	Books	*110*
	Dictionaries	*119*
	Directories	*120*
	Encyclopedias and Handbooks	*130*
	Government Documents	*143*
	Loose-leaf Materials	*143*
	Newsletters	*145*
	Reports	*150*

CHAPTER 4	Where Should I Go to Find Health Information in Computerized Databases?	151
	Alternative Medical Care	*152*
	Associations and Organizations	*152*
	The Body's Structure and Functions	*153*
	Definitions	*153*
	Dental Health	*153*
	The Disabled	*154*
	Diseases	*154*
	Drugs: Use and Abuse	*156*
	Food Facts	*157*
	Geriatrics	*157*
	Health Care Centers and Services	*158*
	Health Care Equipment and Prosthetics	*158*
	Health Care Professionals	*159*
	Health and Matters of Law	*159*
	Mental Health	*160*

Occupational Health and Safety   *161*

Pediatric and Adolescent Diseases   *161*

Physical Fitness   *162*

Rehabilitation   *162*

Sex and Reproduction   *163*

Sports Medicine   *163*

Surgery   *163*

Toxicology   *164*

CHAPTER 5   Descriptive Profiles of Computerized Databases   165

CHAPTER 6   Where Should I Go to Find Health Information in Organizations?   173

Information About Health Centers   *173*

Information About Health Professionals   *174*

Information About Health Problems   *180*

Information About Health Procedures   *192*

Other Health Information   *196*

CHAPTER 7   Health Organizations Listed According to the Type of Medical Question   203

Organizations According to Information About Health Centers   *203*

Organizations According to Information About Health Professionals   *205*

Organizations According to Information About Specific Health Problems   *224*

Organizations According to Information About Specific Health Procedures   *254*

Organizations According to Other Health Information   *263*

CHAPTER 8   Where Should I Go to Find Information in the U.S. Department of Health and Human Services?   277

Information About Health Problems   *278*

Information About Health Procedures   *282*

Other Health-Related Information   *282*

CHAPTER 9   Profiles of Clearinghouses and Information Centers of the U.S. Department of Health and Human Services   285

CHAPTER 10   Guide to State Sources of Health Information   293

APPENDIX I   Directory of Print Publishers   331

APPENDIX II   Directory of Computer Database Publishers and Vendors   339

APPENDIX III   Directory of Non-Governmental Health Organizations   343

Index   *371*

Preface

Here is the layperson's guide to medical and other health information. Although this book is not a substitute for the professional advice of one's personal physician, it will help the would-be patient and patient find information that supplements the doctor's explanation and treatment. Medical care must be personalized; consequently, no publication can replace the care given by a professional health provider.

The authors recognize that no book of this type can address all medical topics; however, many health questions of popular concern have been included. A series of volumes would be necessary for this to be an all-inclusive publication.

The Patient's Desk Reference is a unique presentation of health information sources. Instead of being a traditional annotated bibliography, it provides a more analytical and detailed review. In the process, this book presents many of the commonly recognized publications along with lesser-known ones that may be of equal value in a given search. Due to the diversity of library collections and their varying degrees of completeness, the authors have often informed the reader of several titles to enhance the probability of finding an answer to the medical question.

Until now, it has been difficult to determine the specific and detailed contents of printed reference materials without actually examining them. For books, the researcher has had to consult the publication itself, unlike journal articles on a subject that can be identified by resorting to one of the journal indexing services or a parallel CD-ROM or online service. Knowing the title or general subject of a publication is insufficient because it does not disclose whether a specific information item has been included. Subject card catalogs and traditional annotated bibliographies are of limited value. *The Patient's Desk Reference* seeks to alleviate this situation by revealing significant features of the titles cited by using a series of questions and answers. Each question highlights a different important feature of the information source. In many cases, several sources with the same feature have been cited. For example,

WHERE SHOULD I GO TO FIND . . .	*TRY*
questions to be asked by a patient when being advised by a physician to enter a hospital?	*How to Talk to Your Doctor* [3-34] *Take This Book to the Hospital With You* [3-50]

Thus the reader locates the needed information with this efficient and succinct approach. Supplementing this feature-question format is a brief description of each source and the address and telephone number of its publisher.

The feature-questions have been classified, first, under broad subject areas and, second, under more specific topics. To assist the reader, the feature-questions oftentimes have been placed in more than one category; that is, the question appears wherever the researcher may logically search. This approach will enhance one's ability to locate the information source vis-à-vis the traditional single-entry classification.

The authors understand that no library can shelve every publication in the field of health. For this reason, multiple titles have often been cited in the event that any single one is not available to the researcher. Furthermore, since similar publications still have their individual uniqueness, the listing of several titles expands one's choice and resources.

Following each title in Chapter 2 is a bracketed item entry number. This will aid the reader in locating the title in Chapter 3, where an expanded description will be found. This includes the full bibliographic citation and a more comprehensive description of the contents. (Note: A similar system is used in Chapters 4 and 5 regarding computer databases.) The reader can find the name of the publisher in the citation and then, if necessary, refer to Appendix I for the publisher's address and telephone number.

The item entry number has several components, namely, the chapter number and the title number. Thus 3-1 means Chapter 3, title number 1. Following is a sample feature-question.

Sample

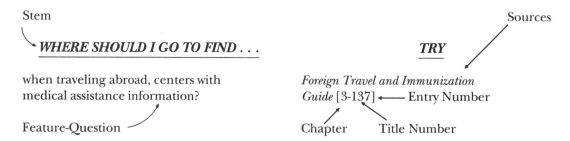

Stem

Sources

WHERE SHOULD I GO TO FIND . . .

TRY

when traveling abroad, centers with medical assistance information?

Foreign Travel and Immunization Guide [3-137] ◀——— Entry Number

Feature-Question

Chapter   Title Number

When using Chapter 2, the reader should first select the proper general category and then proceed to the subcategory. Due to the different approaches that individual authors have taken to common topics, it was necessary to craft carefully the feature-questions. Occasionally, several feature-questions may appear to be repetitive; however, upon closer examination, important technical differences will be discovered. For the most efficient approach to using Chapter 2, the authors suggest reading as a cluster all questions related to the subject being researched. This will broaden the scope of the inquiry and introduce more possibilities for finding the answer.

Some of the reference works contain a diversity of facts, and occasionally there are multiple publications with the same purpose. Although they have a common objective, they usually have subtle differences. If several titles have been listed in response to a feature-question, it is possible that each title may provide different components of the answer. One or more may offer the complete response, while others contain a partial response. All of the titles, either alone or together, will give the full information. This approach permits the reader to identify more materials.

Among the valuable resources for health information are magazines and journals. The former are usually targeted for a nontechnical readership, whereas the latter are written for the health professional. There are numerous magazines in the different health fields. Each has its purpose and its intended audience. Due to the enormous number of magazines and journals, it was decided that they could not be adequately and satisfactorily treated in this volume along with other sources; consequently, the reader is referred to such cumulative indexes as *Reader's Guide to Periodical Literature* [3-4], *Index Medicus* [3-2], *Index to Dental Literature* [3-3], and to other sources cited in "Health Information Source Listings," a section of Chapter 2.

The mention of any single information source should not be interpreted as an endorsement; each citation is meant only to direct the reader's attention to its existence and to the type of information contained within it. Furthermore, the accuracy of the content of each title is the responsibility of the author(s) of that publication. There is no expressed or implied warranty as to the accuracy or completeness of any materials described herein. Nevertheless, the authors of *The Patient's Desk Reference* have endeavored to be diligent in the pursuit of their responsibilities as laypersons as they worked with the publications of others. This collection of information sources should be regarded as only a sample of the health information materials that are available to the public.

While conducting research for this book we profiled the latest edition of each publication; however, due to the time required for the total process of researching, writing, and publishing, newer editions may have been released subsequent to the preparation of any single profile. This was beyond the authors' control.

Whether a reader uses the chapters on printed sources, computer databases, organizations, or government agencies, this book is a place to start. The reader's journey through the literature will reveal many other sources that will be valuable in the search for knowledge about the human body and its state of health.

1

In Search of Health Information

Diagnosing the Problem

Where oh where can I find the answer to my medical question? This dilemma confronts almost everyone at different times in his or her life. With the advent of computers and the explosion of knowledge, we are almost drowning in information. It is everywhere; yet without guidance on where to look, it is nowhere. Whether the inquirer be a professional or a layperson, the challenge is to locate the answer, and in a timely manner. There are so many sources from which to choose. Which one contains the answer? Help is needed! This book is the layperson's guide through this maze of information.

Effective health care is a team effort between the patient and the health-care provider. Each person must share responsibility for his or her health. This obligation involves knowing when and how to select a physician or dentist, being able to carry out the medical instructions issued by the health professional, and practicing responsible self-care at home. In this era of highly sophisticated medical care, information is the essential prescription.

To secure the information that is necessary, the patient and the would-be patient must know where to find it. Even before visiting a physician, an individual must become informed. Oftentimes during and following treatment additional information is wanted. The doctor alone cannot be the sole source. Libraries and bookstores are replete with health-related books. The task is to locate the right publication that contains the relevant information. This is not easily accomplished.

As a consequence of living in the Information Age, we are required to select from multiple information sources. First, we must be aware of the different sources: books, magazines, journals, newsletters, special reports, computerized databases, health organizations, governmental agencies, and the news media. Next, we must be capable of selecting the one(s) that is most likely to have the needed information. Finally, we must identify the specific information source, i.e., the individual title, organization, or agency. Only then can the answer be found. This process can appear to be insurmountable; hence the reason for this book. Its purpose is to assist the layperson in locating answers to health questions.

Medical research is unveiling new truths almost daily. Myths of health care are being superseded with scientific facts. The rate of discovery is challenging the health professional to keep abreast. For the layperson, this pace can be overwhelming. Today's revelation may become obsolete tomorrow.

People are becoming more involved in their own health care than ever before. They are seeking information on how to stay healthy, and when they are not well, they are being assertive and demanding the latest and best that medicine has to offer. Second and third opinions are being sought. Many patients are insisting on being well informed.

The Treatment

Seek and ye shall find: the operating assumption of this admonition is that the precise question is known. If the question is vague, the pursuit of an answer will be difficult. The first step is to know exactly what is needed. General questions produce general answers which usually are not useful.

There are several notable bibliographies of health publications. These are organized by topic; however, it often remains a difficult task to find the right information source. The title-by-subject approach is not focused enough to enable the researcher to determine if a specific item of information is contained in a given title. There is need for the question-and-answer format provided in this book.

The vigorous quest for medical facts coupled with the prolific advances in research has given rise to new information delivery systems. Not only are there the traditional printed materials; access to information can now be made via computerized online and offline databases. Online databases are those that have been stored in a central computer, and access is made via a modem to another computer. Offline databases are stored locally on a disc using a CD-ROM reader accessed by a personal computer. Both types of databases may be updated frequently, thus minimizing the obsolescence of information.

Persons who are searching for medical information are served by various interactive sources. In cases of medical emergency, information may be promptly required. Helplines and hotlines are useful. For both these forms of assistance, use of designated 800-number telephone lines can provide timely information, especially when the emergency involves poisoning, substance abuse, or emergency counseling. These numbers can be found in the local telephone directory or in one of the sources described in this book.

Local, regional, and national health organizations are rich depositories of health information, as are appropriate state and federal agencies. Again, some types of information are not readily available in published form. When this occurs, contact the health organization or government agency that serves the health matter under concern. Where to identify these groups can be found in Chapters 6–10.

It is because the health field is so technical and complex that not all medical information exists in a form that is understandable to the layperson. Scientific terms often confound the reader. To avoid this situation, seek assistance from a reference librarian who can disclose sources that are suitable for the medical nonprofessional. In most cases, this book will lead the reader to materials that do not require specialized education to be understood. Readers with different levels of understanding of medical information will be served by the chapters that follow.

Important for any lay consumer wanting to acquire medical information is knowing the right type of library to visit. There are different kinds of libraries. Some are community libraries that are dedicated to serving the general public. Although some highly technical materials can be found in their collections, most titles are suitable for the majority of lay readers.

There are libraries with collections that have been intended for readers with specialized training. These are known as special libraries. In the case of health, a medical library will usually feature publications that are beyond the understanding of a nonprofessional. The materials are research oriented and require a sophisticated understanding of biological and medical principles and concepts.

Choosing the Medicine

How do you know what to read? In the health field, there are numerous authors of books and magazine articles. Their opinions are diverse and often contradictory, even on matters of life and death. How should you select from among the multiplicity of materials from various authors?

First, recognize that the printed word is not sacrosanct. Understand that albeit medicine is scientific, its practice is also an art. Different scientific approaches can be taken to establish a scientific fact. Authors often write with these different approaches in mind, and this will determine the direction of the writing. Recognize any bias.

What is the author's philosophic school of medicine? Different areas of medicine operate with different philosophies, as is illustrated by traditional medicine vis-à-vis the various nonconventional approaches to health care, such as acupuncture, homeopathy, naturopathy, herbalism, and others. Knowing the underlying conceptual principles will help you to understand the remedies that are being advocated.

For current findings of research, magazines and journals offer the most up-to-date reporting. Again, which publications are suitable depends on the educational level of the reader because many articles require some degree of scientific sophistication to be understood. Specialized newsletters are published that address a specific medical disorder, such as diabetes or Alzheimer's disease, and these, quite often, are intended for lay readers. They discuss matters that are of concern to the patient and to his or her family, such as how to care for the patient at home.

If the search is for the name, address, telephone number, and descriptive information about a health care facility or organization, consult an appropriate directory. This book identifies numerous specialized directories. An example is the *Directory of Pain Treatment Centers in the U.S. and Canada* and *Substance Abuse Residential Treatment Centers for Teens*. If a medical definition is wanted, check a medical dictionary, such as *Dorland's Illustrated Medical Dictionary*. A specialized medical dictionary may offer a more extensive explanation than that which is to be found in a general dictionary.

The amount of information that is being sought will help a reader to decide which publication to choose. If only a cursory overview is needed, refer to a medical encyclopedia, such as the *American Medical Association Encyclopedia of Medicine*. If the need is for more complete information, seek either a book that is devoted to that subject or one that devotes a chapter to it. The treatment of subjects varies. It helps to know what and how much information is wanted before pursuing your search.

Fads abound among health publications. This is especially true for subjects like dieting, weight loss, and exercising. As with any other subject, determine the qualifications of the author. What is his or her educational background and experience?

Has the book been endorsed by a recognized health authority? Know the source of knowledge before you commit to it. In the pursuit of health information, as in any other field, the consumer must be vigilant by discriminating between authority and charlatanism. The selection of medical information sources places a special responsibility with the consumer. Be aware! Be discriminating! Be informed!

2

Where Should I Go to Find Health Information in Printed Sources?

In this chapter is a selection of information sources that have been published in printed form. The medical questions and the sources in which their answers may be found are arranged under twenty-four major sections with each section containing numerous subcategories. For an explanation of the format and methodology of this chapter, see the Preface to this book.

Printed Sources of Information

WHERE SHOULD I GO TO FIND . . .   *TRY*

> **Agencies, Organizations, Associations, Boards, and Companies**

Associations and Organizations

a listing of addresses and telephone numbers for health associations and organizations that focus on the different diseases and disorders and that provide information and self-help services?

See Chapter 7.
AIDS and Women: A Sourcebook [3-5]
AIDS Information Sourcebook [3-67]
American Cancer Society Cancer Book [3-17]
American Medical Association Encyclopedia of Medicine [3-107]
Complete Guide to Early Child Care [3-118]

(*answer continues*)

WHERE SHOULD I GO TO FIND. . .   *TRY*

Associations and Organizations

a listing of addresses and telephone numbers for health associations and organizations that focus on the different diseases and disorders and that provide information and self-help services?

Complete Home Medical Guide [3-124]
Consumer Health Information Source Book [3-8]
Encyclopedia of Associations, Vol. 1 [3-82]
Encyclopedia of Medical Organizations and Agencies [3-83]
Health Care U.S.A. [3-85]
Medical and Health Information Directory, Vol. 1 [3-88]
Once A Month (*re* PMS) [3-41]
Physicians' Desk Reference for Nonprescription Drugs [3-154]
Research Centers Directory [3-97]

the names, addresses, and telephone numbers of organizations that can identify practitioners of various alternative approaches to health care, including osteopathy, acupuncture, holistic medicine, biofeedback, and others?

Natural Health, Natural Medicine [3-39]

a directory of medical organizations for health professionals?

See Chapter 7.
Encyclopedia of Associations, Vol. 1 [3-82]
Encyclopedia of Medical Organizations and Agencies [3-83]
Health Care U.S.A. [3-85]
Medical and Health Information Directory, Vol. 1 [3-88]

a directory of professional dental associations and organizations?

American Dental Directory [3-69]
Encyclopedia of Associations, Vol. 1 [3-82]
Encyclopedia of Medical Organizations and Agencies [3-83]
Family Guide to Dental Health [3-133]
Medical and Health Information Directory, Vol. 1 [3-88]

a bibliography of membership lists of professional health associations?

Medical and Health Information Directory, Vol. 2 [3-89]

the locations and telephone numbers of centers of the International Association for Medical Assistance to Travelers (IAMAT)?

Encyclopedia of Medical Organizations and Agencies [3-83]
Foreign Travel and Immunization Guide [3-137]

WHERE SHOULD I GO TO FIND...	*TRY*
Associations and Organizations	
the locations and telephone numbers of centers of the International Association for Medical Assistance to Travelers (IAMAT)?	*Medical and Health Information Directory,* Vol. 1 [3-88]
a listing of state optometric associations with their addresses and telephone numbers?	*Blue Book of Optometrists* [3-72] *Medical and Health Information Directory,* Vol. 1 [3-88]
an explanation of health maintenance organizations (HMOs) and preferred provider organizations (PPOs)?	*Complete Home Medical Guide* [3-124] *HMOs* [3-32]
a directory of health maintenance organizations (HMOs) with their addresses and telephone numbers?	*HMOs* [3-32] *Medical and Health Information Directory,* Vol. 1 [3-88]
a directory of preferred provider organizations (PPOs) with their addresses and telephone numbers?	*HMOs* [3-32] *Medical and Health Information Directory,* Vol. 1 [3-88]
the names of national health information centers and clearinghouses with their purposes, addresses, and telephone numbers?	See Chapter 9. *Consumer Health Information Source Book* [3-8] *Medical and Health Information Directory,* Vol. 2 [3-89]
a directory of private organizations and government agencies that protect or advocate consumer rights in the health field and distribute information that assists consumers with their rights?	*Consumer Sourcebook* [3-73]
a directory of hospital associations of the individual states?	*Encyclopedia of Medical Organizations and Agencies* [3-88] *Medical and Health Information Directory,* Vol. 1 [3-88]
the names and addresses of organizations that provide information on the legal/civil rights of disabled persons?	*Meeting the Needs of People with Disabilities* [3-144]
a description of many of the private organizations that serve people with disabilities, including the organization's purposes, services, and address?	*Meeting the Needs of People with Disabilities* [3-144]

WHERE SHOULD I GO TO FIND. . .   *TRY*

Associations and Organizations

the names and addresses of organizations that provide information and help for drug abuse?	*Drugs, Alcohol, and Your Children* [3-24]
the names, addresses, and telephone numbers of sports organizations for persons with disabilities?	*Encyclopedia of Medical Organizations and Agencies* [3-83] *Health Care U.S.A.* [3-85] *Medical and Health Information Directory,* Vol. 1 [3-88]
the names, addresses, and telephone numbers of national and regional organizations offering information and services regarding fitness and the prevention of sports injuries?	*Medical and Health Information Directory,* Vol. 1 [3-88] *Research Centers Directory* [3-97] *Sportswise* [3-47]
the addresses and telephone numbers of state associations for learning disabilities?	*Encyclopedia of Medical Organizations and Agencies* [3-83] *Medical and Health Information Directory,* Vol. 1 [3-88]
current information on the National Foundation for Ileitis and Colitis?	*National Foundation for Ileitis and Colitis: Foundation Focus* [3-187]
a directory of organizations that provide services pertaining to AIDS?	*AIDS and Women: A Sourcebook* [3-5] *AIDS Information Sourcebook* [3-67] *Surviving with AIDS* [3-49]
a directory of chapters of the National Chronic Pain Outreach Association?	*Directory of Pain Treatment Centers in the U.S. and Canada* [3-78]
organized by state, a listing of premenstrual syndrome clinics and support groups?	*Once A Month* [3-41]

Certifying and Licensing Boards and Agencies

a listing of state medical licensing boards with their addresses and telephone numbers?	See Chapter 10. *Directory of Medical Specialists* [3-76] *Encyclopedia of Medical Organizations and Agencies* [3-83] *Medical and Health Information Directory,* Vol. 1 [3-88] *State Administrative Officials Classified by Function* [3-98] *The State Executive Directory Annual* [3-99] *Surgery* [3-156]

WHERE SHOULD I GO TO FIND. . .	*TRY*
Certifying and Licensing Boards and Agencies	
the addresses and telephone numbers of state licensing boards for osteopathic physicians?	*Encyclopedia of Medical Organizations and Agencies* [3-83] *Medical and Health Information Directory,* Vol. 1 [3-88] *State Administrative Officials Classified by Function* [3-98] *The State Executive Directory Annual* [3-99] *Yearbook and Directory of Osteopathic Physicians* [3-102]
the address and telephone number of a state's agency that licenses hospitals?	*Encyclopedia of Medical Organizations and Agencies* [3-83] *Medical and Health Information Directory,* Vol. 1 [3-88] *State Administrative Officials Classified by Function* [3-98] *The State Executive Directory Annual* [3-99]
a listing of medical specialty boards that certify medical specialists, citing the address, telephone number, purpose, and certification requirements of each board?	See Chapter 7. *ABMS Compendium of Certified Medical Specialists* [3-66] *Directory of Medical Specialists* [3-76] *Encyclopedia of Associations,* Vol. 1 (excludes certification requirements) [3-82] *Encyclopedia of Medical Organizations and Agencies* (excludes certification requirements) [3-83] *Medical and Health Information Directory,* Vol. 1 (excludes certification requirements) [3-88]
a listing of dental specialty certification boards with their addresses and telephone numbers?	*American Dental Directory* [3-69] *Encyclopedia of Associations,* Vol. 1 [3-82] *Encyclopedia of Medical Organizations and Agencies* [3-83] *Medical and Health Information Directory,* Vol. 1 [3-88]
a listing of osteopathic specialty certification boards with their addresses, telephone numbers, and certification requirements?	*Yearbook and Directory of Osteopathic Physicians* [3-102]
the continuing education requirements of state dental boards for the relicensure of dentists?	*American Dental Directory* [3-69]

WHERE SHOULD I GO TO FIND...   *TRY*

Certifying and Licensing Boards and Agencies

a listing of state and/or regional boards of dental examiners?

American Dental Directory [3-69]
Encyclopedia of Medical Organizations and Agencies [3-83]
Medical and Health Information Directory, Vol. 1 [3-88]
State Administrative Officials Classified by Function [3-98]
The State Executive Directory Annual [3-99]

the addresses and telephone numbers of state nursing home administrator examining boards?

Encyclopedia of Medical Organizations and Agencies [3-83]
Medical and Health Information Directory, Vol. 1 [3-88]

a directory of state optometric boards of examiners, citing their addresses and telephone numbers?

Blue Book of Optometrists [3-72]
Medical and Health Information Directory, Vol. 1 [3-88]

the address and telephone number for obtaining information about the disciplinary record of a physician in a specified state?

9479 Questionable Doctors [3-65]

Drug Regulatory Authorities Abroad

a listing of therapeutic drug regulatory authorities in other countries, along with an overview of their drug approval requirements and protocols?

Drugs Available Abroad [3-131]

Government Departments and Agencies

a directory of private organizations and government agencies that protect or advocate consumer rights in the health field and distribute information that assists consumers with their rights?

Consumer Sourcebook [3-73]

the address and telephone number of a state's department of health?

See Chapter 10.
Encyclopedia of Medical Organizations and Agencies [3-83]
Medical and Health Information Directory, Vol. 1 [3-88]

WHERE SHOULD I GO TO FIND. . .   *TRY*

Government Departments and Agencies

the address and telephone number of a
state's department of health?

National Health Directory [3-94]
*State Administrative Officials Classified by
Function* [3-98]
The State Executive Directory Annual [3-99]

the address and telephone number of a
state's bureau of vital records and statistics?

*Encyclopedia of Medical Organizations and
Agencies* [3-83]
Medical and Health Information Directory,
Vol. 1 [3-88]
*State Administrative Officials Classified by
Function* [3-98]
The State Executive Directory Annual [3-99]

a directory of state vocational rehabilitation
agencies?

Meeting the Needs of People with Disabilities
[3-144]
*State Administrative Officials Classified by
Function* [3-98]

a directory of organizations and
government agencies that provide family
planning services?

Medical and Health Information Directory,
Vol. 3 [3-90]

Health Industry Companies

a directory of commercial insurance
companies that offer individual or group
health insurance plans, citing their
addresses and telephone numbers?

Medical and Health Information Directory,
Vol. 1 [3-88]

a directory of Blue Cross and Blue Shield
Plans with their addresses and telephone
numbers?

Medical and Health Information Directory,
Vol. 1 [3-88]

a directory of Delta Dental Insurance Plans
with their addresses and telephone
numbers?

Medical and Health Information Directory,
Vol. 1 [3-88]

a directory of pharmaceutical
manufacturers abroad with their addresses
and telephone numbers?

Drugs Available Abroad [3-131]
International Directory of Corporate Affiliations
[3-87]
Principal International Businesses [3-95]

a directory of suppliers of medical products?

Medical Device Register [3-91]
(answer continues)

WHERE SHOULD I GO TO FIND. . .	*TRY*
Health Industry Companies	
a directory of suppliers of medical products?	*Medical Device Register: International* Volume [3-92]
the addresses and telephone numbers of manufacturers of food products for allergen-free diets?	*Allergy Encyclopedia* [3-103]
a listing of published business and market research reports on companies in the health care industry?	*Findex* [3-10]
Health Officials	
a listing of state and U.S. territorial directors of dental health?	*American Dental Directory* [3-69]
the names, addresses, and telephone numbers of federal, state, city, and county health officials and members of legislative health committees?	*National Health Directory* [3-94]
Libraries and Research Centers	
the addresses and telephone numbers of libraries with special services for the blind and physically handicapped?	*Medical and Health Information Directory,* Vol. 3 [3-90]
a directory of special library collections in the health sciences that lists the specialties, locations, and other descriptive information?	*Directory of Special Libraries and Information Centers* [3-80] *Medical and Health Information Directory,* Vol. 2 [3-89]
the services that libraries offer to persons with disabilities?	*Meeting the Needs of People with Disabilities* [3-144]
a directory of research centers, institutes, and other nonprofit research organizations in the medical and health sciences?	*Research Centers Directory* [3-97]
Trade Shows	
a directory of medical trade shows, citing their dates, locations, and other descriptive facts?	*Medical Device Register* [3-91]

WHERE SHOULD I GO TO FIND. . .   *TRY*

Aging and the Aged

The Aging Process

a discussion of the aging process and the
disorders and diseases associated with it?

Complete Home Medical Guide [3-124]
Nutrition Almanac [3-150]
Old Enough to Feel Better [3-40]

answers to questions regarding aging skin?

New Family Medical Guide [3-149]
The Look You Like [3-36]

Care Centers

a directory of nursing homes, by state, that
reports for each home the address,
telephone number, name of administrator,
admission requirements, level of care
licensed to provide, size of staff, and other
descriptive information?

Directory of Nursing Homes [3-77]

a checklist of considerations for selecting a
nursing home?

Complete Home Medical Guide [3-124]
Understanding Alzheimer's Disease [3-52]

a directory of continuing-care retirement
communities with a profile of each
community that includes types of facilities
and services offered, fees, nursing care,
accreditation, address, telephone number,
and other descriptive items?

National Continuing Care Directory [3-93]

an explanation of "continuing care" and
what it involves?

National Continuing Care Directory [3-93]

Diets, Medicines, Tests

dietary guidelines for the older person?

Instructions for Patients [3-139]
New Family Medical Guide [3-149]
Nutrition Almanac [3-150]

general guidelines for the use of drugs by
the elderly?

Essential Guide to Prescription Drugs [3-132]
Old Enough to Feel Better [3-40]

WHERE SHOULD I GO TO FIND...	*TRY*

Diets, Medicines, Tests

special precautions and warnings for the elderly regarding the use of specific therapeutic drugs?	*Complete Guide to Prescription and Non-Prescription Drugs* [3-121] *Essential Guide to Prescription Drugs* [3-132] *Guide to Prescription and Over-the-Counter Drugs* [3-138]
medical diagnostic tests that are recommended for healthy older persons, including the frequency for these tests?	*Complete Book of Medical Tests* [3-116] *The People's Book of Medical Tests* [3-152]

Newsletters

a newsletter that keeps its readers current on matters affecting the elderly?	*AARP Bulletin* [3-166] *Aging Action Alert* [3-168]
a newsletter that provides information on how to care for the elderly?	*Caregivers* [3-180]

Alternative Medical Care

NOTE: To learn where to find practitioners of the different schools of alternative medical care, see the section "Health Care Professionals."

Chiropractic Therapy

an explanation of the field of chiropractic health care?	*Alternatives in Healing* [3-105] *Essential Principles of Chiropractic* [3-26] *Everybody's Guide to Chiropractic Health Care* [3-27] *Health and Healing* [3-30] *Health and Healing: Understanding Conventional and Alternative Medicine* [3-31] *The Confusion About Chiropractors* [3-20]
what comprises the education and training of a chiropractor?	*Everybody's Guide to Chiropractic Health Care* [3-27]
guidelines for selecting a chiropractor?	*Everybody's Guide to Chiropractic Health Care* [3-27]

WHERE SHOULD I GO TO FIND. . .	*TRY*

Chiropractic Therapy

a chiropractic explanation of the effects on health of specific spinal vertebrae and disc misalignments?	*Everybody's Guide to Chiropractic Health Care* [3-27]
exercises recommended by chiropractors that strengthen muscles in the neck, back, and abdomen?	*Everybody's Guide to Chiropractic Health Care* [3-27]

Comparing Therapeutic Alternatives

an explanation of alternative approaches to health, such as acupuncture, homeopathy, medical herbalism, and osteopathy?	*Alternatives in Healing* [3-105] *Health and Healing* [3-30] *Health and Healing: Understanding Conventional and Alternative Medicine* [3-31]
a chart that reports the suitability of each of the following therapies for each of a selection of medical conditions: acupuncture, chiropractic, homeopathy, medical herbalism, osteopathy, and conventional medicine?	*Alternatives in Healing* [3-105]
a comparison of how an acupuncturist, chiropractor, homeopath, medical herbalist, osteopath, and conventional physician would each diagnose and treat specific diseases and disorders?	*Alternatives in Healing* [3-105]

Herbal Suppliers

sources of supplier names for organic produce, vitamins and supplements, freeze-dried herbal extracts, herbal pharmaceutical products, and Chinese medicinal herbs?	*Natural Health, Natural Medicine* [3-39]

Natural Medicine

an explanation of alternative approaches to health, including natural medicine?	*Alternatives in Healing* [3-105] *Health and Healing* [3-30] *Health and Healing: Understanding Conventional and Alternative Medicine* [3-31]

WHERE SHOULD I GO TO FIND. . .	*TRY*

Natural Medicine

what is meant by natural medicine and its approach to wellness and self-care?	*Health and Healing* [3-30] *Natural Health, Natural Medicine* [3-39] *The Complete Book of Natural Medicines* [3-117]
treatment programs for specific ailments as advocated by natural medicine practitioners?	*The Complete Book of Natural Medicines* [3-117]

Newsletters

a newsletter that provides information on new discoveries in the field of natural health care?	*Alternatives* [3-172]

Osteopathic Medicine

an explanation of alternative approaches to health, including osteopathy?	*Alternatives in Healing* [3-105] *Health and Healing* [3-30] *Health and Healing: Understanding Conventional and Alternative Medicine* [3-31]
a listing of osteopathic hospitals in the United States with their addresses and telephone numbers?	*Health Care U.S.A.* [3-85]
a chart showing the spinal column and some of the possible medical disorders that, according to osteopathic medicine, could result from the misalignment of certain vertebrae?	*Alternatives in Healing* [3-105]

The Body's Structure and Functions

Anatomical Illustrations and Explanations

drawings and explanations of the bones, muscles, skin, nerves, blood vessels, organs, and other anatomical features of the human body?	*American Medical Association Encyclopedia of Medicine* [3-107] *Anatomy of the Human Body* [3-108] *Atlas of Human Anatomy* (Illustrations only) [3-109] *Dorland's Illustrated Medical Dictionary* [3-58]

WHERE SHOULD I GO TO FIND. . .   *TRY*

Anatomical Illustrations and Explanations

drawings and explanations of the bones, muscles, skin, nerves, blood vessels, organs, and other anatomical features of the human body?	*Melloni's Illustrated Medical Dictionary* [3-63] *New Family Medical Guide* [3-149] *Stedman's Medical Dictionary* [3-64]
an explanation of the different blood groups (types)?	*American Medical Association Encyclopedia of Medicine* [3-107] *Complete Home Medical Guide* [3-124] *Dorland's Illustrated Medical Dictionary* [3-58] *New Family Medical Guide* [3-149] *Stedman's Medical Dictionary* [3-64]
an explanation of the structure of a gene?	*American Medical Association Encyclopedia of Medicine* [3-107] *New Family Medical Guide* [3-149]
a listing of the principal endocrine glands with an explanation of their respective functions?	*American Medical Association Encyclopedia of Medicine* [3-107] *Complete Guide to Early Child Care* [3-118] *New Family Medical Guide* [3-149]
by age, what the normal heart rate should be?	*Warning Symptoms* [3-159]
an explanation of the nervous system and the effects of spinal misalignments according to chiropractic?	*Everybody's Guide to Chiropractic Health Care* [3-27]
the normal physical characteristics of newborn infants?	*Complete Guide to Early Child Care* [3-118]
the growth and development schedule of babies during their first year?	*Complete Guide to Early Child Care* [3-118] *New Family Medical Guide* [3-149]

Dental Features

drawings and explanations of dental features of the mouth?	*Anatomy of the Human Body* [3-108] *Atlas of Human Anatomy* (Illustrations only) [3-109] *Dorland's Illustrated Medical Dictionary* [3-58] *Family Guide to Dental Health* [3-133] *Illustrated Dictionary of Dentistry* [3-60] *Melloni's Illustrated Medical Dictionary* [3-63]

(*answer continues*)

WHERE SHOULD I GO TO FIND. . .	*TRY*

Dental Features

drawings and explanations of dental features of the mouth?	*New Family Medical Guide* [3-149] *Stedman's Medical Dictionary* [3-64] *Tooth and Gum Care* [3-51] *Why Root Canal Therapy?* [3-55]

Childhood and Adolescent Health

Child Care Services

an explanation of the different types of child care arrangements that may be available to working parents?	*Complete Guide to Early Child Care* [3-118]
what to look for and how to evaluate the quality of a child daycare center?	*Complete Guide to Early Child Care* [3-118]
a checklist to be used when selecting a child daycare center?	*Complete Guide to Early Child Care* [3-118]
the questions that parents should ask about safety when considering a daycare center or school for their child?	*Complete Guide to Early Child Care* [3-118]

Diagnostic Tests and Measurements

which medical tests are used to diagnose each of numerous common diseases and common symptoms, followed by an explanation of each test?	*Complete Book of Medical Tests* [3-116]
an explanation of medical diagnostic tests and procedures, including their purpose, risks, reference values of normality, abnormal values, and/or other information?	*American Medical Association Encyclopedia of Medicine* [3-107] *Complete Book of Medical Tests* [3-116] *Complete Guide to Medical Tests* [3-119] *Complete Home Medical Guide* [3-124] *How to Talk to Your Doctor* [3-34] *Medical Tests and Diagnostic Procedures* [3-143] *New Family Medical Guide* (selected information) [3-149] *Patient's Guide to Medical Tests* [3-151]

WHERE SHOULD I GO TO FIND. . .	*TRY*

Diagnostic Tests and Measurements

an explanation of medical diagnostic tests and procedures, including their purpose, risks, reference values of normality, abnormal values, and/or other information?	*People's Book of Medical Tests* [3-152] *Surgery on File: Pediatrics* [3-165]
the estimated average cost of selected medical tests? (Note: Allow for recent escalating increases.)	*Complete Guide to Medical Tests* [3-119] *Patient's Guide to Medical Tests* [3-151] *People's Book of Medical Tests* [3-152]
questions for the patient to ask about diagnostic tests and procedures that have been recommended by a physician?	*How to Talk to Your Doctor* [3-34] *Take This Book to the Hospital with You* [3-50]
for specific diagnostic tests, an explanation of what is meant by an abnormal result?	*Complete Book of Medical Tests* [3-116] *Complete Guide to Medical Tests* [3-119] *Patient's Guide to Medical Tests* [3-151] *People's Book of Medical Tests* [3-152]
an explanation of an electrocardiogram?	*American Medical Association Encyclopedia of Medicine* [3-107] *New Family Medical Guide* [3-149]
an explanation of the APGAR physical examination system for newborn infants?	*Complete Guide to Early Child Care* [3-118] *The Merck Manual of Diagnosis and Therapy* [3-146]
a schedule for pediatric physical examinations and medical tests?	*Complete Book of Medical Tests* [3-116] *People's Book of Medical Tests* [3-152] *The Merck Manual of Diagnosis and Therapy* [3-146]
how to measure the body's temperature and interpret the results?	*Complete Book of Medical Tests* [3-116] *People's Book of Medical Tests* [3-152]
an interpretation of rectal temperatures in young children?	*Complete Guide to Early Child Care* [3-118]
how to measure pulse rate and interpret it?	*Complete Book of Medical Tests* [3-116] *Complete Guide to Medical Tests* [3-119] *Complete Home Medical Guide* [3-124] *New Family Medical Guide* [3-149] *People's Book of Medical Tests* [3-152]
how to use a peak flow meter with an asthmatic child?	*Children with Asthma* [3-19]

WHERE SHOULD I GO TO FIND. . .	*TRY*

Diagnostic Tests and Measurements

for children with asthma, the peak flow rates measured in liters per minute?	*Children with Asthma* [3-19]
an explanation of tests that are used when diagnosing bladder disorders?	*Overcoming Bladder Disorders* [3-43]

Diseases, Disorders, and Their Therapies

an explanation of childhood and adolescent diseases and medical disorders, including their causes, symptoms, diagnoses, and treatment?	*American Cancer Society Cancer Book* [3-17] *American Medical Association Encyclopedia of Medicine* [3-107] *Complete Guide to Early Child Care* [3-118] *Complete Guide to Symptoms, Illness, and Surgery* [3-123] *Complete Home Medical Guide* [3-124] *Complete Parents' Guide to Telephone Medicine* [3-125] *Instructions for Patients* [3-139] *New Family Medical Guide* [3-149] *The Merck Manual of Diagnosis and Therapy* [3-146]
a listing of medical symptoms with the illness or disorder that each may indicate?	*Complete Guide to Symptoms, Illness and Surgery* [3-123]
how physicians treat individual childhood diseases and disorders?	*Current Pediatric Therapy* [3-127]
the immunization schedule for childhood diseases?	*American Medical Association Encyclopedia of Medicine* [3-107] *Complete Book of Medical Tests* [3-116] *Complete Guide to Early Child Care* [3-118] *Complete Guide to Symptoms, Illness and Surgery* [3-123] *Complete Home Medical Guide* [3-124] *Complete Parents' Guide to Telephone Medicine* [3-125] *Countries of the World and Their Leaders* [3-126] *Current Pediatric Therapy* [3-127] *Instructions for Patients* [3-139] *New Family Medical Guide* [3-149] *The Merck Manual of Diagnosis and Therapy* [3-146]

WHERE SHOULD I GO TO FIND. . .	*TRY*
Diseases, Disorders, and Their Therapies	
symptoms that if exhibited by an infant are cause for calling the doctor?	*Complete Guide to Early Child Care* [3-118]
drugs that can cause acne and those that are use to treat it?	*Essential Guide to Prescription Drugs* [3-132] *The Look You Like* [3-36]
an explanation of acne, its causes, and its treatment?	*Complete Guide to Symptoms, Illness and Surgery* [3-123] *Essential Guide to Prescription Drugs* [3-132] *Instructions for Patients* [3-139] *New Family Medical Guide* [3-149] *The Look You Like* [3-36] *The Merck Manual of Diagnosis and Therapy* [3-146]
answers to questions about skin problems and care?	*Complete Guide to Early Child Care* [3-118] *Complete Guide to Symptoms, Illness and Surgery* [3-123] *Instructions for Patients* [3-139] *New Family Medical Guide* [3-149] *The Look You Like* [3-36]
names of drugs that may sensitize the skin to the effects of the sun?	*Complete Guide to Prescription and Non-Prescription Drugs* [3-121] *Complete Home Medical Guide* [3-124] *Essential Guide to Prescription Drugs* [3-132]
a discussion of child and/or adolescent behavioral problems and their modification?	*American Medical Association Encyclopedia of Medicine* [3-107] *Complete Guide to Early Child Care* [3-118] *Complete Home Medical Guide* [3-124] *Current Pediatric Therapy* [3-127]
a discussion of psychological problems that may develop in children and/or adolescents?	*Complete Guide to Early Child Care* [3-118] *Complete Home Medical Guide* [3-124] *Current Pediatric Therapy* [3-127] *New Family Medical Guide* [3-149] *The Merck Manual of Diagnosis and Therapy* [3-146]
medical instructions for patients to follow regarding specific diseases, disorders, or injuries?	*Instructions for Patients* [3-139]

WHERE SHOULD I GO TO FIND...	*TRY*

Diseases, Disorders, and Their Therapies

a discussion of health problems that may occur in newborn infants, and the services of neonatal intensive care units?	*Complete Guide to Early Child Care* [3-118]
how to care for a colicky baby?	*Complete Guide to Early Child Care* [3-118]
why babies get hiccups?	*Complete Guide to Early Child Care* [3-118]
why babies spit up and what is considered normal?	*Complete Guide to Early Child Care* [3-118]
a discussion of Sudden Infant Death Syndrome (SIDS) and its causes?	*American Medical Association Encyclopedia of Medicine* [3-107] *Complete Guide to Early Child Care* [3-118] *Complete Home Medical Guide* [3-124] *The Merck Manual of Diagnosis and Therapy* [3-146]
a discussion of diabetes in children?	*Complete Home Medical Guide* [3-124] *New Family Medical Guide* [3-149] *The Merck Manual of Diagnosis and Therapy* [3-146]
for individual diseases and injuries, when the physician should be called and guidelines for how to talk to the doctor?	*Complete Parents' Guide to Telephone Medicine* [3-125]
what to do to help my child with a specific illness or injury?	*Complete Parents' Guide to Telephone Medicine* [3-125]
guidance that will help decide if a surgical procedure should be undertaken?	*Is Surgery Necessary?* [3-140] *Surgery: Yes or No?* [3-157]
an explanation of diseases and disorders as they affect the athlete, including symptoms, causes, prevention, and treatment?	*Complete Guide to Sports Injuries* [3-122]
the causes of specific sports-related injuries, an explanation of each injury, and the appropriate treatment?	*Complete Guide to Sports Injuries* [3-122] *Sports Health* [3-155]
how long it takes for different types of fractures to heal?	*Complete Guide to Sports Injuries* [3-122] *Sports Health* [3-155]

WHERE SHOULD I GO TO FIND. . .   *TRY*

Diseases, Disorders, and Their Therapies

a description of different types of seizures?

Complete Guide to Early Child Care [3-118]

an explanation of neurological and neuromuscular disorders in children?

Complete Guide to Early Child Care [3-118]

an explanation of Lyme disease, including its symptoms, cause, treatment, and probable outcome?

Complete Guide to Early Child Care [3-118]
Complete Guide to Symptoms, Illness and Surgery [3-123]
Current Pediatric Therapy [3-127]
New Family Medical Guide [3-149]
The Merck Manual of Diagnosis and Therapy [3-146]

how to reduce a fever?

Complete Guide to Symptoms, Illness and Surgery [3-123]
Complete Home Medical Guide [3-124]
Instructions for Patients [3-139]

an explanation of Acquired Immune Deficiency Syndrome (AIDS)?

AIDS: A Self-Care Manual [3-16]
AIDS Information Sourcebook [3-67]
American Medical Association Encyclopedia of Medicine [3-107]
Complete Guide to Early Child Care [3-118]
Complete Guide to Symptoms, Illness and Surgery [3-123]
Complete Home Medical Guide [3-124]
Health Care U.S.A. [3-85]
New Family Medical Guide [3-149]
The Merck Manual of Diagnosis and Therapy [3-146]

the symptoms of AIDS and what the patient should do to manage each symptom?

AIDS: A Self-Care Manual [3-16]

advice regarding the social and psychological concerns for AIDS in children?

AIDS: A Self-Care Manual [3-16]

for common diseases and disorders, the drugs that are used to treat them?

Drug Interactions Guide Book [3-130]

an explanation of allergies in children?

Complete Guide to Early Child Care [3-118]

WHERE SHOULD I GO TO FIND. . .	*TRY*
Diseases, Disorders, and Their Therapies	
brief answers to questions often asked about allergies?	*Allergy Encyclopedia* [3-103]
the causes, symptoms, diagnoses, and treatment of allergy emergencies?	*Allergy Encyclopedia* [3-103]
the allergen characteristics of each region in the United States, including a listing of the pollen-producing trees, grasses, and broad-leafed plants without woody stems that are to be found in each region?	*Allergy Encyclopedia* [3-103]
a map that shows the ragweed density by state?	*Allergy Encyclopedia* [3-103]
a listing of the principal kinds of airborne pollen and spores found in major U.S. cities?	*Allergy Encyclopedia* [3-103]
a pollen calendar for each state?	*Allergy Encyclopedia* [3-103]
answers to questions that are commonly asked about food allergies?	*Allergy Encyclopedia* [3-103] *Eating and Allergy* [3-25] *Food Allergy* [3-28]
an explanation of asthma, how to diagnose it, and how to treat it at home?	*Children with Asthma* [3-19]
an explanation of medications that are frequently prescribed for children with asthma?	*Children with Asthma* [3-19]
ways to minimize dust in the bedroom of the asthmatic child?	*Children with Asthma* [3-19]
a description of inhalation devices used to assist children with asthma, and instructions for their use?	*Children with Asthma* [3-19]
a discussion of the most common serious poisonings of children, including symptoms and treatments?	*The Merck Manual of Diagnosis and Therapy* [3-146]
warning signs of illicit drug experimentation?	*Complete Home Medical Guide* [3-124] *Drugs, Alcohol, and Your Children* [3-24] *New Family Medical Guide* [3-149]

WHERE SHOULD I GO TO FIND. . .   *TRY*

Diseases, Disorders, and Their Therapies

a guidebook for parents who have a child
involved with substance abuse?

Drugs, Alcohol, and Your Children [3-24]

information on bladder disorders?

Overcoming Bladder Disorders [3-43]

a description of those drugs that are often
used for the treatment of bladder disorders?

Overcoming Bladder Disorders [3-43]

a discussion of childhood cancer, including
methods of treatment, cure rates, and
other related information?

American Cancer Society Cancer Book [3-17]

the different side effects of chemotherapy and
external radiation therapy, how to recognize
these side effects, and how to manage them?

*Managing the Side Effects of Chemotherapy and
Radiation* [3-37]

Growth and Development

a typical schedule of the physical, mental,
and social skills growth and development of
a child?

*American Medical Association Encyclopedia of
Medicine* [3-107]
Complete Guide to Early Child Care [3-118]
Complete Home Medical Guide [3-124]
New Family Medical Guide [3-149]
The Merck Manual of Diagnosis and Therapy
[3-146]

a discussion of child and/or adolescent
behavioral problems and their
modification?

*American Medical Association Encyclopedia of
Medicine* [3-107]
Complete Guide to Early Child Care [3-118]
Complete Home Medical Guide [3-124]
Current Pediatric Therapy [3-127]

an explanation of physical, emotional, and
social development during the adolescent
years?

*American Medical Association Encyclopedia of
Medicine* [3-107]
Complete Home Medical Guide [3-124]

weight and height growth charts for boys
and girls?

*American Medical Association Encyclopedia of
Medicine* [3-107]
Complete Guide to Early Child Care [3-118]

the normal physical characteristics of
newborn infants?

Complete Guide to Early Child Care [3-118]
The Merck Manual of Diagnosis and Therapy
[3-146]

WHERE SHOULD I GO TO FIND. . .   TRY

Growth and Development

when a baby can be expected to sleep throughout the night?

Complete Guide to Early Child Care [3-118]

what is normal emotional and intellectual development in infants, toddlers, and preschoolers?

Complete Guide to Early Child Care [3-118]

how a parent should approach the development of a gifted child?

Complete Guide to Early Child Care [3-118]

how to determine when a child's behavioral problem is serious enough to require professional help?

Complete Guide to Early Child Care [3-118]

suggestions for dealing with discipline of toddlers and young children?

Complete Guide to Early Child Care [3-118]

by age, what is the normal heart rate?

Warning Symptoms [3-159]

Medical Care

questions to be asked and guidelines to be followed by parents when selecting a pediatrician?

Complete Guide to Early Child Care [3-118]
Complete Guide to Pregnancy [3-120]
Complete Parent's Guide to Telephone Medicine [3-125]

how parents can prepare a child for hospitalization, and what they should do during the stay?

Complete Guide to Early Child Care [3-118]
New Family Medical Guide [3-149]

an explanation of individual medical specialties and what to expect when visiting a particular type of specialist?

Medical Tests and Diagnostic Procedures [3-143]

suggestions on how to find a medical specialist for a child?

Complete Guide to Early Child Care [3-118]

questions to ask a consulting medical specialist?

How to Talk to Your Doctor [3-34]
Take This Book to the Hospital with You [3-50]

a guide to what is a pediatric emergency, near-emergency, or nonemergency?

Complete Guide to Early Child Care [3-118]

WHERE SHOULD I GO TO FIND. . .	*TRY*
Medical Care	
guidelines on when to call the doctor and what to say when reporting a medical emergency?	*Complete Guide to Early Child Care* [3-118]
what information should be assembled before calling the pediatrician about a specific health problem?	*Complete Parents' Guide to Telephone Medicine* [3-125]
for individual diseases and injuries, when the doctor should be called and guidelines on how to speak with the physician?	*Complete Parents' Guide to Telephone Medicine* [3-125]
how to care for a sick child at home?	*Instructions for Patients* [3-139]
guidelines for providers of home care for AIDS patients?	*AIDS: A Self-Care Manual* [3-16]
a model medical record form that can be used at home?	*Complete Guide to Early Child Care* [3-118]
how to select a doctor for a child with asthma?	*Children with Asthma* [3-19]
how to decide when a second medical opinion should be obtained for an asthmatic condition in a child?	*Children with Asthma* [3-19]
what to do to prepare for a second-opinion visit with an asthma specialist?	*Children with Asthma* [3-19]
Medical Questions	
questions to be asked and guidelines to be followed by parents when selecting a pediatrician?	*Complete Guide to Early Child Care* [3-118] *Complete Guide to Pregnancy* [3-120] *Complete Parents' Guide to Telephone Medicine* [3-125]
how to ask the right questions when I go to my child's pediatrician so I will get the information I need?	*How to Talk to Your Doctor* [3-34]
sample basic questions that I can ask my child's doctor so that I will receive the medical information that I need?	*How to Talk to Your Doctor* [3-34]

WHERE SHOULD I GO TO FIND. . .	TRY

Medical Questions

questions to ask a consulting medical specialist?	*How to Talk to Your Doctor* [3-34] *Take This Book to the Hospital with You* [3-50]
questions to ask following a diagnosis of asthma?	*How to Talk to Your Doctor* [3-34]
questions to ask following a diagnosis of cancer?	*How to Talk to Your Doctor* [3-34]
questions to ask following a diagnosis of diabetes mellitus?	*How to Talk to Your Doctor* [3-34]
questions to ask following a diagnosis of kidney disease?	*How to Talk to Your Doctor* [3-34]

Newsletter

a newsletter that addresses matters of teenage health?	*Adolescent Medicine—Newsletter* [3-167]
a newsletter that disseminates current information on AIDS and issues about it?	*The AIDS Letter* [3-170]
a newsletter that reports on pediatric cancer research news, community activities related to this disease, and fund-raising for children with cancer?	*AROCC Newsletter* [3-174]
a newsletter that reports current information on the prevention and treatment of birth defects?	*Association of Birth Defect Children—Newsletter* [3-175]
newsletters that provide advice for children with allergies?	*Asthma and Allergy Advocate* [3-176] *Living with Allergies* [3-183]
a newsletter that offers suggestions on how to cope with diabetes?	*Diabetes* [3-181]
for cancer patients and their families, a newsletter that promotes a positive attitude, encourages good medical care, and reports information on advances in cancer research?	*The Cancer Challenge* [3-178]

WHERE SHOULD I GO TO FIND. . .	*TRY*

Newsletter

a newsletter that specializes in reporting on the diagnosis and treatment of skin cancer and on related research developments?	*The Melanoma Letter* [3-186]
a newsletter that is dedicated to heart-related topics, such as the prevention of heart disease, surgery, drugs, diet, rehabilitation, and exercise?	*Cardiac Alert* [3-179]
a newsletter that discusses issues, programs, and services pertaining to the donation of human organs and tissues for transplantation?	*Transplant Action* [3-195]

Nutrients and Dietary Guidelines

the amount of nutrients contained in some of the popular mineral and vitamin supplements for children?	*Food and Drug Interaction Guide* [3-135]
the daily Recommended Dietary Allowances (RDAs) for minerals and vitamins?	*American Medical Association Encyclopedia of Medicine* [3-107] *Complete Guide to Early Child Care* [3-118] *Complete Home Medical Guide* [3-124] *Food and Drug Interaction Guide* [3-135] *Food Values of Portions Commonly Used* [3-136] *Guide to Prescription and Over-the-Counter Drugs* [3-138] *Modern Nutrition in Health and Disease* [3-147] *The Merck Manual of Diagnosis and Therapy* [3-146] *Nutrition Almanac* [3-150]
dietary guidelines for infants up to 12 months of age?	*Food Values of Portions Commonly Used* [3-136] *Instructions for Patients* [3-139] *Modern Nutrition in Health and Disease* [3-147] *Nutrition Almanac* [3-150]
guidelines for breast feeding?	*Complete Guide to Early Child Care* [3-118] *Instructions for Patients* [3-139] *The Merck Manual of Diagnosis and Therapy* [3-146]

WHERE SHOULD I GO TO FIND. . .	*TRY*

Nutrients and Dietary Guidelines

for infants, the average number of recommended daily feedings and the average quantity per feeding?	*Instructions for Patients* [3-139]
guidelines for teaching toddlers and preschoolers how to eat, including suggestions on how to manage those "terrible" feeding problems?	*Complete Guide to Early Child Care* [3-118]
for each of the basic food groups, the number of daily servings and the size of each serving recommended for children during the first five years?	*Complete Guide to Early Child Care* [3-118]
the daily calorie requirements of children one to six years of age?	*Complete Guide to Early Child Care* [3-118] *Nutrition Almanac* [3-150]
dietary guidelines for children one to sixteen years of age?	*Food Values of Portions Commonly Used* [3-136] *Instructions for Patients* [3-139] *Nutrition Almanac* [3-150]

Rearing the Child

guidelines for raising the young child, including toilet training, sibling rivalry, bedtime problems, and other behavioral issues?	*Complete Guide to Early Child Care* [3-118]
guidelines for teaching toddlers and preschoolers how to eat, including suggestions on how to manage those "terrible" feeding problems?	*Complete Guide to Early Child Care* [3-118]
a discussion of child abuse, including causes and symptoms?	*American Medical Association Encyclopedia of Medicine* [3-107] *Complete Guide to Early Child Care* [3-118] *The Merck Manual of Diagnosis and Therapy* [3-146]

Safety Guidelines

a checklist for assessing the safety of a home for a child?	*Complete Guide to Early Child Care* [3-118]

WHERE SHOULD I GO TO FIND. . .	*TRY*

Safety Guidelines

tips on how to make a home safe for a toddler?	*Complete Guide to Early Child Care* [3-118] *New Family Medical Guide* [3-149]
a listing of both dangerous and safe toys for children at different ages?	*Complete Guide to Early Child Care* [3-118]
safety standards and guidelines for selecting a baby crib?	*Complete Guide to Early Child Care* [3-118]
instructions for the use of an infant/toddler car seat and a stroller?	*Complete Guide to Early Child Care* [3-118]
a checklist for assessing the safety of a playground?	*Complete Guide to Early Child Care* [3-118]
the questions that parents should ask about safety when considering a daycare center or school for their child?	*Complete Guide to Early Child Care* [3-118]

Things for the Baby

a checklist of items to be purchased for the newborn baby?	*Complete Guide to Early Child Care* [3-118]
safety standards and guidelines for selecting a baby crib?	*Complete Guide to Early Child Care* [3-118]
if pacifiers may be used?	*Complete Guide to Early Child Care* [3-118]
if baby bottles and related equipment should be sterilized?	*Complete Guide to Early Child Care* [3-118]
a listing of both dangerous and safe toys for children at different ages?	*Complete Guide to Early Child Care* [3-118]

Definitions

Abbreviations and Acronyms

an interpretation of the abbreviations and/or terms found in a medical prescription?	*Acronyms, Initialisms, and Abbreviations Dictionary* [3-56] *Complete Home Medical Guide* [3-124]

(*answer continues*)

WHERE SHOULD I GO TO FIND. . .	*TRY*

Abbreviations and Acronyms

an interpretation of the abbreviations and/or terms found in a medical prescription?	*Dorland's Illustrated Medical Dictionary* [3-58] *How to Talk to Your Doctor* [3-34] *Medical Acronyms and Abbreviations* [3-61] *Melloni's Illustrated Medical Dictionary* [3-63] *The Merck Index* [3-145] *The Merck Manual of Diagnosis and Therapy* [3-146] *Stedman's Medical Dictionary* [3-64]
an interpretation of acronyms, abbreviations, initialisms, and contractions used in medicine and the health care industry?	*Acronyms, Initialisms, and Abbreviations Dictionary* [3-56] *Medical Acronyms and Abbreviations* [3-61]

Terms and Phrases

an explanation of medical terms, phrases, and abbreviations?	*Acronyms, Initialisms, and Abbreviations Dictionary* [3-56] *American Medical Association Encyclopedia of Medicine* [3-107] *Complete Home Medical Guide* [3-124] *Dorland's Illustrated Medical Dictionary* [3-58] *Medical Sign Language* [3-62] *Melloni's Illustrated Medical Dictionary* [3-63] *Stedman's Medical Dictionary* [3-64]
a list of AIDS-related terms and their meanings?	*AIDS: A Self-Care Manual* [3-16] *AIDS and Women: A Sourcebook* [3-5] *AIDS Information Sourcebook* [3-67]
a dictionary of food ingredients that cites the functions, properties, and applications of each ingredient?	*Dictionary of Food Ingredients* [3-57]
a glossary of asthma-related terms?	*Children with Asthma* [3-19]
the meaning of drug-related terms?	*Dorland's Illustrated Medical Dictionary* [3-58] *Drugs, Alcohol, and Your Children* [3-24] *Essential Guide to Prescription Drugs* [3-132] *Guide to Prescription and Over-the-Counter Drugs* [3-138] *How to Talk to Your Doctor* [3-34]

WHERE SHOULD I GO TO FIND. . .	*TRY*

Terms and Phrases

the meaning of drug-related terms?	*Melloni's Illustrated Medical Dictionary* [3-63] *Stedman's Medical Dictionary* [3-64]
the different types of phobias and their meanings?	*Stedman's Medical Dictionary* [3-64]
a list of allergy-related terms and their definitions?	*Allergy Encyclopedia* [3-103] [Note: Also see general medical dictionaries cited in this section.]
a definition for each type of disability along with sources for further information on each disability?	*Meeting the Needs of People with Disabilities* [3-144]
the translation of medical and dental terms into American Sign Language for the deaf?	*Medical Sign Language* [3-62]
the definitions of dental terms?	*Dorland's Illustrated Medical Dictionary* [3-58] *Illustrated Dictionary of Dentistry* [3-60] *Melloni's Illustrated Medical Dictionary* [3-63] *Stedman's Medical Dictionary* [3-64]
the meaning of folk names used to designate occupational diseases and other ailments?	*Folk Name and Trade Diseases* [3-59]

Dental Health

Dental Appliances, Implants, Inlays, and Crowns

an explanation of orthodontic appliances and how they work?	*American Medical Association Encyclopedia of Medicine* [3-107] *Family Guide to Dental Health* [3-133] *Tooth and Gum Care* [3-51]
an explanation of dental implants?	*American Medical Association Encyclopedia of Medicine* [3-107] *Change Your Smile* [3-111] *Dental Implants: Are They For Me?* [3-22] *Family Guide to Dental Health* [3-133]

(*answer continues*)

WHERE SHOULD I GO TO FIND. . .	*TRY*

Dental Appliances, Implants, Inlays, and Crowns

an explanation of dental implants?	*Illustrated Dictionary of Dentistry* [3-60] *New Family Medical Guide* [3-149]
an explanation of dental fillings, inlays, and crowns?	*American Medical Association Encyclopedia of Medicine* [3-107] *Change Your Smile* [3-111] *Family Guide to Dental Health* [3-133] *Tooth and Gum Care* [3-51]
how a tooth is filled or crowned?	*Change Your Smile* [3-111] *Family Guide to Dental Health* [3-133]
an explanation of the kinds of bridges and dentures, and how to care for them?	*Change Your Smile* [3-111] *Family Guide to Dental Health* [3-133] *Tooth and Gum Care* [3-51]

Dental Hygiene

suggestions on how to select and use a toothbrush?	*Family Guide to Dental Health* [3-133] *Tooth and Gum Care* [3-51]
how to clean teeth properly?	*Family Guide to Dental Health* [3-133] *Tooth and Gum Care* [3-51]
how to care for the teeth of a child?	*Family Guide to Dental Health* [3-133] *Tooth and Gum Care* [3-51]

Dental Instruments and Materials

an explanation of dental instruments and materials?	*Family Guide to Dental Health* [3-133] *Illustrated Dictionary of Dentistry* [3-60]

Dentists

[*Note:* For the names of dentists and their specialties and location, see the section titled "Health Care Professionals."]

how to evaluate a dentist?	*Complete Home Medical Guide* [3-124] *Family Guide to Dental Health* [3-133]
an explanation of the different dental specialties?	*American Medical Association Encyclopedia of Medicine* [3-107] *Family Guide to Dental Health* [3-133] *Tooth and Gum Care* [3-51]

WHERE SHOULD I GO TO FIND. . .   *TRY*

Diseases, Disorders, and Their Therapies

an explanation of dental diseases, disorders, and treatments?

American Medical Association Encyclopedia of Medicine [3-107]
Complete Guide to Early Child Care [3-118]
Complete Guide to Symptoms, Illness and Surgery [3-123]
Family Guide to Dental Health [3-133]
The Merck Manual of Diagnosis and Therapy [3-146]
Tooth and Gum Care [3-51]
What is Periodontal Disease? [3-53]

what to do for different dental emergencies?

Family Guide to Dental Health [3-133]

how to control my dental fears?

Family Guide to Dental Health [3-133]

a discussion of common medical problems that dictate special care when receiving dental treatment?

Family Guide to Dental Health [3-133]

a listing of drugs that have side effects which affect dental health and treatment?

Family Guide to Dental Health [3-133]

snack foods that are not cariogenic?

Complete Home Medical Guide [3-124]

a classification of dental caries (cavities)?

Dorland's Illustrated Medical Dictionary [3-58]
Illustrated Dictionary of Dentistry [3-60]
Tooth and Gum Care [3-51]

how a tooth is filled or crowned?

Change Your Smile [3-111]
Family Guide to Dental Health [3-133]

how pain is controlled during dental treatment?

Family Guide to Dental Health [3-133]

the location of anesthetic injection sites for the different dental procedures?

Tooth and Gum Care [3-51]

an explanation of root canal therapy?

American Medical Association Encyclopedia of Medicine [3-107]
Family Guide to Dental Health [3-133]
Tooth and Gum Care [3-51]
Why Root Canal Therapy? [3-55]

WHERE SHOULD I GO TO FIND. . .	*TRY*

Diseases, Disorders, and Their Therapies

an explanation of the causes, symptoms, and treatment of periodontal disease?	*American Medical Association Encyclopedia of Medicine* [3-107] *Change Your Smile* [3-111] *Complete Guide to Symptoms, Illness and Surgery* [3-123] *Complete Home Medical Guide* [3-124] *Family Guide to Dental Health* [3-133] *New Family Medical Guide* [3-149] *Tooth and Gum Care* [3-51] *What is Periodontal Disease?* [3-53]
how to conduct a self-examination for oral tumors?	*Tooth and Gum Care* [3-51]
answers to questions about cosmetic dentistry?	*Change Your Smile* [3-111] *Family Guide to Dental Health* [3-133]
a discussion of different treatments for stained teeth, including the relative advantages and disadvantages?	*Change Your Smile* [3-111] *Family Guide to Dental Health* [3-133]
maintenance advice for dental patients who have had composite resin bonding?	*Change Your Smile* [3-111]
the different methods used to extend the life of dental restorations, including their advantages and disadvantages?	*Change Your Smile* [3-111]
how fractured teeth can be repaired?	*Change Your Smile* [3-111] *Family Guide to Dental Health* [3-133]
what to do when a tooth has been knocked out?	*Change Your Smile* [3-111] *Family Guide to Dental Health* [3-133]
what can be done to close gaps between teeth?	*Change Your Smile* [3-111] *Family Guide to Dental Health* [3-133]
solutions to correcting crowded and crooked teeth?	*Change Your Smile* [3-111]
what treatments are available for various bite problems?	*Change Your Smile* [3-111]
how to prevent aesthetic dental problems during childhood?	*Change Your Smile* [3-111]

WHERE SHOULD I GO TO FIND. . .	*TRY*

Diseases, Disorders, and Their Therapies

whether to replace a back tooth that has been extracted?	*Why Replace a Missing Back Tooth?* [3-54]
how wisdom teeth develop, become impacted, and what problems are caused by impacted wisdom teeth?	*Family Guide to Dental Health* [3-133] *The Story of Impacted Wisdom Teeth* [3-48]
the reasons for early removal of impacted wisdom teeth?	*Advantages to Early Removal of Impacted Wisdom Teeth* [3-15] *Family Guide to Dental Health* [3-133]
problems that may occur in middle age or later with wisdom teeth that have been impacted for many years?	*Impacted Wisdom Teeth in the Middle and Later Years* [3-35]
dental care guidelines for persons with AIDS or HIV infection?	*AIDS: A Self-Care Manual* [3-16]
a discussion of dental problems confronted by senior citizens and guidelines for their dental care?	*Family Guide to Dental Health* [3-133]
an explanation of the use of fluorides to protect teeth?	*Family Guide to Dental Health* [3-133]
an explanation of the different types of oral and maxillofacial surgery?	*Change Your Smile* [3-111] *Family Guide to Dental Health* [3-133]
an explanation of temporomandibular disorders (TMDs) and their treatments?	*Family Guide to Dental Health* [3-133]

Oral Features

drawings and explanations of dental features in the human mouth?	*Anatomy of the Human Body* [3-108] *Atlas of Human Anatomy* [drawings only] [3-109] *Dorland's Illustrated Medical Dictionary* [3-58] *Family Guide to Dental Health* [3-133] *Illustrated Dictionary of Dentistry* [3-60] *Melloni's Illustrated Medical Dictionary* [3-63] *New Family Medical Guide* [3-149] *Stedman's Medical Dictionary* [3-64]

(*answer continues*)

WHERE SHOULD I GO TO FIND. . .	*TRY*

Oral Features

drawings and explanations of dental features in the human mouth?	*Tooth and Gum Care* [3-51] *Why Root Canal Therapy?* [3-55]
a diagram depicting the primary and secondary teeth?	*Complete Home Medical Guide* [3-124] *Family Guide to Dental Health* [3-133] *Melloni's Illustrated Medical Dictionary* [3-63] *Tooth and Gum Care* [3-51]
the development schedule of teeth?	*Complete Home Medical Guide* [3-124] *Family Guide to Dental Health* [3-133] *Melloni's Illustrated Medical Dictionary* [3-63] *The Merck Manual of Diagnosis and Therapy* [3-146] *Tooth and Gum Care* [3-51]

The Disabled

Accessibility Standards

standards that are followed to provide an architecturally barrier-free environment for persons with a physical disability?	*American National Standard for Buildings and Facilities—Providing Accessibility and Usability for Physically Handicapped People* [3-197]

Equipment and Devices

a directory of major companies that supply equipment and devices specially designed for use by persons with disabilities?	*Health Care U.S.A.* [3-85]
what computers can do for persons with different types of disabilities?	*Meeting the Needs of People with Disabilities* [3-144]

Living with a Disability

information for the disabled person regarding independent living, clothing, telephone services, traveling, use of pets, and recreation?	*Meeting the Needs of People with Disabilities* [3-144]
suggestions on how to conduct oneself when meeting a person with a disability?	*Meeting the Needs of People with Disabilities* [3-144]

WHERE SHOULD I GO TO FIND. . .	*TRY*

Living with a Disability

guidelines for involving children with disabilities in sports and recreation?	*Sportswise* [3-47]

Newsletters

a newsletter that provides information on how to care for persons with disabilities?	*Caregivers* [3-180]

Schools, Organizations, and Services

an explanation of the rights of disabled children and how to secure special education services as provided by Public Law 94–142?	*Directory of Residential Facilities for Emotionally Handicapped Children and Youth* [3-79]
the names, addresses, and telephone numbers of schools for the blind and for visually impaired children?	*Medical and Health Information Directory,* Vol. 3 [3-90]
the names, addresses, and telephone numbers of schools for the deaf and for hearing-impaired children?	*Medical and Health Information Directory,* Vol. 3 [3-90]
a directory of libraries with special services for the blind and physically disabled?	*Medical and Health Information Directory,* Vol. 3 [3-90]
the addresses and telephone numbers of sports organizations for disabled persons?	*Health Care U.S.A.* [3-85] *Medical and Health Information Directory,* Vol. 1 [3-88]
a directory of summer camps for children with physical or mental disabilities, including for each camp the address, telephone number, name of contact person, and a brief description of facilities and activities?	*Allergy Encyclopedia* [3-103] *Guide to Accredited Camps* [3-84]

Diseases and Disorders of Adults

Diagnostic Tests and Measurements

a schedule for medical checkups?	*New Family Medical Guide* [3-149]

WHERE SHOULD I GO TO FIND...	*TRY*

Diagnostic Tests and Measurements

an explanation of medical diagnostic tests and procedures, including their purposes, their risks, reference values for normality, abnormal values, and/or other information?	*American Medical Association Encyclopedia of Medicine* [3-107] *Complete Book of Medical Tests* [3-116] *Complete Guide to Medical Tests* [3-119] *Complete Home Medical Guide* [3-124] *How to Talk to Your Doctor* [3-34] *Medical Tests and Diagnostic Procedures* [3-143] *New Family Medical Guide* [3-149] *Old Enough to Feel Better* [3-40] *Patient's Guide to Medical Tests* [3-151] *People's Book of Medical Tests* [3-152] *Surgery On File: General Surgery* [3-162] *Surgery On File: Eye, Ear, Nose, and Throat Surgery* [3-161] *Surgery On File: Obstetrics and Gynecology* [3-163] *Surgery On File: Orthopedics and Trauma Surgery* [3-164]
questions for a patient to ask about diagnostic tests and procedures that have been recommended by a physician?	*How to Talk to Your Doctor* [3-34] *Take This Book to the Hospital With You* [3-50]
answers to general questions that are commonly asked about medical tests?	*Complete Book of Medical Tests* [3-116]
the estimated average cost of specific medical tests? [Note: Allow for recent escalating increases.]	*Complete Guide to Medical Tests* [3-119] *Patient's Guide to Medical Tests* [3-151] *People's Book of Medical Tests* [3-152]
for specific diagnostic tests, an interpretation of what is considered to be abnormal?	*Complete Book of Medical Tests* [3-116] *Complete Guide to Medical Tests* [3-119] *Patient's Guide to Medical Tests* [3-151] *People's Book of Medical Tests* [3-152]
an explanation of the body imaging methods of X-rays, CAT or CT scanning, MRI scanning, and PET scanning?	*American Medical Association Encyclopedia of Medicine* [3-107] *Complete Book of Medical Tests* [3-116] *Complete Home Medical Guide* [3-124] *How to Talk to Your Doctor* [3-34] *Medical Tests and Diagnostic Procedures* [3-143] *New Family Medical Guide* [3-149]

WHERE SHOULD I GO TO FIND...	*TRY*

Diagnostic Tests and Measurements

an explanation of the body imaging methods of X-rays, CAT or CT scanning, MRI scanning, and PET scanning?	*Patient's Guide to Medical Tests* [3-151] *People's Book of Medical Tests* [3-152]
an explanation of an electrocardiogram?	*American Medical Association Encyclopedia of Medicine* [3-107] *New Family Medical Guide* [3-149]
how to conduct a home vision test, including eye charts?	*People's Book of Medical Tests* [3-152]
how to measure body temperature and interpret the results?	*Complete Book of Medical Tests* [3-116] *Patient's Guide to Medical Tests* [3-151] *People's Book of Medical Tests* [3-152]
how to measure pulse rate and interpret it?	*Complete Book of Medical Tests* [3-116] *Complete Guide to Medical Tests* [3-119] *Complete Home Medical Guide* [3-124] *New Family Medical Guide* [3-149] *People's Book of Medical Tests* [3-152]
how to monitor blood pressure and general guidelines for interpreting it?	*Complete Book of Medical Tests* [3-116] *Complete Guide to Medical Tests* [3-119] *New Family Medical Guide* [3-149] *Patient's Guide to Medical Tests* [3-151] *People's Book of Medical Tests* [3-152]
a discussion of self-diagnostic tests that can be performed at home, including an explanation of the reason for each test, procedure, and results?	*Complete Book of Medical Tests* [3-116] *People's Book of Medical Tests* [3-152]
medical diagnostic tests that are recommended for healthy adolescents and adults?	*Complete Book of Medical Tests* [3-116] *People's Book of Medical Tests* [3-152]
an explanation of tests that are used for the diagnosis of bladder disorders?	*Overcoming Bladder Disorders* [3-43]
a questionnaire and/or charts that can be completed by a woman for the purpose of helping her determine if she is suffering from PMS?	*Once A Month* [3-41] *PMS: A Positive Program to Gain Control* [3-44] *Self-Help for Premenstrual Syndrome* [3-46]

WHERE SHOULD I GO TO FIND. . .	*TRY*

Diagnostic Tests and Measurements

a rating scale that helps assess changes in behavior of the Alzheimer patient and assists with determining the progression of this disease?	*Caring for the Alzheimer Patient* [3-18]

Diseases, Disorders, and Their Therapies

an explanation of diseases and various medical disorders, including their causes, symptoms, diagnoses, and treatments?	*American Cancer Society Cancer Book* [3-17] *American Medical Association Encyclopedia of Medicine* [3-107] *Complete Guide to Symptoms, Illness and Surgery* [3-123] *Complete Home Medical Guide* [3-124] *Health Care U.S.A.* [3-85] *Instructions for Patients* [3-139] *The Merck Manual of Diagnosis and Therapy* [3-146] *New Family Medical Guide* [3-149] *Nutrition Almanac* [3-150] *Old Enough to Feel Better* [3-40]
a discussion of selected chronic medical disorders with an explanation of the drugs often used to treat them and how these drugs work in the body?	*Complete Home Medical Guide* [3-124] *Essential Guide to Prescription Drugs* [3-132] *Guide to Prescription and Over-the-Counter Drugs* [3-138]
medical instructions for patients to follow regarding individual diseases, disorders, and injuries?	*Instructions for Patients* [3-139]
a listing of medical symptoms with a disclosure of the illness or disorder that each symptom may indicate?	*Complete Guide to Symptoms, Illness and Surgery* [3-123]
medical symptoms, their causes, and what to do about them?	*Warning Symptoms* [3-159]
a diagnostic chart of some infectious diseases that reports for each disease its infective agent, transmission, incubation period, symptoms, and treatment?	*American Medical Association Encyclopedia of Medicine* [3-107]
the symptoms, causes, complications, and treatment of diabetes?	*American Medical Association Encyclopedia of Medicine* [3-107]

WHERE SHOULD I GO TO FIND. . .   *TRY*

Diseases, Disorders, and Their Therapies

the symptoms, causes, complications, and treatment of diabetes?	*Complete Guide to Symptoms, Illness and Surgery* [3-123]
	Complete Home Medical Guide [3-124]
	Diabetes Type II [3-23]
	Health Care U.S.A. [3-85]
	Instructions for Patients [3-139]
	The Merck Manual of Diagnosis and Therapy [3-146]
	New Family Medical Guide [3-149]
	Nutrition Almanac [3-150]
	Old Enough to Feel Better [3-40]
how blood glucose levels are regulated by insulin and other hormones?	*Diabetes Type II* [3-23]
the step-by-step procedure for measuring blood sugar?	*Diabetes Type II* [3-23]
descriptive information on over-the-counter blood glucose monitoring kits?	*Physicians' Desk Reference for Nonprescription Drugs* [3-154]
information about the different insulins, including their strengths, care, and approximate action times?	*Diabetes Type II* [3-23]
how to mix and inject insulin?	*Complete Home Medical Guide* [3-124]
	Diabetes Type II [3-23]
	Instructions for Patients [3-139]
how to perform the numerical computations that are used in the process of normalizing blood sugars in diabetics?	*Diabetes Type II* [3-23]
a list of sources of supplies for diabetics in the treatment of their illness?	*Diabetes Type II* [3-23]
how to prevent extreme blood sugar variations during the menstrual cycle?	*Diabetes Type II* [3-23]
the causes, symptoms, and treatment of hypoglycemia?	*Diabetes Type II* [3-23]
	Nutrition Almanac [3-150]
a listing of visual impairments and the drugs that may cause them?	*Essential Guide to Prescription Drugs* [3-132]

WHERE SHOULD I GO TO FIND. . .	*TRY*

Diseases, Disorders, and Their Therapies

health risks that are associated with specific industrial chemicals?	*Complete Home Medical Guide* [3-124]
an explanation of high and low blood cholesterol, and how to lower it?	*Complete Book of Medical Tests* [3-116] *Complete Home Medical Guide* [3-124] *Food and Drug Interaction Guide* [3-135] *New Family Medical Guide* [3-149] *Nutrition Almanac* [3-150] *Patient's Guide to Medical Tests* [3-151]
nutritional disorders caused by specific drugs, including their symptoms and treatment?	*Food and Drug Interaction Guide* [3-135]
the nature, causes, treatment, and prevention of osteoporosis?	*American Medical Association Encyclopedia of Medicine* [3-107] *New Family Medical Guide* [3-149] *Osteoporosis: The Silent Thief* [3-42]
the symptoms of alcoholism?	*Complete Home Medical Guide* [3-124] *How to Defeat Alcoholism* [3-33] *New Family Medical Guide* [3-149]
the truth about alcoholism and what happens in the body?	*How to Defeat Alcoholism* [3-33]
examples of proper therapeutic procedures for the different symptoms of alcoholism?	*How to Defeat Alcoholism* [3-33]
the names of drugs that have an adverse interaction with alcohol and what that effect may be?	*Complete Guide to Prescription and Non-Prescription Drugs* [3-121] *Complete Home Medical Guide* [3-124] *Essential Guide to Prescription Drugs* [3-132] *Guide to Prescription and Over-the-Counter Drugs* [3-138]
drugs that may sensitize the skin to the effects of the sun?	*Complete Guide to Prescription and Non-Prescription Drugs* [3-121] *Complete Home Medical Guide* [3-124] *Essential Guide to Prescription Drugs* [3-132]
answers to questions about skin problems and their care?	*Complete Guide to Symptoms, Illness and Surgery* [3-123] *Instructions for Patients* [3-139]

WHERE SHOULD I GO TO FIND. . .   *TRY*

Diseases, Disorders, and Their Therapies

answers to questions about skin problems and their care?	*The Look You Like* [3-36] *The Merck Manual of Diagnosis and Therapy* [3-146] *New Family Medical Guide* [3-149]
an explanation of skin conditions associated with AIDS?	*The Look You Like* [3-36]
methods that are used to remove tattoos?	*The Look You Like* [3-36]
answers to questions about hair problems and care?	*The Look You Like* [3-36]
how to stop smoking?	*Complete Home Medical Guide* [3-124]
an explanation of coronary heart disease, heart attack, angina, heart valve disease, and other cardiovascular diseases, along with methods of treatment?	*American Medical Association Encyclopedia of Medicine* [3-107] *Complete Guide to Symptoms, Illness and Surgery* [3-123] *Complete Home Medical Guide* [3-124] *The Merck Manual of Diagnosis and Therapy* [3-146] *New Family Medical Guide* [3-149] *Old Enough to Feel Better* [3-40]
the relative effectiveness of different methods of exercising for achieving cardiovascular fitness?	*Complete Home Medical Guide* [3-124]
an explanation of different blood and blood vessel disorders?	*American Medical Association Encyclopedia of Medicine* [3-107] *Complete Home Medical Guide* [3-124] *New Family Medical Guide* [3-149]
an explanation of the different types of cancer, including causes, symptoms, treatment, and other essential information?	*American Cancer Society Cancer Book* [3-17] *Complete Home Medical Guide* [3-124] *Complete Guide to Symptoms, Illness and Surgery* [3-123] *Health Care U.S.A.* [3-85] *The Merck Manual of Diagnosis and Therapy* [3-146] *New Family Medical Guide* [3-149] *Old Enough to Feel Better* [3-40]

WHERE SHOULD I GO TO FIND...	*TRY*

Diseases, Disorders, and Their Therapies

the five-year disease-free survival rates of different cancers treated by different therapies?	*The Merck Manual of Diagnosis and Therapy* [3-146]
the side effects of chemotherapy and external radiation therapy, how to recognize these effects, and how to manage each effect?	*Managing the Side Effects of Chemotherapy and Radiation* [3-37]
what is Acquired Immune Deficiency Syndrome (AIDS)?	*AIDS: A Self-Care Manual* [3-16] *AIDS and Women: A Sourcebook* [3-5] *AIDS Information Sourcebook* [3-67] *American Medical Association Encyclopedia of Medicine* [3-107] *Complete Guide to Symptoms, Illness and Surgery* [3-123] *Complete Home Medical Guide* [3-124] *Health Care U.S.A.* [3-85] *New Family Medical Guide* [3-149] *The Merck Manual of Diagnosis and Therapy* [3-146]
the symptoms of AIDS and what the patient should do to manage each symptom?	*AIDS: A Self-Care Manual* [3-16]
a nutritional program that helps to manage the chronic malnutrition that accompanies AIDS?	*AIDS: A Self-Care Manual* [3-16] *Surviving with AIDS* [3-49]
the effects of the deficiency of specific nutrients on the human immune system?	*Surviving with AIDS* [3-49]
symptoms that suggest gynecological disorders and an explanation of each symptom?	*Complete Home Medical Guide* [3-124]
an explanation of the causes, symptoms, and treatment of various female disorders?	*American Medical Association Encyclopedia of Medicine* [3-107] *Complete Guide to Symptoms, Illness and Surgery* [3-123] *Complete Home Medical Guide* [3-124] *Instructions for Patients* [3-139]

WHERE SHOULD I GO TO FIND. . .   *TRY*

Diseases, Disorders, and Their Therapies

an explanation of the causes, symptoms, and treatment of various female disorders?	*The Merck Manual of Diagnosis and Therapy* [3-146] *New Family Medical Guide* [3-149]
an explanation of the causes, symptoms, and treatment of various male disorders?	*American Medical Association Encyclopedia of Medicine* [3-107] *Complete Guide to Symptoms, Illness and Surgery* [3-123] *Complete Home Medical Guide* [3-124] *The Merck Manual of Diagnosis and Therapy* [3-146] *New Family Medical Guide* [3-149]
the causes and symptoms of cataracts and an explanation and illustration of the procedure(s) for removing them?	*American Medical Association Encyclopedia of Medicine* [3-107] *Complete Guide to Symptoms, Illness and Surgery* [3-123] *Consumer Guide to Modern Cataract Surgery* [3-21] *New Family Medical Guide* [3-149]
the causes, symptoms, treatment, and related information on the different types of arthritis?	*American Medical Association Encyclopedia of Medicine* [3-107] *Complete Guide to Symptoms, Illness and Surgery* [3-123] *Complete Home Medical Guide* [3-124] *Health Care U.S.A.* [3-85] *Instructions for Patients* [3-139] *The Merck Manual of Diagnosis and Therapy* [3-146] *New Family Medical Guide* [3-149] *Nutrition Almanac* [3-150] *Old Enough to Feel Better* [3-40]
the causes, symptoms, and treatment of various diseases of the brain and nervous system, including Huntington's disease, Parkinson's disease, epilepsy, and others?	*American Medical Association Encyclopedia of Medicine* [3-107] *Complete Guide to Symptoms, Illness and Surgery* [3-123] *Complete Home Medical Guide* [3-124] *Health Care U.S.A.* [3-85] *Instructions for Patients* [3-139] *The Merck Manual of Diagnosis and Therapy* [3-146]

(*answer continues*)

WHERE SHOULD I GO TO FIND. . .   *TRY*

Diseases, Disorders, and Their Therapies

the causes, symptoms, and treatment of various diseases of the brain and nervous system, including Huntington's disease, Parkinson's disease, epilepsy, and others?	*New Family Medical Guide* [3-149] *Old Enough to Feel Better* [3-40]
the causes of specific sports-related injuries, an explanation of each injury, and the appropriate treatment?	*Complete Guide to Sports Injuries* [3-122] *Sports Health* [3-155]
an explanation of diseases and other medical disorders that affect the athlete, including symptoms, causes, prevention, and treatment?	*Complete Guide to Sports Injuries* [3-122]
answers to questions frequently asked about allergies?	*Allergy Encyclopedia* [3-103]
answers to questions that are commonly asked about food allergies?	*Allergy Encyclopedia* [3-103] *Eating and Allergy* [3-25] *Food Allergy* [3-28]
how to distinguish allergies from different respiratory illnesses?	*New Family Medical Guide* [3-149]
the causes, symptoms, diagnoses, and treatment of allergy emergencies?	*Allergy Encyclopedia* [3-103]
a map that discloses ragweed density by state?	*Allergy Encyclopedia* [3-103]
a pollen calendar for each state?	*Allergy Encyclopedia* [3-103]
a listing of the principal kinds of airborne pollen and spores found in major U.S. cities?	*Allergy Encyclopedia* [3-103]
the allergen characteristics of each region in the United States, including a listing of the pollen-producing trees, grasses, and broad-leafed plants without woody stems that are to be found in each region?	*Allergy Encyclopedia* [3-103]
for specific ailments, treatment programs that are advocated by natural-medicine practitioners?	*The Complete Book of Natural Medicines* [3-117]

WHERE SHOULD I GO TO FIND. . .	*TRY*
Diseases, Disorders, and Their Therapies	
for common diseases and disorders, the drugs that are used to treat them?	*Drug Interactions Guide Book* [3-130]
information on the diagnosis, treatment, and prevention of bladder disorders?	*Overcoming Bladder Disorders* [3-43]
a description of those drugs that are often used in the treatment of bladder disorders?	*Overcoming Bladder Disorders* [3-43]
a discussion of headaches, including their types, causes, and treatments?	*American Medical Association Encyclopedia of Medicine* [3-107] *Complete Guide to Symptoms, Illness and Surgery* [3-123] *Complete Home Medical Guide* [3-124] *Instructions for Patients* [3-139] *The Merck Manual of Diagnosis and Therapy* [3-146] *New Family Medical Guide* [3-149]
an explanation of sleep disorders?	*American Medical Association Encyclopedia of Medicine* [3-107] *Complete Guide to Symptoms, Illness and Surgery* [3-123] *Complete Home Medical Guide* [3-124] *Health Care U.S.A.* [3-85] *The Merck Manual of Diagnosis and Therapy* [3-146]
an explanation of Lyme disease, including its symptoms, cause, treatment, and probable outcome?	*Complete Guide to Symptoms, Illness and Surgery* [3-123] *The Merck Manual of Diagnosis and Therapy* [3-146] *New Family Medical Guide* [3-149]
literature that explains premenstrual syndrome (PMS), helps to determine if a woman is suffering from it, and tells what to do to control it?	*The Merck Manual of Diagnosis and Therapy* [3-146] *Once A Month* [3-41] *PMS: A Positive Program to Gain Control* [3-44] *Self-Help for Premenstrual Syndrome* [3-46]
guidelines for preventing recurrent back pain?	*Complete Guide to Symptoms, Illness and Surgery* [3-123]

WHERE SHOULD I GO TO FIND. . .	*TRY*

Diseases, Disorders, and Their Therapies

rules for proper care of the back?	*Instructions for Patients* [3-139]
exercises to perform during and after back pain?	*Complete Guide to Symptoms, Illness and Surgery* [3-123]
a guide to Alzheimer's disease with answers to many questions families ask, including how to care for the patient?	*Caring for the Alzheimer Patient* [3-18] *Understanding Alzheimer's Disease* [3-52]
symptoms of Alzheimer's disease, and how they are revealed in routine activities?	*Caring for the Alzheimer Patient* [3-18] *New Family Medical Guide* [3-149] *Understanding Alzheimer's Disease* [3-52]
suggestions on how to help the Alzheimer patient eat and maintain an adequate intake of food?	*Caring for the Alzheimer Patient* [3-18]
ways to improve nutrition, hygiene, communication, safety, and body elimination for the Alzheimer patient?	*Caring for the Alzheimer Patient* [3-18]
warning signs of illicit drug experimentation?	*Complete Home Medical Guide* [3-124] *Drugs, Alcohol, and Your Children* [3-24] *New Family Medical Guide* [3-149]
guidelines that will help to decide when to consider a second medical opinion?	*How to Talk to Your Doctor* [3-34]
guidance that will help decide if a surgical procedure should be undertaken?	*Is Surgery Necessary?* [3-140] *Surgery: Yes or No?* [3-157]
advice on how to cope with a long-term illness?	*How to Talk to Your Doctor* [3-34]

Health Standards

weight and height standards for men and women?	*American Medical Association Encyclopedia of Medicine* [3-107] *Complete Home Medical Guide* [3-124] *Modern Nutrition in Health and Disease* [3-147] *New Family Medical Guide* [3-149] *Nutrition Almanac* [3-150]
how long it takes for different types of fractures and other injuries to heal?	*Complete Guide to Sports Injuries* [3-122] *Sports Health* [3-155]

WHERE SHOULD I GO TO FIND...	*TRY*

Health Standards

what is the normal heart rate?	*Warning Symptoms* [3-159]

Health Information for Travelers

guidelines for determining immunizations needed when traveling?	*American Medical Association Encyclopedia of Medicine* [3-107] *Complete Home Medical Guide* [3-124] *Countries of the World and Their Leaders* [3-126] *Foreign Travel and Immunization Guide* [3-137]
health information and recommendations for the international traveler regarding diseases, potential health risks in specified countries, and other health tips for travel abroad?	*Countries of the World and Their Leaders* [3-126] *Foreign Travel and Immunization Guide* [3-137]
the allergens that are to be found in individual countries, and the time of the year when certain pollens and molds are active in those countries?	*Allergy in the World* [3-104]
a map that discloses the ragweed density in the United States by state?	*Allergy Encyclopedia* [3-103]
a pollen calendar for each state?	*Allergy Encyclopedia* [3-103]
a listing of the principal kinds of airborne pollen and spores found in major U.S. cities?	*Allergy Encyclopedia* [3-103]
the allergen characteristics of each region in the United States, including a listing of the pollen-producing trees, grasses, and broad-leafed plants without woody stems that are to be found in each region?	*Allergy Encyclopedia* [3-103]

Medical Care

guidelines for providers of home care for AIDS patients?	*AIDS: A Self-Care Manual* [3-16]

WHERE SHOULD I GO TO FIND. . .   *TRY*

Medical Care

guidance that will help decide if a surgical procedure should be undertaken?

Is Surgery Necessary? [3-140]
Surgery: Yes or No? [3-157]

guidelines that will help one decide when to consider seeking a second medical opinion?

How to Talk to Your Doctor [3-34]

advice on how to cope with a long-term illness?

How to Talk to Your Doctor [3-34]

Medical Questions

questions to be asked by a patient regarding diagnostic tests and procedures that have been recommended by a doctor?

How to Talk to Your Doctor [3-34]
Take This Book to the Hospital with You [3-50]

how to ask the right questions about my medical concerns so that I will receive the information I need?

How to Talk to Your Doctor [3-34]

sample basic questions that will elicit information that I need regarding my medical condition?

How to Talk to Your Doctor [3-34]

questions to be asked by a patient following a diagnosis of one of the following:
   arthritis
   asthma
   cancer
   coronary artery disease
   diabetes mellitus
   emphysema/chronic bronchitis
   hepatitis and/or cirrhosis of the liver
   high blood pressure
   kidney disease
   stroke
   ulcers

How to Talk to Your Doctor [3-34]

questions to be asked by a patient when a consulting specialist is to become involved with the medical care?

How to Talk to Your Doctor [3-34]
Take This Book to the Hospital with You [3-50]

questions for a patient to ask the physician, surgeon, and anesthesiologist before undergoing surgery?

Take This Book to the Hospital with You [3-50]

WHERE SHOULD I GO TO FIND. . .	*TRY*

Newsletters

a newsletter that publishes tips on the care of Alzheimer patients and reports new developments in research on this disease?	*Alzheimer's Research Review* [3-173]
a newsletter that keeps its readers abreast of matters pertaining to arthritis?	*AHPA Newsletters* [3-169]
a newsletter that disseminates current information on AIDS and issues related to it?	*The AIDS Letter* [3-170]
a newsletter that discusses the use of health foods and nutritional products in the prevention and treatment of disease?	*Alternatives* [3-172]
a newsletter that reports on allergies, including treatments and research findings?	*Asthma and Allergy Advocate* [3-176] *Living with Allergies* [3-183]
a newsletter that provides current information on the prevention, treatment, rehabilitation, and compensation of back problems?	*Back Pain Monitor* [3-177]
for cancer patients and their families, a newsletter that promotes a positive attitude, encourages good medical care, and provides information on advances in cancer research?	*The Cancer Challenge* [3-178]
a newsletter that reports on heart-related topics?	*Cardiac Alert* [3-179]
a newsletter that provides suggestions on how to cope with diabetes?	*Diabetes* [3-181]
a newsletter that specializes in reporting on the diagnosis, treatment, and research developments concerning skin cancer?	*The Melanoma Letter* [3-186]
a newsletter that is dedicated to the treatment of and research on ileitis (Crohn's disease) and ulcerative colitis?	*National Foundation for Ileitis and Colitis—Foundation Focus* [3-187]

WHERE SHOULD I GO TO FIND...	*TRY*

Newsletters

a newsletter that discusses the causes and treatment of headaches?	*National Headache Foundation—Newsletter* [3-188]
a newsletter that keeps patients of Parkinson's disease current on research developments and treatments available?	*Parkinson's Disease Foundation—Newsletter* [3-191]
a newsletter that publishes information about spinal cord injuries and their treatment?	*Spinal Cord Injury Life* [3-193]
a newsletter that discusses issues, programs, and services regarding the donation of human organs and tissues for transplantation?	*Transplant Action* [3-195]

Drugs: Use and Abuse

INTRODUCTION: In recent years, the term "drug" has assumed a negative connotation, that is, illicit and abusive use of either bona fide medicines or other substances. It is sometimes forgotten that our therapeutic chemicals are legitimate medicines (drugs) and most are being properly prescribed by physicians and correctly dispensed by pharmacists. Thus the term "drug" should continue to evoke an accepting attitude. In this section, the authors address both the professional use of drugs (medicines) and the consequences of the illicit use. Regarding the latter, the focus is on treatment programs and related matters. Thus the reader should recognize that attention is being given to both aspects of drugs; the medical perspective is the purpose in both cases.

Description of Medicine

| descriptions of prescription and/or non-prescription drugs that includes their purpose, ingredients, usage, dosage, precautions, adverse reactions, chemical interactions with other drugs, warnings, or other information? | *Complete Guide to Prescription and Non-Prescription Drugs* [3-121] *Drug Evaluations Annual* [3-129] *Drugs Available Abroad* [3-131] *Essential Guide to Prescription Drugs* [3-132] *Guide to Prescription and Over-the-Counter Drugs* [3-138] *Martindale, the Extra Pharmacopoeia* [3-142] *Physicians' Desk Reference* [3-153] *Physicians' Desk Reference for Nonprescription Drugs* [3-154] *U.S. Pharmacopeia Drug Information for the Consumer* [3-158] |

WHERE SHOULD I GO TO FIND. . .	*TRY*

Description of Medicine

descriptive monographs of drugs, chemicals, and biological substances that offer chemical, pharmacological, and clinical information; toxicity data; titles of review articles; and other explanations?	*The Merck Index* [3-145]
a colored pictorial identification chart of capsules, tablets, medicinal tubes and bottles, injection devices, and other drug-product packages?	*Guide to Prescription and Over-the-Counter Drugs* (capsules and tablets only) [3-138] *Physicians' Desk Reference* [3-153] *Physicians' Desk Reference for Nonprescription Drugs* [3-154] *U.S. Pharmacopeia Drug Information for the Consumer* (capsules and tablets only) [3-158]
the names and descriptions of therapeutic drugs that have been approved by foreign regulatory authorities and are in use abroad but are not generally available in the United States?	*Drugs Available Abroad* [3-131]
the alcohol content of selected medications?	*Drug Evaluations Annual* [3-129] *How to Defeat Alcoholism* [3-33] *Physicians' Desk Reference* [3-153]
a list of alcohol-free medications?	*How to Defeat Alcoholism* [3-33]
an indication of a drug's potential for abuse?	*Essential Guide to Prescription Drugs* [3-132] *Guide to Prescription and Over-the-Counter Drugs* [3-138] *Physicians' Desk Reference* [3-153]
the calorie content of different pharmaceuticals?	*The Calorie Factor* [3-110]
an explanation of the basic ingredients commonly found in cold medicines?	*Complete Guide to Early Child Care* [3-118]
an explanation of drugs used to treat allergic diseases, including side effects and precautions?	*Allergy Encyclopedia* [3-103] *Martindale, The Extra Pharmacopoeia* [3-142]
an explanation of drugs frequently prescribed for children with asthma?	*Children with Asthma* [3-19]

WHERE SHOULD I GO TO FIND. . .	*TRY*

Description of Medicine

drugs that have been found to alter the blood glucose level, along with their individual mechanisms and the probability and level of response?	*Diabetes Type II* [3-23]
a description of those drugs that are often used for the treatment of bladder disorders?	*Overcoming Bladder Disorders* [3-43]

Drug Abuse and Treatment

an explanation of the different types of drugs that are often abused and their effects?	*Complete Guide to Prescription and Non-Prescription Drugs* [3-121] *Complete Home Medical Guide* [3-124] *Guide to Prescription and Over-the-Counter Drugs* [3-138] *Health Care U.S.A.* [3-85] *How to Defeat Alcoholism* [3-33]
an indication of a drug's potential for abuse?	*Essential Guide to Prescription Drugs* [3-132] *Guide to Prescription and Over-the-Counter Drugs* [3-138] *Physicians' Desk Reference* [3-153]
warning signs of drug experimentation?	*Complete Home Medical Guide* [3-124] *Drugs, Alcohol, and Your Children* [3-24] *New Family Medical Guide* [3-149]
a guidebook for parents who are confronted with their child's substance abuse?	*Drugs, Alcohol, and Your Children* [3-24]
guidelines for parents and coaches as they work with young athletes involved with drugs?	*Sportswise* [3-47]
a national directory of programs that offer prevention, education, and early intervention services for substance abuse among children, with a description of each program?	*Substance Abuse and Kids* [3-100]
a listing, by state, of drug treatment programs for adolescents, citing addresses and telephone numbers?	*Health Care U.S.A.* [3-85] *Substance Abuse Residential Treatment Centers for Teens* [3-101]

WHERE SHOULD I GO TO FIND. . .   *TRY*

Drug Abuse and Treatment

a directory of self-help and information   *Health Care U.S.A.* [3-85]
organizations targeting drug abuse rehab?   *Medical and Health Information Directory*, Vol. 3
                                                 [3-90]

Effects of Drugs

a guide to adverse drug interactions that   *Drug Interactions Guide Book* [3-130]
reports the uses of the drugs involved,
which drug's action is increased or
decreased during the interaction, and what
to do to prevent or reduce the interaction
effect?

how likely it is that an adverse interaction   *Drug Interactions Guide Book* [3-130]
will occur between two specified drugs?

a comprehensive discussion of the   *Food and Drug Interaction Guide* [3-135]
interaction between prescription or
non-prescription drugs and the body's
nutritional system, including possible side
effects, recommendations for dietary
practices while taking a specific drug, and
an explanation of the symptoms and
treatment for nutritional interactions?

the possible interaction effect between an   *Complete Guide to Prescription and
individual drug and foods, beverages,   Non-Prescription Drugs* [3-121]
tobacco, cocaine, and marijuana?   *Drug Interactions Guide Book* (foods and
                                                 beverages only) [3-130]

how drugs work in the body?   *American Medical Association Encyclopedia of
                                                 Medicine* [3-107]
                                                 *Guide to Prescription and Over-the-Counter
                                                 Drugs* [3-138]
                                                 The Merck Manual of Diagnosis and Therapy
                                                 [3-146]

a listing of drugs that have side effects that   *Family Guide to Dental Health* [3-133]
affect dental health and treatment?

the possible effects of a drug on sexual   *Essential Guide to Prescription Drugs* [3-132]
function?   *Martindale, The Extra Pharmacopoeia*
                                                 [3-142]

WHERE SHOULD I GO TO FIND. . .	*TRY*

Effects of Drugs

a listing of drugs that have been reported to cause emotional and/or behavioral disturbances?	*Essential Guide to Prescription Drugs* [3-132]
drugs that may cause impairment to vision?	*Essential Guide to Prescription Drugs* [3-132]
drugs that may sensitize the skin to the effects of the sun?	*Complete Guide to Prescription and Non-Prescription Drugs* [3-121] *Complete Home Medical Guide* [3-124] *Essential Guide to Prescription Drugs* [3-132]
the effects that drugs most commonly used by athletes have on the body?	*Complete Guide to Sports Injuries* [3-122]
the negative side effects of steroids?	*Sportswise* [3-47]
a table of drug-nutrient interactions that are associated with the treatment of AIDS?	*Surviving with AIDS* [3-49]
drugs that have an adverse interaction with alcohol, and what that interaction effect may be?	*Complete Guide to Prescription and Non-Prescription Drugs* [3-121] *Complete Home Medical Guide* [3-124] *Essential Guide to Prescription Drugs* [3-132] *Guide to Prescription and Over-the-Counter Drugs* [3-138]
the truth of what alcoholism is and what happens within the body?	*How to Defeat Alcoholism* [3-33]
the symptoms of alcoholism?	*Complete Home Medical Guide* [3-124] *How to Defeat Alcoholism* [3-33] *New Family Medical Guide* [3-149]

Generic and Brand-Name Drugs

a glossary of generic-name drugs with an explanation of their purposes?	*American Medical Association Encyclopedia of Medicine* [3-107] *Guide to Prescription and Over-the-Counter Drugs* [3-138]
the generic name of a brand-name drug?	*American Medical Association Encyclopedia of Medicine* [3-107] *Complete Guide to Prescription and Non-Prescription Drugs* [3-121]

WHERE SHOULD I GO TO FIND...	*TRY*

Generic and Brand-Name Drugs

the generic name of a brand-name drug?	*Drug Interactions Guide Book* [3-130] *Drugs Available Abroad* [3-131] *Essential Guide to Prescription Drugs* [3-132] *Food and Drug Interaction Guide* [3-135] *Guide to Prescription and Over-the-Counter Drugs* [3-138] *Martindale, The Extra Pharmacopoeia* [3-142] *The Merck Index* [3-145] *Physicians' Desk Reference* [3-153] *Physicians' Desk Reference for Nonprescription Drugs* [3-154] *U. S. Pharmacopeia Drug Information for the Consumer* [3-158]
the brand name(s) of a generic drug?	*Complete Guide to Prescription and Non-Prescription Drugs* [3-121] *Drug Interactions Guide Book* [3-130] *The Merck Index* [3-145] *The Merck Manual of Diagnosis and Therapy* [3-146] *U.S. Pharmacopeia Drug Information for the Consumer* [3-158]

Newsletters

a newsletter that provides information from medical journals and other sources about the use and effects of all kinds of drugs and the trends in their treatment of drug abuse?	*Drug Abuse Update* [3-182]

Prescriptions

an interpretation of the abbreviations and/or terms found in a medical prescription?	*Acronyms, Initialisms, and Abbreviations Dictionary* [3-56] *Complete Home Medical Guide* [3-124] *Dorland's Illustrated Medical Dictionary* [3-58] *How to Talk to Your Doctor* [3-34] *Medical Acronyms and Abbreviations* [3-61] *Melloni's Illustrated Medical Dictionary* [3-63] *The Merck Index* [3-145] *The Merck Manual of Diagnosis and Therapy* [3-146] *Stedman's Medical Dictionary* [3-64]

WHERE SHOULD I GO TO FIND. . .   *TRY*

Uses of Medicinal Drugs
(Also see "Descriptions of Medicines")

medicinal drugs arranged by categories of use?

Complete Guide to Prescription and Non-Prescription Drugs [3-121]
Essential Guide to Prescription Drugs [3-132]
Guide to Prescription and Over-the-Counter Drugs [3-138]
Martindale, The Extra Pharmacopoeia [3-142]
The Merck Index [3-145]
Physicians' Desk Reference [3-153]
Physicians' Desk Reference for Nonprescription Drugs [3-154]
U.S. Pharmacopeia Drug Information for the Consumer [3-158]

which drugs are used to treat selected chronic health disorders and how they work in the body?

Complete Home Medical Guide [3-124]
Essential Guide to Prescription Drugs [3-132]
Guide to Prescription and Over-the-Counter Drugs [3-138]
Martindale, The Extra Pharmacopoeia [3-142]

questions to be asked by a patient regarding the use of drugs being prescribed for the treatment of a medical condition?

How to Talk to Your Doctor [3-34]

an explanation of the U.S. drug testing program and why many foreign drugs are not available in the United States?

Drugs Available Abroad [3-131]

information about the use of specific medicines during pregnancy?

Complete Guide to Prescription and Non-Prescription Drugs [3-121]
Essential Guide to Prescription Drugs [3-132]
Guide to Prescription and Over-the-Counter Drugs [3-138]
Martindale, The Extra Pharmacopoeia [3-142]
Physicians' Desk Reference [3-153]
U.S. Pharmacopeia Drug Information for the Consumer [3-158]

FDA safety ratings for the use of individual drugs during pregnancy?

Essential Guide to Prescription Drugs [3-132]
Physicians' Desk Reference [3-153]

information about the use of specific drugs during breast feeding?

Complete Guide to Early Child Care [3-118]
Complete Guide to Prescription and Non-Prescription Drugs [3-121]

WHERE SHOULD I GO TO FIND...	*TRY*

Uses of Medicinal Drugs
(Also see "Descriptions of Medicines")

information about the use of specific drugs during breast feeding?	*Essential Guide to Prescription Drugs* [3-132] *Guide to Prescription and Over-the-Counter Drugs* [3-138] *Martindale, The Extra Pharmacopoeia* [3-142] *Physicians' Desk Reference* [3-153] *U.S. Pharmacopeia Drug Information for the Consumer* [3-158]
general guidelines for the use of drugs by the elderly?	*Essential Guide to Prescription Drugs* [3-132] *Old Enough to Feel Better* [3-40]
special precautions and warnings for the elderly regarding the use of specific drugs?	*Complete Guide to Prescription and Non-Prescription Drugs* [3-121] *Essential Guide to Prescription Drugs* [3-132] *Guide to Prescription and Over-the-Counter Drugs* [3-138]
drugs that have been found to alter the blood glucose level, along with their individual mechanisms and the probability and level of response?	*Diabetes Type II* [3-23]
a description of those drugs that are often used for the treatment of bladder disorders?	*Overcoming Bladder Disorders* [3-43]
the drugs that are used to treat specific diseases and disorders?	*Drug Interactions Guide Book* [3-130]

First Aid

Assessment and Reporting

how to assess a medical emergency situation?	*First Aid Book* [3-134]
guidelines for when to call the doctor and what to say when reporting a medical emergency?	*Complete Guide to Early Child Care* [3-118]
a guide to what is a pediatric emergency, near-emergency, or non-emergency?	*Complete Guide to Early Child Care* [3-118]

WHERE SHOULD I GO TO FIND. . .	***TRY***
Diagnostics	
how to take your own blood pressure?	*Complete Home Medical Guide* [3-124]
an interpretation of rectal temperatures in young children?	*Complete Guide to Early Child Care* [3-118]
Emergency Procedures and Actions	
an explanation of first-aid procedures for emergency medical situations?	*American Medical Association Encyclopedia of Medicine* [3-107] *Complete Guide to Early Child Care* [3-118] *Complete Guide to Symptoms, Illness and Surgery* [3-123] *Complete Home Medical Guide* [3-124] *First Aid Book* [3-134] *New Family Medical Guide* [3-149]
what to do to help a child for a specific illness or injury?	*Complete Parents' Guide to Telephone Medicine* [3-125]
the procedure to follow during an emergency childbirth?	*American Medical Association Encyclopedia of Medicine* [3-107]
how to administer CPR (cardiopulmonary resuscitation)?	*American Medical Association Encyclopedia of Medicine* [3-107] *Complete Guide to Early Child Care* [3-118] *Complete Home Medical Guide* [3-124]
how to reduce a fever?	*Complete Guide to Early Child Care* [3-118] *Complete Guide to Symptoms, Illness and Surgery* [3-123] *Complete Home Medical Guide* [3-124]
the causes, symptoms, diagnoses, and treatment of allergy emergencies?	*Allergy Encyclopedia* [3-103]
what to do for different dental emergencies?	*Family Guide to Dental Health* [3-133]
First Aid Preparation	
what to include in a family's home first-aid kit?	*Complete Home Medical Guide* [3-124] *First Aid book* [3-134] *New Family Medical Guide* [3-149]

WHERE SHOULD I GO TO FIND. . .	*TRY*

| **Food Facts** | |

Allergens and Foods

guidelines for a food-sensitive diet?	*Instructions for Patients* [3-139]
a classification of foods that will reveal those foods that are related and that may contain a common allergen?	*Eating and Allergy* [3-25] *Food Allergy* [3-28]

Dietary Guidelines for Age Groups

dietary guidelines for infants up to 12 months of age?	*Food Values of Portions Commonly Used* [3-136] *Instructions for Patients* [3-139] *Modern Nutrition in Health and Disease* [3-147] *Nutrition Almanac* [3-150] *Recommended Dietary Allowances* [3-45]
for infants, the average number of recommended daily feedings and the average quantity per feeding?	*Instructions for Patients* [3-139]
dietary guidelines for children one to 16 years of age?	*Food Values of Portions Commonly Used* [3-136] *Instructions for Patients* [3-139] *Nutrition Almanac* [3-150] *Recommended Dietary Allowances* [3-45]
the daily calorie requirements for children one to six years of age?	*Complete Guide to Early Child Care* [3-118] *Nutrition Almanac* [3-150]
for each of the basic food groups, the number of daily servings and the size of each serving recommended for children during the first five years?	*Complete Guide to Early Child Care* [3-118]
guidelines for teaching toddlers and preschoolers how to eat, including suggestions on how to manage those "terrible" feeding problems?	*Complete Guide to Early Child Care* [3-118]
the recommended daily energy allowances for infants, children, and adults?	*Food Values of Portions Commonly Used* [3-136] *Recommended Dietary Allowances* [3-45]

WHERE SHOULD I GO TO FIND. . .	*TRY*

Dietary Guidelines for Age Groups

dietary guidelines for the older person?

Food Values of Portions Commonly Used [3-136]
Instructions for Patients [3-139]
Nutrition Almanac [3-150]
Recommended Dietary Allowances [3-45]

Food Additives

the major types of food additives and an explanation of why each is used?

Complete Home Medical Guide [3-124]
Dictionary of Food Ingredients [3-57]
Eating and Allergy [3-25]
Food Allergy [3-28]
Guide to Prescription and Over-the-Counter Drugs [3-138]

a listing of substances that are used to deliver the different types of additives to foods, along with the foods in which they are to be found and the possible adverse effects or risks?

Guide to Prescription and Over-the-Counter Drugs [3-138]

guidelines for the use of food additives, indicating which ones are safe and which should either be avoided or used with caution?

Complete Home Medical Guide [3-124]

Food Ingredients and Calories

the calorie content of different fast foods, vending machine foods, and airline menus?

The Calorie Factor [3-110]
Food Values of Portions Commonly Used [fast foods only] [3-136]

the calorie content of various foods?

The Calorie Factor [3-110]
Food Values of Portions Commonly Used [3-136]
Nutrition Almanac [3-150]

the calorie content of special weight-loss and weight-gain food products?

The Calorie Factor [3-110]

the calorie content of infant formulas and baby foods by brand?

The Calorie Factor [3-110]
Food Values of Portions Commonly Used [3-136]

the calorie content of dietary supplements and different medicinal drugs?

The Calorie Factor [3-110]

WHERE SHOULD I GO TO FIND. . .	*TRY*
Food Ingredients and Calories	
the calorie content of alcoholic beverages?	*The Calorie Factor* [3-110] *Food Values of Portions Commonly Used* [3-136] *Nutrition Almanac* [3-150]
an explanation of the different vitamins and minerals, including their roles in health, dietary sources, normal daily requirements, and information regarding deficiency and its treatment?	*Complete Home Medical Guide* [3-124] *Dorland's Illustrated Medical Dictionary* [vitamins only] [3-58] *Guide to Prescription and Over-the-Counter Drugs* [3-138] *The Merck Manual of Diagnosis and Therapy* [3-146] *Nutrition Almanac* [3-150] *Recommended Dietary Allowances* [3-45]
the vitamin and mineral content of foods?	*Food Values of Portions Commonly Used* [3-136] *Nutrition Almanac* [3-150]
the amount of nutrients contained in some of the popular mineral and vitamin supplements for children and adults?	*Food and Drug Interaction Guide* [3-135]
an explanation of cholesterol in the diet, how it works, and the names of cholesterol-rich foods with measurements per serving?	*Complete Home Medical Guide* [3-124] *Food and Drug Interaction Guide* [3-135] *Nutrition Almanac* [3-150]
the cholesterol content of foods?	*Food Values of Portions Commonly Used* [3-136] *Nutrition Almanac* [3-150]
the fiber content of foods?	*Food Values of Portions Commonly Used* [3-136] *Nutrition Almanac* [3-150]
foods that are high in potassium?	*Instructions for Patients* [3-139] *Nutrition Almanac* [3-150]
the caffeine, salicylate, and sugar contents of foods?	*Foods Values of Portions Commonly Used* [3-136] *Nutrition Almanac* [3-150]
the carbohydrate, fat, and protein content per serving for common foods?	*The Calorie Factor* [carbohydrates only] [3-110] *Complete Home Medical Guide* [3-124] (*answer continues*)

WHERE SHOULD I GO TO FIND. . .	*TRY*

Food Ingredients and Calories

the carbohydrate, fat, and protein content per serving for common foods?	*Food Values of Portions Commonly Used* [3-136] *Nutrition Almanac* [3-150]
the alcohol content of alcoholic beverages?	*Food Values of Portions Commonly Used* [3-136]

Food Poisoning

an explanation of food poisoning?	*American Medical Association Encyclopedia of Medicine* [3-107] *The Merck Manual of Diagnosis and Therapy* [3-146] *New Family Medical Guide* [3-149] *Nutrition Almanac* [3-150]

Food Sources

tables that report major food sources for selected nutrients, including vitamins and minerals?	*American Medical Association Encyclopedia of Medicine* [3-107] *Complete Home Medical Guide* [3-124] *Food and Drug Interaction Guide* [3-135] *Guide to Prescription and Over-the-Counter Drugs* [3-138] *The Merck Manual of Diagnosis and Therapy* [3-146] *New Family Medical Guide* [3-149] *Nutrition Almanac* [3-150]
an illustration of the different retail cuts of beef and from where each is derived?	*The Calorie Factor* [3-110]

Food and Drug Interactions

the interaction effect between individual drugs and specific foods, and what should be done to relieve unwanted effects and correct the resulting condition?	*Drug Interactions Guide Book* [3-130] *Food and Drug Interaction Guide* [3-135]
the effects of drugs on food intake and nutrient requirements?	*Modern Nutrition in Health and Disease* [3-147]
a table of drug-nutrient interactions that are associated with the treatment of AIDS?	*Surviving with AIDS* [3-49]

WHERE SHOULD I GO TO FIND. . .	*TRY*

Manufacturers and Suppliers

the names, addresses, and telephone numbers of manufacturers of food products for allergen-free diets?	*Allergy Encyclopedia* [3-103]
sources of suppliers for organic produce, vitamins and supplements, freeze-dried herbal extracts, herbal pharmaceutical products, and Chinese medicinal herbs?	*Natural Health, Natural Medicine* [3-39]

Newsletters

a newsletter that discusses the uses of nutritional and health food products as an alternative to the use of drugs and surgery in the prevention and treatment of diseases and disorders?	*Alternatives* [3-172]

Nutrition: Disorders and Diseases

an explanation of nutritional disorders and the effects of nutrition on different diseases?	*American Medical Association Encyclopedia of Medicine* [3-107] *Complete Guide to Symptoms, Illness and Surgery* [3-123] *Complete Home Medical Guide* [3-124] *The Merck Manual of Diagnosis and Therapy* [3-146] *Modern Nutrition in Health and Disease* [3-147] *Nutrition Almanac* [3-150]
information about diet and nutrition in the prevention and treatment of disease?	*Modern Nutrition in Health and Disease* [3-147] *Nutrition Almanac* [3-150]
dietary guidelines for women with premenstrual syndrome?	*Self-Help for Premenstrual Syndrome* [3-46]
a nutritional program that helps to manage the chronic malnutrition that accompanies AIDS?	*AIDS: A Self-Care Manual* [3-16] *Surviving with AIDS* [3-49]

WHERE SHOULD I GO TO FIND...	*TRY*

Nutrition: Disorders and Diseases

a table of drug-nutrient interactions that are associated with the treatment of AIDS?	*Surviving with AIDS* [3-49]
suggestions on how to help the Alzheimer patient eat and maintain a sufficient intake of food?	*Caring for the Alzheimer Patient* [3-18]
a guide for selecting the right kinds of foods and the proper portions for achieving a balanced daily diet for the Alzheimer patient?	*Caring for the Alzheimer Patient* [3-18]
nutritional guidelines and recipes for cancer patients?	*Managing the Side Effects of Chemotherapy and Radiation* [3-37]
nutritional guidelines and recipes that may reduce the risk of cancer, according to the American Cancer Society?	*American Cancer Society Cookbook* [3-106]
a nutritional program designed to aid in the treatment of alcoholism?	*How to Defeat Alcoholism* [3-33]

Nutritional Standards

the daily Recommended Dietary Allowances (RDAs)?	*American Cancer Society Cookbook* [3-106] *American Medical Association Encyclopedia of Medicine* [3-107] *Complete Guide to Early Child Care* [3-118] *Complete Home Medical Guide* [3-124] *Food and Drug Interaction Guide* [3-135] *Food Values of Portions Commonly Used* [3-136] *Guide to Prescription and Over-the-Counter Drugs* [3-138] *The Merck Manual of Diagnosis and Therapy* [3-146] *Modern Nutrition in Health and Disease* [3-147] *Nutrition Almanac* [3-150] *Recommended Dietary Allowances* [3-45]
the Recommended Dietary Allowances (RDAs) during pregnancy?	*Complete Guide to Early Child Care* [3-118] *Complete Guide to Pregnancy* [3-120] *Food Values of Portions Commonly Used* [3-136] *Recommended Dietary Allowances* [3-45]

WHERE SHOULD I GO TO FIND. . .	**TRY**

Nutritional Standards

the Estimated Safe and Adequate Daily Dietary Intakes for selected vitamins and minerals?	*Food Values of Portions Commonly Used* [3-136] *Recommended Dietary Allowances* [3-45]
the four basic food groups with an explanation of the recommended daily servings?	*American Cancer Society Cookbook* [3-106] *American Medical Association Encyclopedia of Medicine* [3-107] *Complete Guide to Early Child Care* [3-118] *Complete Guide to Symptoms, Illness and Surgery* [3-123] *Complete Home Medical Guide* [3-124] *Instructions for Patients* [3-139] *New Family Medical Guide* [3-149]
how much fiber should be consumed per day?	*Complete Home Medical Guide* [3-124] *Recommended Dietary Allowances* [3-45]
weight and height standards for men and women?	*American Medical Association Encyclopedia of Medicine* [3-107] *Complete Home Medical Guide* [3-124] *Modern Nutrition in Health and Disease* [3-147] *Nutrition Almanac* [3-150]
how to calculate the number of calories needed per day according to sex, weight, and type of physical activity?	*Complete Home Medical Guide* [3-124]
the daily calorie requirements of children one to six years of age?	*Complete Guide to Early Child Care* [3-118] *Nutrition Almanac* [3-150]
the recommended daily energy allowances for infants, children, and adults?	*Food Values of Portions Commonly Used* [3-136] *Recommended Dietary Allowances* [3-45]
nutrition guidelines for athletes?	*Complete Guide to Sports Injuries* [3-122] *Sports Health* [3-155] *Sportswise* [3-47]

Special Diets and Controls

the proper nutritional practices during pregnancy?	*Complete Guide to Early Child Care* [3-118] *Complete Guide to Symptoms, Illness and Surgery* [3-123] *Complete Home Medical Guide* [3-124]

(answer continues)

WHERE SHOULD I GO TO FIND. . .	*TRY*

Special Diets and Controls

the proper nutritional practices during pregnancy?	*Instructions for Patients* [3-139] *Modern Nutrition in Health and Disease* [3-147] Nutrition Almanac [3-150]
guidelines for breast feeding?	*Complete Guide to Early Child Care* [3-118] *Instructions for Patients* [3-139] *The Merck Manual of Diagnosis and Therapy* [3-146]
how to reduce the intake of calories?	*Complete Home Medical Guide* [3-124]
suggestions for a weight-reduction diet?	*Complete Guide to Symptoms, Illness and Surgery* [3-123] *Instructions for Patients* [3-139]
guidelines for lowering cholesterol and fat levels?	*Complete Guide to Symptoms, Illness and Surgery* [3-123] *Complete Home Medical Guide* [3-124] *Food and Drug Interaction Guide* [3-135] *Instructions for Patients* [3-139] *New Family Medical Guide* [3-149] *Nutrition Almanac* [3-150]
recipes that emphasize natural ingredients, thereby resulting in wholesome foods?	*Nutrition Almanac* [3-150]
a milk-restricted diet, i.e., one that is used to treat lactose intolerance and milk allergy?	*Complete Guide to Symptoms, Illness and Surgery* [3-123] *Instructions for Patients* [3-139]
a gluten-restricted diet, i.e., one that must be free of gluten because of gastrointestinal disease?	*Complete Guide to Symptoms, Illness and Surgery* [3-123] *Instructions for Patients* [3-139]
a liquid diet for patients who cannot chew or swallow solid foods?	*Complete Guide to Symptoms, Illness and Surgery* [3-123] *Instructions for Patients* [3-139]
guidelines for a low-salt diet?	*Complete Guide to Symptoms, Illness and Surgery* [3-123] *Instructions for Patients* [3-139]

WHERE SHOULD I GO TO FIND. . .   *TRY*

Special Diets and Controls

sample high-calcium menus?	*Osteoporosis: The Silent Thief* [3-42]
suggestions for a soft diet?	*Complete Guide to Symptoms, Illness and Surgery* [3-123] *Instructions for Patients* [3-139]
a modified low-protein diet?	*Instructions for Patients* [3-139]
guidelines for a high-protein diet?	*Instructions for Patients* [3-139]
guidelines for a diet that is high in fiber and bulk?	*Instructions for Patients* [3-139]
a suggested bland diet for ambulatory patients?	*Instructions for Patients* [3-139]
guidelines for a food-sensitive (allergy) diet?	*Instructions for Patients* [3-139]
suggestions for cooking allergy-free meals, including recipes?	*Allergy Encyclopedia* [3-103] *Food Allergy* [3-28]
dietary guidelines for women with premenstrual syndrome?	*Self-Help for Premenstrual Syndrome* [3-46]
a nutritional program that helps to manage the chronic malnutrition that accompanies AIDS?	*AIDS: A Self-Care Manual* [3-16] *Surviving with AIDS* [3-49]
recipes for low-carbohydrate meals?	*Diabetes Type II* [3-23]
nutritional guidelines and recipes for cancer patients?	*Managing the Side Effects of Chemotherapy and Radiation* [3-37]
nutritional guidelines and recipes that may reduce the risk of cancer, according to the American Cancer Society?	*American Cancer Society Cookbook* [3-106]
a nutritional program designed to aid in the treatment of alcoholism?	*How to Defeat Alcoholism* [3-33]

WHERE SHOULD I GO TO FIND. . .   *TRY*

Health and Matters of Law

Drug Abuse

the legal responsibilities of parents and   *Drugs, Alcohol, and Your Children* [3-24]
children regarding the use of drugs and
alcohol by children?

Legal Protections and Rights

the rights of patients?   *Family Guide to Dental Health* [3-133]
                                                   How to Talk to Your Doctor [3-34]
                                                   Take This Book to the Hospital with You
                                                   [3-50]
                                                   Understanding Alzheimer's Disease [3-52]

a survey of legal-medical issues, including   *Medicine and the Law* [3-38]
abortion, rights of patients, and standards?

a sample of a Living Will and a Durable   *Complete Home Medical Guide* [3-124]
Power of Attorney?

a summary of federal laws that enhance the   *Meeting the Needs of People with Disabilities*
field of rehabilitation of the disabled?   [3-144]

an explanation of the special civil rights of   *Meeting the Needs of People with Disabilities*
people with disabilities, including   [3-144]
enforcement provisions to prevent
discrimination against them?

a general interpretation of the Education   *Directory of Residential Facilities for Emotionally*
of All Handicapped Act (P.L. 94–142)   *Handicapped Children and Youth* [3-79]
which explains the rights of handicapped
children and how to secure special
education services?

answers to legal questions about caring for   *Understanding Alzheimer's Disease* [3-52]
the patient with Alzheimer's disease?

guidance for patients with AIDS regarding   *AIDS: A Self-Care Manual* [3-16]
a Durable Power of Attorney for Health Care?

a discussion of premenstrual syndrome as a   *Once A Month* [3-41]
defense in court?

WHERE SHOULD I GO TO FIND. . .	*TRY*
Newsletters	
a newsletter that reports on laws, regulations, and political developments regarding AIDS?	*AIDS Policy and Law* [3-171]
a newsletter that reports on current key decisions and pleadings involving medical malpractice?	*Medical Malpractice Litigation Reporter* [3-184]
a newsletter that follows current medical malpractice cases, including new rulings, docket numbers, names of counsel, and the names of expert witnesses in each case?	*Medical Malpractice: Verdicts, Settlements, and Experts* [3-185]
a newsletter that reports current decisions, legislation, standards, enforcement, and other activities of federal and state regulatory agencies regarding occupational safety and health?	*Occupational Safety and Health Reporter* [3-189]
Safety Standards	
the health and safety standards of the U.S. Occupational Safety and Health Administration (OSHA)?	*29 Code of Federal Regulations* [3-160]
Vaccination Requirements	
the vaccination requirements of individual countries?	*Countries of the World and Their Leaders* [3-126]

Health Care Centers and Services

Child Care Services	
an explanation of the different types of child care arrangements that may be available to working parents?	*Complete Guide to Early Child Care* [3-118]
what to look for and how to evaluate the quality of a daycare center?	*Complete Guide to Early Child Care* [3-118]

WHERE SHOULD I GO TO FIND. . .	*TRY*
Child Care Services	
a checklist to be used when selecting a daycare center?	*Complete Guide to Early Child Care* [3-118]
Continuing Care Retirement Communities	
an explanation of *continuing care* and what it involves?	*National Continuing Care Directory* [3-93]
a checklist of what to consider when searching for the *right* continuing care retirement community?	*National Continuing Care Directory* [3-93]
a checklist that helps to analyze and compare service packages offered by continuing care retirement communities?	*National Continuing Care Directory* [3-93]
a cost-comparison worksheet that will assist the retiree in determining the affordability of a continuing care plan?	*National Continuing Care Directory* [3-93]
a directory of continuing care retirement communities with a descriptive profile of each community that includes types of facilities and services offered, fees, nursing care, accreditation, address, telephone number, and other helpful information?	*National Continuing Care Directory* [3-93]
a listing of continuing care retirement communities arranged by metropolitan area and non-metropolitan area?	*National Continuing Care Directory* [3-93]
Drug Treatment Programs	
guidelines for selecting treatment centers for alcohol, drug, or other addictive disorders?	*Drug, Alcohol, and Other Addictions: A Directory of Treatment Centers and Prevention Programs Nationwide* [3-81] *How to Defeat Alcoholism* [3-33]
a directory of alcohol, drug, and other behavioral disorder addiction treatment centers and prevention programs that includes the address, telephone number, contact person's name, addictions treated, treatment methods, and other information about each program or center?	*Drug, Alcohol, and Other Addictions: A Directory of Treatment Centers and Prevention Programs Nationwide* [3-81] *Medical and Health Information Directory,* Vol. 3 [selected information] [3-90]

WHERE SHOULD I GO TO FIND. . .	*TRY*

Drug Treatment Programs

a descriptive and evaluative profile of selected drug and alcohol rehabilitation centers in the United States, explaining the treatment program, staff size and qualifications, facilities, cost, aftercare services, and other information about each center?	*REHAB* [3-96]
a national directory of residential and in-patient treatment programs for alcohol, drug, and behavioral disorders among preteens and teenagers that provides a descriptive profile of each treatment center?	*Substance Abuse Residential Treatment Centers for Teens* [3-101]
a directory of programs that offer prevention, education, and early intervention services for substance abuse among children, with a description of each program?	*Substance Abuse and Kids* [3-100]

Home Health Care

a listing of certified home health care agencies with their addresses and telephone numbers?	*Medical and Health Information Directory,* Vol. 3 [3-90]
guidelines for providers of home care for AIDS patients?	*AIDS: A Self-Care Manual* [3-16]

Hospitals

how to select a hospital?	*Take This Book to the Hospital with You* [3-50]
information that a patient should know about how hospitals function and what to expect and not expect?	*Take This Book to the Hospital with You* [3-50]
guidelines to follow when selecting an outpatient facility?	*Take This Book to the Hospital with You* [3-50]
descriptive profiles of hospitals that have been designated as being among the best in America, including their specialties, admission policies, and approximate charges?	*Best Hospitals in America* [3-71]

WHERE SHOULD I GO TO FIND...	*TRY*
Hospitals	
an exposé of what really goes on behind the scenes at hospitals throughout America, reporting reprehensible conditions that victimize patients?	*The Great White Lie* [3-29]
a listing of osteopathic hospitals with their addresses and telephone numbers?	*Health Care U.S.A.* [3-85]
a listing of selected hospitals and clinics that specialize in sports medicine?	*Best Hospitals in America* [3-71] *Medical and Health Information Directory,* Vol. 3 [3-90]
a listing of selected hospitals and clinics that specialize in geriatrics?	*Best Hospitals in America* [3-71]
a listing of selected hospitals and clinics that specialize in severe pediatric illnesses?	*Best Hospitals in America* [3-71]
a listing of selected hospitals that specialize in dental care?	*Best Hospitals in America* [3-71]
questions for parents to ask when in the process of selecting a hospital for the birth of their child?	*Complete Guide to Early Child Care* [3-118]
a discussion of the services of a neonatal intensive care unit, including a clarification of common fears and myths about this unit?	*Complete Guide to Early Child Care* [3-118]
how parents can prepare their child for hospitalization, and what parents should do during the child's stay?	*Complete Guide to Early Child Care* [3-118] *New Family Medical Guide* [3-149]
questions to be asked by a patient when being advised by a physician to enter a hospital?	*How to Talk to Your Doctor* [3-34] *Take This Book to the Hospital with You* [3-50]
questions to ask and what to do when preparing to check into a hospital?	*Take This Book to the Hospital with You* [3-50]
what to do about specific problem situations that may arise while being hospitalized?	*Take This Book to the Hospital with You* [3-50]

WHERE SHOULD I GO TO FIND. . .	**_TRY_**

Hospitals

how and where to register a complaint about services received in a hospital?	*Take This Book to the Hospital with You* [3-50]
guidance on matters pertaining to leaving a hospital?	*Take This Book to the Hospital with You* [3-50]

Hotlines and Helplines

health care hotline and/or helpline telephone numbers?	*AIDS: A Self-Care Manual* [3-16] *AIDS and Women: A Sourcebook* [3-5] *American Medical Association Encyclopedia of Medicine* [3-107] *Consumer Health Information Source Book* [3-8] *Drug, Alcohol, and Other Addictions: A Directory of Treatment Centers and Prevention Programs Nationwide* [3-81] *Drugs, Alcohol, and Your Children* [3-24] *Health Care U.S.A.* [3-85] *Health Hotlines* [3-86] *How to Defeat Alcoholism* [3-33] *Substance Abuse and Kids* [3-100] *Substance Abuse Residential Treatment Centers for Teens* [3-101] *Surviving with AIDS* [3-49] Note: See also your local telephone directory.

Insurance

guidelines for deciding if a Health Maintenance Organization (HMO) should be joined?	*Complete Home Medical Guide* [3-124]
guidelines on how to select an HMO?	*HMOs* [3-32]
an explanation of Medicare and Medicaid?	*Complete Home Medical Guide* [3-124]
the address and telephone number to be used for filing a complaint with the Medicare sanctions program about a health care provider?	*9479 Questionable Doctors* [3-65]

WHERE SHOULD I GO TO FIND. . .	TRY

Insurance

| information about federal and state insurance disability benefits that are available to persons with AIDS? | *AIDS: A Self-Care Manual* [3-16] |
| an explanation of dental insurance issues? | *Family Guide to Dental Health* [3-133] |

Newsletters

| a newsletter that provides information on how to care for the elderly and the handicapped? | *Caregivers* [3-180] |

Nursing Homes

a checklist of considerations for selecting a nursing home?	*Caring for the Alzheimer Patient* [3-18] *Complete Home Medical Guide* [3-124] *Understanding Alzheimer's Disease* [3-52]
a directory of nursing homes, by state, that reports for each the address, telephone number, name of administrator, admission requirements, level of care licensed to provide, size of staff, and other helpful information?	*Directory of Nursing Homes* [3-77]
nursing homes classified by their affiliation (e.g., religious, fraternal, etc.)?	*Directory of Nursing Homes* [3-77]
the addresses and telephone numbers of the headquarters of corporate nursing homes?	*Directory of Nursing Homes* [3-77]

Poison Control Centers

| a directory of poison control centers with their addresses and emergency telephone numbers? | *Complete Guide to Early Child Care* [3-118]
 Complete Home Medical Guide [3-124]
 Current Pediatric Therapy [3-127]
 Health Hotlines [3-86]
 Physicians' Desk Reference [3-153]
 Physicians' Desk Reference for Nonprescription Drugs [3-154]
 Note: See also your local telephone directory. |

WHERE SHOULD I GO TO FIND. . .	*TRY*

Self-Help Organizations

| the addresses and telephone numbers of self-help organizations and support groups? | *AIDS and Women: A Sourcebook* [3-5]
 AIDS Information Sourcebook [3-67]
 American Cancer Society Cancer Book [3-17]
 American Medical Association Encyclopedia of Medicine [3-107]
 Health Care U.S.A. [3-85]
 Health Hotlines [3-86]
 How to Defeat Alcoholism [3-33]
 Medical and Health Information Directory, Vol. 3 [3-90] |
| information sources on AIDS, including addresses and telephone numbers? | *AIDS: A Self-Care Manual* [3-16]
 AIDS and Women: A Sourcebook [3-5]
 AIDS Information Sourcebook [3-67]
 Consumer Health Information Source Book [3-8]
 Health Care U.S.A. [3-85]
 Health Hotlines [3-86]
 Medical and Health Information Directory, Vol. 3[3-90]
 Surviving with AIDS [3-49] |

Summer Camps

| a directory of summer camps for children with physical or emotional disabilities that reports for each camp the address, telephone number, name of contact person, and a brief description of the facilities and activities? | *Allergy Encyclopedia* [3-103]
 Guide to Accredited Camps [3-84] |

Travelers' Health Services

| centers with medical assistance information when traveling abroad? | *Foreign Travel and Immunization Guide* [3-137] |

Treatment Centers and Other Health Providers

| for individual diseases and medical disorders, the names, addresses, and telephone numbers of special treatment centers, clinics, hospital-based services, transplant centers, federal health agencies, and/or other health-care providers? | See Chapters 6, 7, and 8.
 AIDS Information Sourcebook [3-67]
 American Cancer Society Cancer Book [3-17]
 Best Hospitals in America [3-71]
 Directory of Medical Rehabilitation Programs [3-75] |

(*answer continues*)

WHERE SHOULD I GO TO FIND. . .	*TRY*

Treatment Centers and Other Health Providers

for individual diseases and medical disorders, the names, addresses, and telephone numbers of special treatment centers, clinics, hospital-based services, transplant centers, federal health agencies, and/or other health-care providers?	*Directory of Pain Treatment Centers in the U.S. and Canada* [3-78] *Health Care U.S.A.* [3-85] *Medical and Health Information Directory,* Vol. 3 [3-90]
a listing of hospice services?	*Health Care U.S.A.* [3-85] *Medical and Health Information Directory,* Vol. 3 [3-90]
how to receive treatment from the National Institutes of Health?	*Health Care U.S.A.* [3-85]
a directory of *in-vitro* fertilization centers and sperm banks, listed by state?	*Health Care U.S.A.* [3-85]
information sources on AIDS, including addresses and telephone numbers?	*AIDS: A Self-Care Manual* [3-16] *AIDS and Women: A Sourcebook* [3-5] *AIDS Information Sourcebook* [3-67] *Consumer Health Information Source Book* [3-8] *Health Care U.S.A.* [3-85] *Health Hotlines* [3-86] *Medical and Health Information Directory,* Vol. 3 [3-90] *Surviving with AIDS* [3-49]
the names, addresses, and telephone numbers of mental retardation treatment and/or research centers?	*Health Care U.S.A.* [3-85] *Medical and Health Information Directory,* Vol. 3 [3-90]
a listing of schools specially designed to serve children with dyslexia that reports for each school the address, telephone number, ages of children accepted, and other information?	*Health Care U.S.A.* [3-85]
a listing of Comprehensive Cancer Centers (CCC), as designated by the National Cancer Institute, reporting their addresses and telephone numbers?	*American Cancer Society Cancer Book* [3-17] *Complete Home Medical Guide* [3-124] *Health Care U.S.A.* [3-85]
health care centers that specialize in the treatment of cancer in children?	*Best Hospitals in America* [3-71] *Health Care U.S.A.* [3-85]

WHERE SHOULD I GO TO FIND. . .   *TRY*

Treatment Centers and Other Health Providers

a directory of facilities and programs that serve patients with Alzheimer's disease and their families, including addresses, telephone numbers, and descriptive profiles?	*Directory of Alzheimer's Disease Treatment Facilities and Home Health Care Programs* [3-74]
the names, addresses, and telephone numbers of schools for the blind and for visually impaired children?	*Medical and Health Information Directory,* Vol. 3 [3-90]
the names, addresses, and telephone numbers of schools for the deaf and for hearing-impaired children?	*Medical and Health Information Directory,* Vol. 3 [3-90]
a listing of rehabilitation programs in audiology or speech-language pathology?	*Medical and Health Information Directory,* Vol. 3 [3-90]
the names, addresses, and telephone numbers of certified eye banks that have tissue for use in corneal transplantation?	*Medical and Health Information Directory,* Vol. 3 [3-90]
the names, addresses, and telephone numbers of agencies that provide family planning services?	*Medical and Health Information Directory,* Vol. 3 [3-90]
a directory of genetic diagnostic and counseling centers?	*Health Care U.S.A.* [3-85] *Medical and Health Information Directory,* Vol. 3 [3-90]
the names, addresses, and telephone numbers of agencies and institutions that provide mental health services?	*Medical and Health Information Directory,* Vol. 3 [3-90]
a listing of medical facilities that provide evaluation, treatment, or follow-up services for children who are mentally retarded?	*Medical and Health Information Directory,* Vol. 3 [3-90]
a listing of major allergy and/or asthma centers and clinics in the United States?	*Allergy Encyclopedia* [3-103] *Health Care U.S.A.* [3-85]
the names and descriptive profiles of medical rehabilitation programs and facilities in the United States?	*Directory of Medical Rehabilitation Programs* [3-75]

WHERE SHOULD I GO TO FIND. . .	*TRY*

Treatment Centers and Other Health Providers

guidelines for finding and applying to residential treatment facilities for children with emotional handicaps and behavior disorders?	*Directory of Residential Facilities for Emotionally Handicapped Children and Youth* [3-79]
a national directory that describes individual residential treatment facilities for children with emotional handicaps and behavior disorders?	*Directory of Residential Facilities for Emotionally Handicapped Children and Youth* [3-79]
guidelines to follow when selecting an outpatient facility?	*Take This Book to the Hospital with You* [3-50]
a directory of pain treatment centers with descriptive information for each center?	*Directory of Pain Treatment Centers in the U.S. and Canada* [3-78]
a directory of chapters of the National Chronic Pain Outreach Association?	*Directory of Pain Treatment Centers in the U.S. and Canada* [3-78]

Health Care Equipment and Prosthetics

Assessments

a listing of market research reports on medical equipment and supplies?	*Findex* [3-10]

Crutches

how to use crutches safely?	*Complete Guide to Sports Injuries* [3-122]

Electronic Aids

developments in robotics intended for use in rehabilitation of persons who have disabilities?	*Meeting the Needs of People with Disabilities* [3-144]
what computers can do for persons with different types of disabilities?	*Meeting the Needs of People with Disabilities* [3-144]

WHERE SHOULD I GO TO FIND...	*TRY*
Suppliers	
a directory of major companies that supply equipment and devices specially designed for persons with disabilities?	*Health Care U.S.A.* [3-85]
the titles of directories that contain the names and addresses of manufacturers and providers of health care products?	*Medical and Health Information Directory,* Vol. 2 [3-89]
a listing of rehabilitation engineering centers that develop technological aides for the handicapped?	*Health Care U.S.A.* [3-85]
suppliers of specified medical products with the addresses, telephone numbers, and product information of these companies?	*Medical Device Register* [3-91] *Medical Device Register: International Volume* [3-92]
a directory of optical supply houses and manufacturers?	*Blue Book of Optometrists* [3-72]

Health Care Professionals

Chiropractors: Listings

a national listing of chiropractors containing their addresses and telephone numbers and arranged by city within state?	*American Chiropractic Association, Membership Directory* [3-68]

Dentists: Listings and Specialties

the names of dentists, citing for each his/her office address, specialty, dental school from which graduated, and other biographical information?	*American Dental Directory* [3-69]
the names of certified dental specialists by city and according to their dental specialty?	*American Dental Directory* [3-69]

WHERE SHOULD I GO TO FIND. . .	*TRY*

Dentists: Listings and Specialties

an explanation of the purposes of the individual dental specialties?	*American Medical Association Encyclopedia of Medicine* [3-107] *Tooth and Gum Care* [3-51]

Natural Medicine Practitioners

sources for names of practitioners who practice alternative approaches to health care, including osteopathy, holistic medicine, homeopathy, naturopathic medicine, acupuncture, ayurvedic medicine, biofeedback, Trager work, Feldenkrais work, and others?	*Natural Health, Natural Medicine* [3-39]

Optometrists: Listings

a directory of optometrists in the United States, Puerto Rico, and Canada that reports for each person his/her specialty, education, address, telephone number, and other descriptive information?	*Blue Book of Optometrists* [3-72]

Physician Rights and Responsibilities

the rights and responsibilities of the physician?	*How to Talk to Your Doctor* [3-34]

Physicians and Surgeons: Listings and Specialties

a listing of physicians (not arranged by specialty) which cites for each his/her professional address, education, specialty practiced, and other descriptive information?	*American Medical Directory* [3-70]
the names of medical specialists, arranged by specialty, with the address, telephone number, and biographical information for each physician?	*ABMS Compendium of Certified Medical Specialists* [3-66] *Directory of Medical Specialists* [3-76] *Health Care U.S.A.* [addresses and telephone numbers only] [3-85]
the names of well-known medical specialists at each of the better hospitals in America?	*Best Hospitals in America* [3-71]

WHERE SHOULD I GO TO FIND. . .   *TRY*

Physicians and Surgeons: Listings and Specialties

a national directory of osteopathic physicians that reports the specialty, address, and other biographical information for each physician?

Yearbook and Directory of Osteopathic Physicians [3-102]

the purpose of individual medical specialties and what to expect when visiting a particular type of specialist?

Medical Tests and Diagnostic Procedures [3-143]

a bibliography of membership directories of professional health care associations?

Directories in Print [3-9]
Medical and Health Information Directory, Vol. 2 [3-89]

a listing of centers around the world, including their telephone numbers, where information on English-speaking doctors in different countries can be obtained?

Foreign Travel and Immunization Guide [3-137]

Professional Training

the educational and professional training of a physician?

ABMS Compendium of Certified Medical Specialists [3-66]
American Medical Directory [3-70]
Directory of Medical Specialists [3-76]

what comprises the education and professional training of a chiropractor?

Everybody's Guide to Chiropractic Health Care [3-27]

Quality Control

a summary explanation of the U.S. quality control system for health providers?

9479 Questionable Doctors [3-65]

the names and information about individual doctors, arranged by state, who have been disciplined for reasons related to their medical practices?

9479 Questionable Doctors [3-65]

Selecting a Health Professional

tips on how to check a physician's qualifications?

9479 Questionable Doctors [3-65]

WHERE SHOULD I GO TO FIND. . .	*TRY*
Selecting a Health Professional	
questions to ask when interviewing a doctor I am considering using as my personal physician?	*How to Talk to Your Doctor* [3-34]
suggestions on when and how to change doctors?	*How to Talk to Your Doctor* [3-34]
guidelines to follow and/or questions to be asked by parents when selecting a pediatrician?	*Complete Guide to Early Child Care* [3-118] *Complete Guide to Pregnancy* [3-120] *Complete Parents' Guide to Telephone Medicine* [3-125]
suggestions on how to find a medical specialist for a child?	*Complete Guide to Early Child Care* [3-118]
how to choose a doctor for a child with asthma?	*Children with Asthma* [3-19]
how to prepare for a second-opinion visit with an asthma specialist for a child?	*Children with Asthma* [3-19]
guidelines for selecting an obstetrician/ gynecologist?	*Complete Guide to Pregnancy* [3-120] *Complete Home Medical Guide* [3-124]
guidelines for selecting a cosmetic surgeon?	*Complete Book of Cosmetic Surgery* [3-115]
guidelines for selecting an eye surgeon and questions to ask in the process?	*Consumer Guide to Modern Cataract Surgery* [3-21]
guidelines for selecting a chiropractor?	*Everybody's Guide to Chiropractic Health Care* [3-27]
how to find a dentist?	*Tooth and Gum Care* [3-51]
guidelines for evaluating a dentist?	*Complete Home Medical Guide* [3-124]

Health Information Source Listings

---

a listing of books, periodicals, and other serials in print in the health sciences and allied fields?	*Books in Print* [3-7] *Medical and Health Care Books and Serials in Print* [3-11] *Ulrich's International Periodicals Directory* [3-14]

WHERE SHOULD I GO TO FIND. . .	*TRY*
evaluative descriptions of specific health information sources, such as books, magazines, newsletters, and organizations?	*Consumer Health Information Source Book* [3-8]
a bibliography of review journals that summarize the state of the art for individual medical specialties?	*Medical and Health Information Directory,* Vol. 2 [3-89]
a bibliography of journals in the biomedical and health sciences with the addresses and telephone numbers of their publishers?	*Medical and Health Information Directory,* Vol. 2 [3-89]
a bibliography of indexing and abstracting services for published literature in the medical and health-related sciences?	*Medical and Health Information Directory,* Vol. 2 [3-89]
an index to health and/or medical articles that have been published in periodicals, citing the bibliographic information necessary to locate each article?	*Consumer Health and Nutrition Index* [3-1] *Index Medicus* [3-2] *Readers' Guide to Periodical Literature* [3-4]
an index to periodical literature in dentistry with bibliographic citations to individual articles?	*Index Medicus* [3-2] *Index to Dental Literature* [3-3] *Readers' Guide to Periodical Literature* [3-4]
a bibliography of medical and health-related newsletters with the addresses and telephone numbers of their publishers?	*Medical and Health Information Directory,* Vol. 2 [3-89] *Newsletters in Print* [3-12] *Oxbridge Directory of Newsletters* [3-13]
a bibliography of directories that contain names, addresses, and telephone numbers of health care practitioners, health and medical programs, clinics, services, companies in the health care industry, and membership lists of professional associations?	*Directories in Print* [3-9] *Medical and Health Information Directory,* Vol. 2 [3-89]
a bibliography of online and offline computer databases that provide health-related information?	*Medical and Health Information Directory,* Vol. 2 [3-89]
a comprehensive bibliography of information sources on topics regarding persons with disabilities, including books, journals, newsletters, and organizations?	*Meeting the Needs of People with Disabilities* [3-144]

WHERE SHOULD I GO TO FIND. . .	*TRY*
an annotated bibliography of literature on AIDS?	*AIDS and Women: A Sourcebook* [3-5] *AIDS Information Sourcebook* [3-67]
a listing of publications on asthma in children?	*Children with Asthma* [3-19]

Mental Health

Crisis Centers

a listing, by state, of suicide prevention centers with their addresses and crisis telephone numbers?	*Health Care U.S.A.* [3-85]

Diagnostics

a classification of mental disorders with descriptive information that facilitates diagnoses?	*Diagnostic and Statistical Manual of Mental Disorders* [3-128] *The Merck Manual of Diagnosis and Therapy* [3-146]
a test that measures vulnerability to certain types of stress?	*Complete Home Medical Guide* [3-124]
a rating scale that helps assess changes in behavior of the Alzheimer patient and that assists with determining the progression of this disease?	*Caring for the Alzheimer Patient* [3-18]

Diseases and Disorders

an explanation of the different types of psychoses, including causes, symptoms, and treatment?	*American Medical Association Encyclopedia of Medicine* [3-107] *Complete Home Medical Guide* [3-124] *New Family Medical Guide* [3-149]
the causes, symptoms, and treatment of various diseases of the brain and nervous system, including Parkinson's disease, Huntington's disease, and epilepsy?	*American Medical Association Encyclopedia of Medicine* [3-107] *Complete Guide to Symptoms, Illness and Surgery* [3-123] *Complete Home Medical Guide* [3-124] *Health Care U.S.A.* [3-85]

WHERE SHOULD I GO TO FIND. . .	*TRY*
Diseases and Disorders	
the causes, symptoms, and treatment of various diseases of the brain and nervous system, including Parkinson's disease, Huntington's disease, and epilepsy?	*New Family Medical Guide* [3-149] *Old Enough to Feel Better* [3-40]
a listing of the different types of phobias and their definitions?	*Stedman's Medical Dictionary* [3-64]
a listing of emotional and/or behavioral disturbances and the drugs that have been reported to cause them?	*Essential Guide to Prescription Drugs* [3-132]
the causes, signs, and treatment of depression?	*American Medical Association Encyclopedia of Medicine* [3-107] *Complete Guide to Early Child Care* [3-118] *Complete Guide to Symptoms, Illness and Surgery* [3-123] *Complete Home Medical Guide* [3-124] *New Family Medical Guide* [3-149]
a discussion of psychological problems that may develop in children and adolescents?	*Complete Guide to Early Child Care* [3-118] *Complete Home Medical Guide* [3-124] *Current Pediatric Therapy* [3-127]
a discussion of child and/or adolescent behavioral problems and their modification?	*American Medical Association Encyclopedia of Medicine* [3-107] *Complete Guide to Early Child Care* [3-118] *Complete Home Medical Guide* [3-124] *Complete Parents' Guide to Telephone Medicine* [3-125] *Current Pediatric Therapy* [3-127]
an explanation of sleep disorders?	*American Medical Association Encyclopedia of Medicine* [3-107] *Complete Guide to Early Child Care* [3-118] *Complete Guide to Symptoms, Illness and Surgery* [3-123] *Complete Home Medical Guide* [3-124] *Current Pediatric Therapy* [3-127] *New Family Medical Guide* [3-149]
guidance on how to cope with and control the emotional and psychological aspects of premenstrual syndrome?	*PMS: A Positive Program to Gain Control* [3-44]

WHERE SHOULD I GO TO FIND. . .	*TRY*

Diseases and Disorders

a guide to Alzheimer's disease with answers to many of the questions that families ask about this disease, including how to care for the patient?	*Caring for the Alzheimer Patient* [3-18] *Understanding Alzheimer's Disease* [3-52]
symptoms of Alzheimer's disease and how they are expressed during routine activities?	*Caring for the Alzheimer Patient* [3-18] *New Family Medical Guide* [3-149] *Understanding Alzheimer's Disease* [3-52]
methods for improving nutrition, hygiene, communication, safety, and body elimination for the Alzheimer patient?	*Caring for the Alzheimer Patient* [3-18]
suggestions for helping the Alzheimer patient eat and maintain an adequate intake of food?	*Caring for the Alzheimer Patient* [3-18]

Mental Development

what is normal emotional and intellectual development in infants, toddlers, and preschoolers?	*Complete Guide to Early Child Care* [3-118]
how to determine when the behavior of a child is a serious problem that needs professional help?	*Complete Guide to Early Child Care* [3-118]
how a parent should approach the development of a gifted child?	*Complete Guide to Early Child Care* [3-118]

Mental Health Services: Directory

the names, addresses, and telephone numbers of agencies and institutions that provide mental health services?	*Medical and Health Information Directory,* Vol. 3 [3-90]

Mental Retardation

a discussion of mental retardation, including its causes, symptoms, and treatment?	*American Medical Association Encyclopedia of Medicine* [3-107] *Complete Guide to Early Child Care* [3-118]

WHERE SHOULD I GO TO FIND. . .	*TRY*

Mental Retardation

a discussion of mental retardation, including its causes, symptoms, and treatment?	*Complete Home Medical Guide* [3-124] *Current Pediatric Therapy* [3-127]
a listing, by state, of mental retardation and developmental disabilities diagnostic and treatment centers?	*Health Care U.S.A.* [3-85] *Medical and Health Information Directory,* Vol. 3 [3-90]
the names, addresses, and telephone numbers of mental retardation research centers?	*Health Care U.S.A.* [3-85]

Newsletters

a newsletter that reports on the treatment and services for pain and phobic disorders?	*Phobia Society of America—Newsletter* [3-192]
a newsletter that offers information about occupational stress and provides legal recourse for this condition?	*Occupational Stress* [3-190]
a newsletter that publishes tips on the care of Alzheimer's patients and reports new developments in research on this disease?	*Alzheimer's Research Review* [3-173]

Treatment and Rehabilitation Centers

a directory of specialists and treatment centers for depression?	*Health Care U.S.A.* [3-85]
guidelines for finding and applying to residential treatment facilities for children with emotional handicaps and behavior disorders?	*Directory of Residential Facilities for Emotionally Handicapped Children and Youth* [3-79]
a listing, by state, of infant and early childhood developmental programs at rehabilitation centers?	*Health Care U.S.A.* [3-85]
a listing, by state, of mental retardation and developmental disabilities diagnostic and treatment centers?	*Health Care U.S.A.* [3-85] *Medical and Health Information Directory,* Vol. 3 [3-90]

WHERE SHOULD I GO TO FIND. . .   *TRY*

Occupational Health and Safety

Industrial Chemicals

a listing of selected industrial chemicals and the health risks associated with each chemical?

Complete Home Medical Guide [3-124]

Legislation and Judicial Cases

the health and safety standards of the U.S. Occupational Safety and Health Administration (OSHA)?

29 Code of Federal Regulations [3-160]

a newsletter that reports current decisions, legislation, enforcement, standards, and other activities of federal and state regulatory agencies regarding occupational health and safety?

Occupational Safety and Health Reporter [3-189]

a summary of major cases that appear before the federal OSHA concerning complaints, citations, and decisions?

The Workers Bi-Weekly [3-196]

a newsletter that offers information about occupational stress and provides legal recourse for this condition?

Occupational Stress [3-190]

Tension Relief

exercises that can be performed at an office desk to relieve tightness, tension, or strain?

Complete Home Medical Guide [3-124]

Physical Fitness and Sports

The Body and Sports

descriptive drawings and an explanation of how different parts of the body function, especially as related to activities in sports?

Sports Health [3-155]

WHERE SHOULD I GO TO FIND. . .	*TRY*
The Body and Sports	
nutrition guidelines for athletes?	*Complete Guide to Sports Injuries* [3-122] *Sports Health* [3-155] *Sportswise* [3-47]
Children in Sports	
answers to questions that parents often ask about children's participation in sports?	*Sportswise* [3-47]
guidance for adults who are involved in organized sports for children?	*Sportswise* [3-47]
how to involve handicapped children and those with chronic illnesses in sports and recreation?	*Sportswise* [3-47]
suggestions on how to modify team sports to accommodate children with disabilities?	*Sportswise* [3-47]
Diseases, Disorders, and Injuries	
an explanation of diseases and medical disorders that affect the athlete, including symptoms, causes, prevention, and treatment?	*Complete Guide to Sports Injuries* [3-122]
medical conditions that may temporarily or permanently disqualify a person from participating in sports?	*Complete Guide to Sports Injuries* [3-122] *Sportswise* [3-47]
the causes of specific sports-related injuries, an explanation of each injury, and the appropriate treatment?	*Complete Guide to Sports Injuries* [3-122] *Sports Health* [3-155]
injuries that are common to different sports?	*Complete Guide to Sports Injuries* [3-122]
a discussion of the nature, prevention, control, and treatment of overuse injuries in sports?	*Sportswise* [3-47]
how to prevent sports injuries through strength and flexibility training?	*Sportswise* [3-47]

WHERE SHOULD I GO TO FIND. . .	*TRY*

Diseases, Disorders, and Injuries

an explanation of the role of stress and psychological injuries in sports?	*Sportswise* [3-47]
answers to questions concerning sports-related skin problems?	*The Look You Like* [3-36]

Drugs and Athletes

the effects that drugs most commonly used by athletes have on the body?	*Complete Guide to Sports Injuries* [3-122]
guidelines for parents and coaches as they work with young athletes who are involved with drug abuse?	*Sportswise* [3-47]
the negative side effects of steroids?	*Sportswise* [3-47]

Exercise

how to perform different types of conditioning exercises?	*Complete Guide to Sports Injuries* [3-122] *Sports Health* [3-155]
guidelines for designing a cardiovascular fitness program?	*Complete Home Medical Guide* [3-124]
the relative effectiveness of different methods of exercising for achieving cardiovascular fitness?	*Complete Home Medical Guide* [3-124]
the heart rate, by age, that an exercise program should be designed to achieve?	*Complete Home Medical Guide* [3-124] *People's Book of Medical Tests* [3-152]
exercises that can be performed at an office desk to relieve tightness, tension, or strain?	*Complete Home Medical Guide* [3-124]
the effects of exercise on the outcome of medical tests?	*Complete Home Medical Guide* [3-124]
exercises to perform for maintenance of the back?	*Complete Guide to Symptoms, Illness, and Surgery* [3-123]
exercises recommended by chiropractors that strengthen muscles in the neck, back, and abdomen?	*Everybody's Guide to Chiropractic Health Care* [3-27]

WHERE SHOULD I GO TO FIND. . .	*TRY*

Exercise

physical exercises that will help increase bone mass?	*Osteoporosis: The Silent Thief* [3-42]

Newsletters

a newsletter that specializes in the prevention, treatment, and rehabilitation of sports injuries?	*Sports Medicine Digest* [3-194]

Women in Sports

answers to questions about health issues and the participation of girls and women in sports?	*Sportswise* [3-47]

Poisons and Non-Toxins

Non-Toxic Substances

a listing of substances that usually are not toxic when ingested?	*The Merck Manual of Diagnosis and Therapy* [3-146]

Poison Control Centers

a directory of poison control centers with their addresses and emergency telephone numbers?	See your local telephone directory. *Complete Guide to Early Child Care* [3-118] *Complete Home Medical Guide* [3-124] *Current Pediatric Therapy* [3-127] *Health Hotlines* [3-86] *Physicians' Desk Reference* [3-153] *Physicians' Desk Reference for Nonprescription Drugs* [3-154]

Toxic Substances

a discussion of the most common serious poisonings of children, including symptoms and treatment?	*The Merck Manual of Diagnosis and Therapy* [3-146]

WHERE SHOULD I GO TO FIND. . .	*TRY*

Toxic Substances

the symptoms resulting from ingestion of specific poisons and the treatments administered *by physicians* for these poisons?

The Merck Manual of Diagnosis and Therapy [3-146]

a listing of toxic herbs and their effects?

Complete Home Medical Guide [3-124]

a listing of the important poisonous snakes around the world, with information about where they are to be found, their types of venom, and other characteristics?

Dorland's Illustrated Medical Dictionary [3-58]

Rehabilitation

Equipment and Devices

developments in robotics intended for use in rehabilitation of persons who have disabilities?

Meeting the Needs of People with Disabilities [3-144]

what computers can do for persons with different types of disabilities?

Meeting the Needs of People with Disabilities [3-144]

a listing of Rehabilitation Engineering Centers that develop technological aides for the handicapped?

Health Care U.S.A. [3-85]

Exercise

how to perform different types of rehabilitation exercises?

Complete Guide to Sports Injuries [3-122]
Sports Health [3-155]

the relative effectiveness of different methods of exercising for achieving cardiovascular fitness?

Complete Home Medical Guide [3-124]

Newsletters

a newsletter that reports current information on the rehabilitation of birth defects?

Association of Birth Defect Children—Newsletter [3-175]

WHERE SHOULD I GO TO FIND. . .	*TRY*

Newsletters

a newsletter that publishes information on the rehabilitation of persons with back problems?	*Back Pain Monitor* [3-177]
a newsletter that specializes in the prevention, treatment, and rehabilitation of sports injuries?	*Sports Medicine Digest* [3-194]

Rehab Developments

an overview of the changes in concepts and approaches to rehabilitation over the years and important current movements in the field of rehabilitation?	*Meeting the Needs of People with Disabilities* [3-144]

Treatment Centers

the names and descriptive profiles of medical rehabilitation programs and facilities?	*Directory of Medical Rehabilitation Programs* [3-75]
a listing of inpatient physical rehabilitation centers and brain-injury centers?	*Health Care U.S.A.* [3-85]
a listing of rehabilitation programs in audiology or speech-language pathology?	*Medical and Health Information Directory,* Vol. 3 [3-90]
a descriptive and evaluative profile of selected drug and alcoholism rehabilitation centers, explaining for each the treatment program, staff size and qualifications, facilities, cost, aftercare services, and other essential information?	*REHAB* [3-96]

Sexuality, Reproduction, and Genetics

Genetics

an explanation of genetic disorders, including the likelihood of occurrence and options?	*American Medical Association Encyclopedia of Medicine* [3-107]

(*answer continues*)

WHERE SHOULD I GO TO FIND...	*TRY*

Genetics

an explanation of genetic disorders, including the likelihood of occurrence and options?	*Complete Guide to Pregnancy* [3-120] *New Family Medical Guide* [3-149]
how traits are inherited?	*American Medical Association Encyclopedia of Medicine* [3-107] *New Family Medical Guide* [3-149]
an explanation of the structure of a gene?	*American Medical Association Encyclopedia of Medicine* [3-107] *New Family Medical Guide* [3-149]
a directory of genetic diagnostic and counseling centers?	*Health Care U.S.A.* [3-85] *Medical and Health Information Directory,* Vol. 3 [3-90]
how DNA fingerprints are used to establish paternity?	*American Medical Association Encyclopedia of Medicine* [3-107]

Reproduction

a listing, by state, of *in vitro* fertilization centers with their addresses and telephone numbers?	*Health Care U.S.A.* [3-85]
a listing, by state, of sperm banks with their addresses and telephone numbers?	*Health Care U.S.A.* [3-85]
a directory of organizations and agencies that provide family planning services?	*Medical and Health Information Directory,* Vol. 3 [3-90]
descriptive information for over-the-counter pregnancy test products?	*Physicians' Desk Reference for Nonprescriptive Drugs* [3-154]
how to perform and interpret a home pregnancy test?	*Complete Book of Medical Tests* [3-116] *People's Book of Medical Tests* [3-152]
the signs of pregnancy?	*American Medical Association Encyclopedia of Medicine* [3-107] *Complete Guide to Pregnancy* [3-120] *Complete Home Medical Guide* [3-124] *The Merck Manual of Diagnosis and Therapy* [3-146] *New Family Medical Guide* [3-149]

WHERE SHOULD I GO TO FIND. . .	*TRY*

Reproduction

how to calculate the due date for birth?	*Complete Guide to Pregnancy* [3-120] *Complete Home Medical Guide* [3-124] *The Merck Manual of Diagnosis and Therapy* [3-146]
an explanation of methods for preventing pregnancy?	*Complete Home Medical Guide* [3-124] *New Family Medical Guide* [3-149]
the causes and treatment of infertility?	*American Medical Association Encyclopedia of Medicine* [3-107] *Complete Guide to Pregnancy* [3-120] *Complete Home Medical Guide* [3-124] *The Merck Manual of Diagnosis and Therapy* [3-146] *New Family Medical Guide* [3-149]
a checklist of information that a woman should provide her obstetrician during the prenatal visit?	*Complete Guide to Pregnancy* [3-120]
a description of embryonic and fetal developments during each of the trimesters of pregnancy?	*American Medical Association Encyclopedia of Medicine* [3-107] *Complete Guide to Pregnancy* [3-120] *Complete Home Medical Guide* [3-124]
an explanation of the physical and emotional changes and discomforts that are to be expected during pregnancy?	*American Medical Association Encyclopedia of Medicine* [3-107] *Complete Guide to Pregnancy* [3-120] *Complete Home Medical Guide* [3-124] *New Family Medical Guide* [3-149]
an explanation of the medical tests that are given during the different phases of pregnancy?	*American Medical Association Encyclopedia of Medicine* [3-107] *Complete Book of Medical Tests* [3-116] *Complete Guide to Medical Tests* [3-119] *Complete Guide to Pregnancy* [3-120] *Complete Home Medical Guide* [3-124] *Patient's Guide to Medical Tests* [3-151] *People's Book of Medical Tests* [3-152]
the weight gain that should be expected during the various stages of pregnancy?	*American Medical Association Encyclopedia of Medicine* [3-107] *Complete Guide to Pregnancy* [3-120]

(answer continues)

WHERE SHOULD I GO TO FIND. . .	*TRY*

Reproduction

the weight gain that should be expected during the various stages of pregnancy?	*Complete Home Medical Guide* [3-124] *The Merck Manual of Diagnosis and Therapy* [3-146] *New Family Medical Guide* [3-149]
the proper nutritional practices during pregnancy?	*Complete Guide to Early Child Care* [3-118] *Complete Guide to Pregnancy* [3-120] *Complete Guide to Symptoms, Illness and Surgery* [3-123] *Complete Home Medical Guide* [3-124] *Instructions for Patients* [3-139]
the recommended dietary allowances during pregnancy?	*Complete Guide to Early Child Care* [3-118] *Complete Guide to Pregnancy* [3-120] *Food Values of Portions Commonly Used* [3-136] *Recommended Dietary Allowances* [3-45]
the relationship between the level of alcohol consumption and its risk to the fetus?	*New Family Medical Guide* [3-149]
information about the use of specific medicines during pregnancy?	*Complete Guide to Early Child Care* [3-118] *Complete Guide to Prescription and Non-Prescription Drugs* [3-121] *Essential Guide to Prescription Drugs* [3-132] *Guide to Prescription and Over-the-Counter Drugs* [3-138] *The Merck Manual of Diagnosis and Therapy* [3-146] *Physicians' Desk Reference* [3-153] *U.S. Pharmacopeia Drug Information for the Consumer* [3-158]
the Federal Drug Administration (FDA) safety ratings for the use of individual drugs during pregnancy?	*Essential Guide to Prescription Drugs* [3-132] *Physicians' Desk Reference* [3-153]
a discussion of possible complications during pregnancy?	*American Medical Association Encyclopedia of Medicine* [3-107] *Complete Guide to Pregnancy* [3-120] *Complete Guide to Symptoms, Illness and Surgery* [3-123] *The Merck Manual of Diagnosis and Therapy* [3-146] *New Family Medical Guide* [3-149]

WHERE SHOULD I GO TO FIND. . .	*TRY*

Reproduction

a list of some warning signs during pregnancy for which a doctor should be consulted?	*Complete Guide to Pregnancy* [3-120]
how to reduce sickness during pregnancy?	*Complete Guide to Pregnancy* [3-120]
a discussion of factors that may cause a high-risk pregnancy?	*Complete Guide to Pregnancy* [3-120]
the dos and don'ts of exercising during pregnancy?	*Complete Guide to Pregnancy* [3-120]
the difference between the contractions of true labor and of false labor?	*Complete Guide to Pregnancy* [3-120]
a discussion of childbirth, including stages of labor, complications, and other related matters?	*American Medical Association Encyclopedia of Medicine* [3-107] *Complete Guide to Pregnancy* [3-120] *Complete Home Medical Guide* [3-124] *The Merck Manual of Diagnosis and Therapy* [3-146] *New Family Medical Guide* [3-149] *Surgery On File: Obstetrics and Gynecology* [3-163]
the procedure to follow during an emergency childbirth?	*American Medical Association Encyclopedia of Medicine* [3-107]

Selecting Professional Care

guidelines for choosing a maternity care provider?	*Complete Guide to Pregnancy* [3-120]
questions to ask an obstetrician that one is considering using as one's personal physician?	*Complete Guide to Pregnancy* [3-120]
questions for a couple to ask when in the process of selecting a hospital for the birth of their child?	*Complete Guide to Early Child Care* [3-118]

Sexuality

a listing of leading sexual dysfunction clinics, citing addresses and phone numbers?	*Health Care U.S.A.* [3-85]

WHERE SHOULD I GO TO FIND. . .	*TRY*

Sexuality

the possible effects of a drug on sexual function?	*Essential Guide to Prescription Drugs* [3-132]
a discussion of the relationship between sexuality and premenstrual syndrome (PMS)?	*Self-Help for Premenstrual Syndrome* [3-46]

Surgery

Cosmetic Surgery

an explanation of the different types of cosmetic surgery, including for each procedure the realistic expectations, risks, what the operation involves, length of both the operation and the healing process, cost, insurance coverage, and other related information?	*Complete Book of Cosmetic Surgery* [3-115] *Complete Guide to Symptoms, Illness and Surgery* [nothing on cost and insurance] [3-123] *Surgery: Yes or No?* [3-157]
information that will help one decide whether to undergo cosmetic surgery?	*Complete Book of Cosmetic Surgery* [3-115]
guidelines for selecting a cosmetic surgeon?	*Complete Book of Cosmetic Surgery* [3-115]

Deciding on Surgery

a discussion of surgical and non-surgical approaches to specific medical disorders?	*Surgery: A Layman's Guide to Common Operations* [3-156]
guidance that will help one decide if a surgical procedure should be undertaken?	*Is Surgery Necessary?* [3-140] *Surgery: Yes or No?* [3-157]
questions for a patient to ask a physician when being advised to enter a hospital for the purpose of undergoing surgery?	*How to Talk to Your Doctor* [3-34]

Surgical Procedures

an explanation of different surgical procedures, including for each the purpose, technique, advantages, possible complications, postoperative care, and other important information?	*American Medical Association Encyclopedia of Medicine* [3-107] *Complete Guide to Symptoms, Illness and Surgery* [3-123] *New Family Medical Guide* [3-149]

WHERE SHOULD I GO TO FIND. . .	*TRY*

Surgical Procedures

an explanation of different surgical procedures, including for each the purpose, technique, advantages, possible complications, postoperative care, and other important information?	*Surgery On File: Eye, Ear, Nose and Throat Surgery* [3-161] *Surgery On File: General Surgery* [3-162] *Surgery On File: Obstetrics and Gynecology* [3-163] *Surgery On File: Orthopedics and Trauma Surgery* [3-164] *Surgery On File: Pediatrics* [3-165]
an explanation and illustration of the surgical procedure for removing cataracts?	*American Medical Association Encyclopedia of Medicine* [3-107] *Complete Guide to Symptoms, Illness and Surgery* [3-123] *Surgery On File: Eye, Ear, Nose and Throat Surgery* [3-161]
an explanation of different kinds of oral and maxillofacial surgery?	*Family Guide to Dental Health* [3-133]
illustrations of the different types of surgical sutures?	*Dorland's Illustrated Medical Dictionary* [3-58] *Melloni's Illustrated Medical Dictionary* [3-63] *Stedman's Medical Dictionary* [3-64]

CHAPTER

3

Descriptive Profiles of Printed Sources

Having selected in Chapter 2 the title of the publication that contains the answer to the question being researched, the reader should now turn to Chapter 3 for the complete bibliographic citation and a brief description of the publication. The profiles in this chapter expand on the contents of the printed sources, thereby permitting the reader better to judge the suitability of the material that has been targeted. These printed sources have been categorized as follows:

> Abstracts and Indexes
> Bibliographies
> Books
> Dictionaries
> Directories
> Encyclopedias and Handbooks
> Government Documents
> Loose-leaf Materials
> Newsletters
> Reports

The classification of a title has been based more on what the publication actually is than on the title it bears. The use of terms in titles sometimes is inconsistent with the standard meaning of the term. Examples include "directory," "encyclopedia," and "handbook." Terms like these are often used in titles without regard to technical or traditional definitions. Again, the authors have endeavored to categorize publications according to their contents; consequently, you may find an "encyclopedia" actually listed under "Directories." There will be some publications that do not fit neatly into any given category.

Readers can purchase a copy of a cited publication through a bookstore or, sometimes, directly from the publisher. Appendix I provides the addresses and telephone numbers of the publishing houses represented in this chapter.

The item entry numbers in Chapter 2 correspond to those printed in Chapter 3. The use of these numbers will make it easier for readers to find the descriptive profiles.

ABSTRACTS AND INDEXES

[3-1] *Consumer Health and Nutrition Index.* Edited by Alan M. Rees. Phoenix: Oryx Press. Published quarterly and cumulated annually.

An index that specializes in identifying for the layperson articles that appear in health and general magazines and in newsletters. These publications focus on diseases, disorders, drugs, nutrition, dental care, exercise, medical care, and other health-related topics. Indexed by subject, the article entries include title, author, name of periodical, volume number, issue number, page number, special notes about the article, and other information. A separate section contains citations to reviews of books and audiovisuals.

[3-2] *Index Medicus.* Two Parts. National Library of Medicine. Washington, DC: Superintendent of Documents. Published monthly and cumulated annually.

A comprehensive index to the biomedical journals of the United States and foreign countries. In addition to indexing articles in medical and health-science periodicals, there are representative journals from such related fields as botany, chemistry, physics, and zoology. Part 1 of each monthly issue is the *Subject Section,* which contains the titles of articles arranged by terms selected from *Medical Subject Headings.* For each article there is cited the author's name, abbreviation of the journal's title, date of publication, volume, issue, and inclusive pages. For articles originally published in a non-English language, an abbreviation appears indicating the language.

Part 2 contains the *Author Section* and the *Bibliography of Medical Reviews.* The alphabetical listing of names includes those of authors, co-authors, and biographees. Following an author's name are the bibliographic elements described in the *Subject Section.* Arrangement of *Bibliography of Medical Reviews* is by subject heading. *Index Medicus* concentrates on the professional literature vis-à-vis popular magazines.

[3-3] *Index to Dental Literature.* Chicago: American Dental Association. Published quarterly.

A guide to articles on dentistry that have been published in dental and non-dental professional journals throughout the world. An example of the latter are medical articles relevant to dentistry but published in medical periodicals. Indexed by subject and names. Also includes bibliographies of dental reviews, dissertations and theses, and dental books.

[3-4] *Readers' Guide to Periodical Literature.* New York: H. W. Wilson Co. Published monthly (January, February, May, June, July, August, and November) and semimonthly (September, October, December, March, and April). Cumulated quarterly and annually.

A subject-author index of periodicals that are of a general public interest vis-à-vis professional and technical journals. Articles that are indexed span a broad range of subjects, including those on health and medicine. Useful for those interested in finding articles concerning diseases, health care, nutrition, mental health, dentistry, and other topics that have been published in popular magazines. Since these periodicals usually are not indexed in the professional medical indexes, the *Readers' Guide to Periodical Literature* serves as a supplementary indexing source.

BIBLIOGRAPHIES

[3-5] ***AIDS and Women: A Sourcebook.*** Sarah B. Watstein and Robert A. Laurich. Phoenix: Oryx Press, 1991.

The main purpose of this publication is to provide an annotated bibliography of literature on women and AIDS. The authors have assembled a collection of source materials on the different aspects of HIV/AIDS as women are impacted by it. Encompassed are such topics as transmission of AIDS heterosexually, transmission through intravenous drug use and via blood and blood products, perinatal transmission, and the risk of sexual contact with hemophiliacs. Since the emphasis is on women, chapters are devoted to the myths and potential for the transmission and spread of AIDS through women, the incidence of AIDS in different sectors of the female population, and ways of preventing AIDS in women.

In addition to providing an annotated bibliography, there is a synthesis of facts or advice on the various topics of AIDS and women. Each topic is introduced with a brief summary of pertinent information. Also presented is a directory of AIDS-related national and state hotlines and the addresses and telephone numbers of organizations that will be of interest to women in their search for information about HIV and AIDS.

AIDS Information Sourcebook. 3rd edition. Edited by H. Robert Malinowsky and Gerald J. Perry. Phoenix: Oryx Press, 1991.

See "Directories," [3-67]

[3-7] ***Books in Print.*** New York: R. R. Bowker Company, 1992. Published annually and updated six months after publication via *Books in Print Supplement*.

A bibliography of U.S. books in print or soon to be published. Covers most subjects, including those that are health related. The books must be available to the trade or general public for purchase. Excludes bibles, textbooks, *professional* medical and law books, pamphlets, subscription-only titles, and other books not accessible to the public. Indexed in three ways: namely, by author, title, and subject. Also includes a listing of book publishers with their addresses and telephone numbers. The bibliographic data contains title, author, editor, number of volumes, edition number, Library of Congress catalog number, ISBN (International Standard Book Number), price, number of pages, publication date, name of publisher, and other bibliographic information.

[3-8] *The Consumer Health Information Source Book.* 3rd edition. Alan M. Rees and Catherine Hoffman. Phoenix: Oryx Press, 1990. Published approximately every four years.

A bibliography of books, magazines, newsletters, and pamphlets on health-related topics. Entries consist of bibliographical citations and descriptive evaluations. For many titles, the authors indicate whether they recommend the publication. Topics for which information sources are provided include various diseases and disorders; nutrition; weight control diets; health of children, the elderly, and women; surgery and second opinions; physical fitness and exercise; pregnancy; and other health-related subjects. Also contains a directory of health hotline telephone numbers, national health information centers and clearinghouses, and a selected list of health organizations.

[3-9] *Directories in Print.* 9th edition. Edited by Charles B. Montney. 2 Volumes. Detroit: Gale Research Company, 1992. Published annually. Formerly titled *Directory of Directories.*

An annotated guide to national, regional, and some international directories in numerous fields, including medicine and health care services. These directories are of many kinds, including directories of the medical specialty boards, manufacturers of medical equipment, and organizations providing health services. It embraces such areas as traditional medicine, osteopathy, dentistry, chiropractic care, mental health, pharmacy, hospitals and clinics, health insurance, and services for the disabled. Profiles of directories report the title, publisher, address, telephone number, scope of the directory, frequency of publication, price, associated online database, and other bibliographic information. Contains subject and title/keyword indexes.

[3-10] *Findex: The Directory of Market Research Reports, Studies, and Surveys.* 12th edition. Edited by JoAnne DuChez. Bethesda, MD: Cambridge Information Group Directories, Inc., 1990. Published annually and updated mid-year.

An annotated bibliography of published business and market research reports, U.S. and foreign. These reports come from many sources and concern both domestic and foreign economies. The focus of these research reports is on the operations of individual companies and on industries and their specific products. Health care is one of the targeted industries, and it includes market research reports related to disease, drugs, medical care facilities, and other health matters. The profile of each market report includes the title, publication date, publisher, summary, number of pages in the report, price, and a report identification number. This is a major source for identifying commercially available market research reports and for learning where to obtain copies.

[3-11] *Medical and Health Care Books and Serials in Print.* 2 Vols. New Providence, NJ: R. R. Bowker, 1991. Published annually.

A bibliography of books in the health sciences and allied fields that are in print or soon to be published or distributed in the U.S. Also contains international coverage of serial titles in the health sciences that includes journals, newsletters, and other serials, These serials are either published more than once a year and at regular intervals, or they are issued irregularly and less frequently (as with an annual).

Books are indexed by title, subject, and author, whereas the serials are indexed by subject and title. Bibliographic data for books include title, author, editor, number of volumes, edition, Library of Congress number, year of publication, International Standard Book Number (ISBN), publisher's name, price, and other information.

Profiles of serials contain full bibliographic information, including where the periodical is indexed and abstracted. Serials that are available online are noted along with their respective vendors; and their addresses and telephone numbers.

Medical and Health Information Directory: Vol. 2, Publications, Libraries, and Other Information Services. 5th ed. Edited by Karen Backus. Detroit: Gale Research Company, 1990.

See "Directories," [3-89]

[3-12] *Newsletters in Print.* 5th ed. Edited by Robert J. Huffman and John Krol. Detroit: Gale Research, Inc., 1990. Formerly titled *Newsletters Directory.* Published biennially.

A guide to newsletters published in the United States and Canada. Includes a broad range of publications—both newsletters *per se* and publications that are only loosely considered to be newsletters. These encompass bulletins, digests, some journals, updates, and other serials that are of a national or regional (not local) interest and that are available to the public (i.e., that are not merely in-house organs). Contains both printed and electronic (online) newsletters. Among the subject categories are medicine and medical care.

Profiles of these newsletters report the title; publisher's name, address, and telephone number; editor's name; description of the purpose, scope, and subjects covered; intended audience; frequency of issues; circulation size; price; whether accessible via online computer; and other descriptive information.

[3-13] *Oxbridge Directory of Newsletters.* 8th ed. Edited by Fay Shapiro. New York: Oxbridge Communications, Inc., 1990. Published annually.

Arranged by subject, this is a bibliography of newsletters with a brief description of each publication. Health, medicine, dentistry, and pharmaceuticals are among the areas for which newsletters are listed. Within each newsletter's profile are the title; publisher's name, address, and telephone number; description of content; frequency of issue; subscription rate; circulation size; primary readership; whether available in microform or online; and other descriptive information.

[3-14] *Ulrich's International Periodicals Directory.* 29th edition. 3 Vols. New York: R. R. Bowker Company, 1990. Published annually. Updated quarterly by *Ulrich's Update.*

Ulrich's includes all serial publications that were formerly reported in *Ulrich's* and in *Irregular Serials and Annuals.* Thus, the scope now encompasses periodicals and other serials that are currently being published and that are being issued regularly and more than once a year. It also includes such serials as annual reviews, monograph series, yearbooks, and proceedings that appear regularly as annuals or less frequently, or which are published irregularly.

The coverage of serials is international, and its range of subjects embraces the medical sciences, nutrition, pharmacy, physical fitness, and the non-health fields.

Within these broad categories are to be found serial titles on cancer, cardiovascular diseases, chiropractic care, osteopathy, dentistry, orthopedics, pediatrics, sports medicine, surgery, and other topics.

Ulrich's provides full bibliographic information, including where the periodical is indexed and abstracted. It also states whether a serial is available online or on CD-ROM. If there is online access to the serial, the publisher, vendor, and file names are given. The addresses and telephone numbers of the publishers and vendors are also reported. All serials that are refereed are listed alphabetically in a separate section along with the publisher's name, address, and telephone number.

The three volumes are divided into ten sections; namely, "The Classified List of Serials," "Refereed Serials," "Serials Available on CD-ROM," "Serials Available On-line," "Producer Listing/Serials on CD-ROM," "Vendor Listing/Serials Online," "Cessations" (of titles), "Index to Publications of International Organizations," "ISSN (International Standard Serial Number) Index," and "Title Index."

BOOKS

[3-15] *Advantages to the Early Removal of Impacted Wisdom Teeth.* Chicago: Quintessence Publishing Co., 1979.

Reasons are given for not delaying the removal of impacted wisdom teeth. Explains the complications that can be avoided by not procrastinating. Includes compelling illustrations.

[3-16] *AIDS: A Self-Care Manual.* 3rd edition. Edited by BettyClare Moffatt, Judith Spiegel, et al. Santa Monica, CA: IBS Press, 1989.

Persons who have been infected with the HIV virus or who have AIDS need much information and many special services. A myriad of questions require answering. The general community, too, needs to be educated about this disease, including what it is and what it isn't. How can AIDS be treated? This book serves as a guide for everyone, especially the AIDS patient. Covering all aspects of this topic, including the medical, social, psychological, business, legal, insurance, and spiritual issues, *AIDS: A Self-Care Manual* is an important guide for anyone concerned about AIDS.

[3-17] *The American Cancer Society Cancer Book: Prevention, Detection, Diagnosis, Treatment, Rehabilitation, Cure.* Edited by Arthur I. Holleb. Garden City, NY: Doubleday, 1986.

Contains a collection of articles (chapters) on cancer, written by experts in cancer research and treatment. Addresses prevention, detection, diagnosis, treatment, rehabilitation, and cure. The largest portion of this book is devoted to specific forms of cancer and their treatments. For each type, consideration is given to the causes, symptoms, diagnosis, and treatment. There is an explanation of the anatomical parts that are involved. Many questions of the cancer patient are answered. A directory is provided that lists numerous cancer resource organizations, such as the addresses of state divisions of the American Cancer Society, Comprehensive Cancer

Centers, and a variety of organizations that offer services for patients with specific kinds of cancer.

[3-18] *Caring for the Alzheimer Patient: A Practical Guide.* 2nd edition. Edited by Raye L. Dippel and J. Thomas Hutton. Buffalo, NY: Prometheus Books, 1991.

Caring for the Alzheimer patient requires knowledge of many complex issues. Both families and secondary caregivers need guidance. *Caring for the Alzheimer Patient* serves as a guidebook for such care. It addresses such topics as the characteristics and symptoms of the disease; how to assess it; how to improve the patient's safety, hygiene, body elimination, nutrition, and communication; and techniques for enhancing memory. Legal and ethical considerations are discussed, as are guidelines for selecting a nursing home. An important feature is this book's explanation of support services that are available to caregivers of Alzheimer patients. The emphasis is on practical information for those who provide care to patients with this debilitating disease.

[3-19] *Children with Asthma: A Manual for Parents.* 2nd edition. Thomas F. Plaut. Amherst, MA: Pedipress, 1988.

Parents who have a child who suffers from asthma often need help managing this disease. What are the four signs of asthma? What should be done to keep the child functional? When should a doctor be consulted? What medications are used, and how do they work? How should a doctor be chosen for treating this disease? *Children With Asthma* addresses these questions. As a guidebook for parents, it offers a straightforward approach that is couched in language sensitive to the needs of parents who often develop anxiety when they witness their child in distress.

[3-20] *The Confusion About Chiropractors.* Richard deRoeck. Danbury, CT: Impulse Publishing, 1989.

Explains the field of chiropractic. Coverage includes the purpose, educational preparation of chiropractors, and the practice of chiropractic care. Answers many of the questions often asked about this profession. Provides a directory of chiropractic colleges in North America.

[3-21] *Consumer Guide to Modern Cataract Surgery.* William F. Maloney, Lincoln Grindle, and Donald E. Pearcy. Fallbrook, CA: La Senda Publishers, 1986.

Presents a simple and comprehensive explanation of the causes, symptoms, and treatment of cataracts. Addresses the questions most often asked by patients. Provides guidance on how to make the decision to have cataract surgery; offers suggestions on how to select the eye surgeon; and cites ways to reduce cost while receiving quality care.

[3-22] *Dental Implants: Are They For Me?* Thomas D. Taylor. Chicago: Quintessence Publishing Co., 1990.

This book explains dental implant therapy. It includes the different types of dental implants, the nature of the procedure, and how to care for dental implants. Also, there is a discussion of who should undergo this form of dental treatment and what risks are involved. Colorful illustrations enhance the text.

[3-23] *Diabetes Type II: Living a Long, Healthy Life Through Blood Sugar Normalization.* Richard K. Bernstein. New York: Prentice-Hall, 1990.

Written as a guidebook for the person who is trying to control diabetes. Focuses primarily on maturity onset or Type II diabetes vis-à-vis Type I or juvenile onset diabetes; however, the latter is addressed. Presents a treatment plan for normalizing blood sugars. Discusses the full range of topics regarding this disease. This book provides a practical guide to procedures and explains the dynamics of diabetes and offers a regimen for treating it. Included is a list of drugs that have been found to affect levels of blood glucose. Sample recipes for low-carbohydrate meals are included.

[3-24] *Drugs, Alcohol, and Your Children: How to Keep Your Family Substance-Free.* Geraldine Youcha and Judith S. Seixas. New York: Crown, 1989.

One of the greatest shocks and frustrations of parents is when they discover that their child has been involved with illicit drugs. How should they respond? What should they do? Where can they find help? This book is the parent's guide to answers to these and other questions. It is a "how-to" guide.

[3-25] *Eating and Allergy.* Robert Eagle. Garden City, NY: Doubleday, 1981.

Explains food allergies—their causes, diagnoses, and treatments. Discusses the relationship between foods and different diseases, such as moodiness, depression, arthritis, migraine headaches, and hyperactivity. Provides a table of food groups that discloses related foods which may be allergenic.

[3-26] *Essential Principles of Chiropractic.* Virgil V. Strang. Davenport, IA: Palmer College of Chiropractic, 1984.

Here is a book that explains the philosophy and fundamental principles of chiropractic health care. The reader will learn about chiropractic's view of health and disease, and its approach to patient care.

[3-27] *Everybody's Guide to Chiropractic Health Care.* Nathaniel Altman. Los Angeles: Jeremy P. Tarcher, 1990.

An introduction to the field of chiropractic. This book explains what chiropractic is and what it is not. Distinctions are made between this and other health systems. The reader is told what to expect when visiting a chiropractor. Guidelines are provided that help with the selection of the right chiropractor. From the chiropractic perspective, there is a discussion of the proper exercise and diet. For those contemplating a first visit to a chiropractor, here is preparation for that visit.

[3-28] *Food Allergy.* Frederic Speer. Littleton, MA: PSG Publishing Co., 1978.

Explains the dynamics of food allergies and their mechanisms. Includes the different types of food allergies, addresses the detection of food allergens, and explains the treatment. There is a chapter on individual foods. The encyclopedic approach offers interesting tidbits of useful information. Of value to the sufferer of food allergies are the tables that report the biological classification of foods. This permits the reader to determine which foods are related biologically. Such information enables one to know which foods are in the same food family. If one member of a family is an allergen, probably others in that family should be avoided.

The chapter on cooking serves as a guide to preparing meals for the person who is sensitive to food allergens.

[3-29] *The Great White Lie: How America's Hospitals Betray Our Trust and Endanger Our Lives.* New York: Simon and Schuster, 1991.

This is an exposé of what goes on behind the scenes in some hospitals across America. It discloses unprofessional, unethical, and incompetent health care practices and unseemly billing operations. From unsanitary conditions to careless operations due to greed, incompetence, personnel shortages, indifference, and other reasons, the author discloses real situations that have cost patients their money and even their lives. These revelations challenge the confidence that Americans have placed in their health care institutions.

[3-30] *Health and Healing.* Andrew Weil. Boston: Houghton Mifflin, 1988.

This is an update of Dr. Weil's 1983 publication titled *Health and Healing: Understanding Conventional and Alternative Medicine* [3-31]. Here he provides further explanation of alternative or non-allopathic medicine. He discusses homeopathy, osteopathy, chiropractic, naturopathy, Chinese medicine, holistic medicine, and other approaches to healing. Dr. Weil also explains how conventional medicine works and places it in the scheme of therapeutic systems. The author discusses the phenomenon of health, what it is, and how it is to be achieved. He offers ten guiding principles of health and illness.

This book expands the reader's intellectual horizon of health, illness, and healing. A variety of non-traditional approaches to health are presented.

[3-31] *Health and Healing: Understanding Conventional and Alternative Medicine.* Andrew Weil. Boston: Houghton Mifflin, 1983.

Traditional Western (allopathic) medicine is but one health system. There are numerous others, each with its own views as to how the human body functions and what approach should be taken to maintain and/or restore a healthy equilibrium. Dr. Weil explains allopathic medicine, homeopathy, osteopathy, chiropractic, naturopathy, Chinese medicine, psychic healing, shamanism, holistic medicine, and other therapeutic alternatives. Each offers a different approach to disease and treatment. This book motivates the reader to rethink attitudes and beliefs about the healing process.

[3-32] *HMOs: What They Are, How They Work, and Which One Is Best for You.* Jill Bloom. Tucson, AZ: The Body Press, 1987.

A guide to the HMO industry. Explains the different types of HMOs, provides tips on how to select the proper one for you, and contains a national directory of HMO organizations. Written as a consumer's guide.

[3-33] *How to Defeat Alcoholism: Nutritional Guidelines for Getting Sober.* Joseph D. Beasley. New York: Random House, 1989.

Discusses the nature, symptoms, and treatment of alcoholism. Helps the reader identify the alcoholic syndrome, and focuses on what can be done within the family and professionally. Offers a nutritional program along with vitamin and mineral supplementation for treating alcoholism. Provides guidance on how to select an alcoholic treatment facility. Discusses long-term recovery. Also discusses other drugs that are often abused. The author is a physician who operates an alcoholic treatment clinic.

[3-34] *How to Talk to Your Doctor: The Questions to Ask.* Janet R. Maurer. New York: Simon and Schuster, 1986.

Being an informed patient necessitates knowing the right questions to ask. This is often difficult because a patient may feel overwhelmed, suffer from anxiety, and/or not know enough to ask the necessary questions. *How to Talk to Your Doctor* comes to the patient's rescue.

Within its pages are basic questions that often should be asked. Of course, depending on the circumstances, other, more focused questions will also be appropriate. This is the patient's guidebook to inquiries that he/she should make concerning specific illnesses, the patient's rights and responsibilities, the physician's rights and responsibilities, diagnostic tests and procedures, seeking a second opinion, role of the specialist consultant, changing doctors, hospitalization, and coping with a chronic illness.

[3-35] *Impacted Wisdom Teeth in the Middle and Late Years.* Chicago: Quintessence Publishing Co., 1979.

What happens when impacted wisdom teeth are kept into middle age or later years? What special problems arise? The author explains these problems and discourages procrastination. Drawings help the reader to understand.

[3-36] *The Look You Like: Medical Answers to 400 Questions on Skin and Hair Care.* Linda A. Schoen and Paul Lazar. New York: Marcel Dekker, 1990.

This is the layperson's guide to the care of skin and hair. It contains 400 questions and their answers regarding the causes and treatment of skin problems, such as acne, blemishes, cancer, infections, and others. Similarly, issues of hair loss, excessive hair, dandruff, hair waving or straightening, and other matters related to the hair are covered. Discusses hair-coloring products, shampoos, and conditioners. Answers are given to questions pertaining to body odor, sports-related skin problems, treatment of insect bites, nail care, and the effects of the sun on the skin.

[3-37] *Managing the Side Effects of Chemotherapy and Radiation.* Marylin J. Dodd. New York: Prentice-Hall, 1991.

This is the cancer patient's guide for managing and alleviating the side effects of chemotherapy and external radiation therapy. The author describes all of the different side effects of these therapies and suggests how each can be managed. Also includes nutritional suggestions for cancer patients.

Forty-eight commonly used chemotherapeutic drugs are listed. For each drug there is cited its side effects and the signs and symptoms for recognizing each effect. Also, suggestions are given on how to manage each effect. This explanation includes a description of the effect, its duration, self-care measures, other measures which can be taken but which require professional services, and when to contact a physician or nurse.

The section on external radiation therapy includes thirty-four side effects that may develop and advice for managing each of these effects.

[3-38] *Medicine and the Law.* Neil Grauer. New York: Chelsea House, 1989.

This book presents a brief overview of the legal history of medicine and a discussion of some of the controversial medical issues of our time. Patient rights, infertility, abortion, physician responsibilities, and other issues are among those addressed.

[3-39] *Natural Health, Natural Medicine: A Comprehensive Manual for Wellness and Self-Care.* Andrew Weil. Boston: Houghton Mifflin, 1990.

The body has its built-in mechanism for maintaining health, and its own recuperative powers. What are the strategies that enable us to use this innate healing power? How can we best use proper eating, rest, and exercise to achieve and maintain wellness? What practices of self-care can we follow that will promote good health without our resorting to synthetic chemicals? These and other questions are answered by Dr. Weil from the perspective of natural medicine.

This book is a fresh approach to health care as it introduces the reader to a lifestyle that emphasizes the proper use of our bodies and the use of vitamins and herbs. It advocates preventive steps and remedial measures that activate the body's own processes and encourage nature's assistance.

[3-40] *Old Enough to Feel Better: A Medical Guide for Seniors.* Michael Gordon. Radnor, PA: Chilton Book Co., 1981.

Here is a friendly guide to aging—its social, medical, and psychological dimensions. It is a ready-reference for the senior citizen. Within its pages are informative and sensitive discussions of how to explain your medical symptoms to your doctor, how to select a surgeon, psychological aspects of aging, nutrition for the aged, and an explanation of medical diagnostic tests that are often performed on older people.

An especially valuable section discusses a variety of health complaints, diseases, and disorders that afflict senior citizens. It explains how the body normally functions and what may go wrong. Methods of diagnosis and treatment are covered for specific ailments. Also discussed are living arrangements, work, recreation, and exercise for the senior citizen.

[3-41] *Once A Month: The Original Premenstrual Syndrome Handbook.* 4th revised edition. Katharina Dalton. Claremont, CA: Hunter House, 1990.

This is the fourth edition of the first and classical book on premenstrual syndrome (PMS). It describes PMS with an intended readership of both men and women. There is an explanation of the menstrual cycle, monthly mood swings and headaches, water retention, and other physical and psychological symptoms of PMS. Most important, there is a discussion of what a woman with PMS can do to help herself and what her physician can do for her. In the appendix appears a directory of PMS clinics and support groups, organized by state and by zip code within each state. In summary, this is a publication for learning about PMS and how to deal with it.

[3-42] *Osteoporosis: The Silent Thief.* William A. Peck and Louis V. Avioli. American Association of Retired Persons. Glenview, IL: Scott, Foresman, 1988.

An informative book on osteoporosis that explains this disease, how to prevent its occurrence, and how to treat it. Discusses the causes, risk factors, and protective factors. Offers sample high-calcium menus and the calcium content of foods in the four basic food groups. Discusses how bone mass is measured. Covers methods of treatment, including estrogen therapy.

[3-43] *Overcoming Bladder Disorders.* Rebecca Chalker and Kristene E. Whitmore. New York: Harper & Row, 1990.

Provides information on the diagnosis, treatment, and prevention of bladder disorders: namely, incontinence, cystitis, prostate problems, and bladder cancer. Explains each disorder and how it is diagnosed and treated. Also includes an index of tests that are commonly used in the diagnosis of bladder problems. The purpose of each test is explained, and the reader is informed as to what should be expected when undergoing the test. Presents a glossary of drugs frequently used in the treatment of bladder disorders and profiles each drug, including the use, side effects, and adverse drug interactions.

[3-44] *PMS: A Positive Program to Gain Control.* Stephanie DeGraff Bender and Kathleen Kelleher. Tucson, AZ: The Body Press, 1986.

A self-help guide for coping with premenstrual syndrome (PMS). Explains PMS, helps a woman ascertain if she has it, and explains what to do if she does. Emphasizes how to regain control. Focuses on the emotional and psychological dimensions of PMS.

This is more than just a book to be read. It is a workbook that provides charts for the reader to complete following self-analysis. Furthermore, it offers self-help exercises and suggestions on how to control PMS. Guidance is given for improving relationships between the PMS woman and her family and friends.

[3-45] *Recommended Dietary Allowances.* 10th edition. National Research Council. Food and Nutrition Board. Washington, DC: National Academy Press, 1989.

This is the authoritative guide for daily nutritional requirements and maintaining good health. Prepared by the Food and Nutrition Board since 1941, it gives the reader the definitive explanation of nutrients and their daily recommended dietary allowances (RDAs). For those nutrients with insufficient research data, Estimated Safe and Adequate Daily Dietary Intake values are provided. Reported for each nutrient is its function, sources of food, customary dietary intake, and the consequences of deficiencies and excessive consumption. Recommended allowances are explained. Also includes recommended daily energy allowances for infants, children, and adults. RDAs are widely recognized as the standard for daily nutrient allowances, and this book is the definitive source for that guide.

[3-46] *Self-Help for Premenstrual Syndrome.* Michelle Harrison. New York: Random House, 1982.

Written by a woman physician who specializes in PMS, this book focuses on the physical and emotional aspects of premenstrual syndrome. It answers questions about the symptoms and causes of PMS, and it discusses treatment. Under the latter, the author addresses diet, exercise, vitamins, minerals, progesterone, psychotherapy, acupuncture, and support groups.

[3-47] *Sportswise: An Essential Guide for Young Adult Athletes, Parents, and Coaches.* Lyle J. Micheli and Mark D. Jenkins. Boston: Houghton Mifflin, 1990.

As the title states, athletes, parents, and coaches will benefit from the counsel offered concerning how safely to involve children in sports. He explains how to minimize sports injuries by following proper conditioning, nutrition, and coaching. A key chapter responds to many of the questions often asked by parents about health concerns for their children who want to be active in organized sports. Attention is given to stress and psychological injuries in sports, overuse injuries, health issues related to female athletes, and other important topics. Also addressed are guidelines for involving handicapped children and those with chronic illnesses in organized sports. This book is helpful to parents who want what is right for their children in fitness, exercise, and sports.

[3-48] *The Story of Impacted Wisdom Teeth.* Chicago: Quintessence Publishing Co., 1979.

Explains how wisdom teeth develop and how they become impacted. Also discusses the problems that are caused by impacted wisdom teeth. The explanations are clarified by ample illustrations.

[3-49] *Surviving with AIDS: A Comprehensive Program of Nutritional Co-Therapy.* C. Wayne Callaway with Catherine Whitney. Boston: Little, Brown, 1991.

Although this book does not address how to cure AIDS, it does discuss how to manage the chronic malnutrition that accompanies it. There is offered a nutritional co-therapy for ameliorating malnutrition and for restoring the AIDS patient to a functional life with an acceptable level of human dignity. The nutritional co-therapy described is not an alternative therapy; instead, it must be used in conjunction with medical treatment. This nutritional treatment program is solely to redress the dietary problems of AIDS: namely, insufficient nutrient intake, poor nutrient absorption, and abnormal nutrient metabolism.

Surviving with AIDS is a practical guide to eating for the person with AIDS. Based on a low-fat, high-calorie regimen, it offers a 21-day meal plan with recipes. Other features include information on drug/nutrient interactions, recommended dietary allowances (RDAs), how to make a nutritional inventory, and other helpful assistance.

[3-50] *Take This Book to the Hospital With You.* Charles B. Inlander and Ed Weiner. Emmaus, PA: Rodale Press, 1985.

Here is the hospital patient's guidebook. Contained within its pages are guidelines, tips, and advice. It is an orientation to a stay in the hospital. The reader's naiveté will be transformed so that if hospitalized, he/she will be knowledgeable about his/her rights and will know what goes on in many hospitals around the nation.

[3-51] *Tooth and Gum Care.* Densie Hatfield. American Family Health Institute. Springhouse, PA: Springhouse Corporation, 1986.

This is the layperson's guide to dental health. It answers many of the questions commonly asked about dental care. From how to select and use a toothbrush to treating cavities and gum disease and wearing bridges and dentures, this book is a one-stop source for dental information.

[3-52] *Understanding Alzheimer's Disease: What It Is; How to Cope With It; Future Directions.* Edited by Miriam K. Aronson. New York: Scribner's, 1988.

Many questions about Alzheimer's disease are addressed in this book. What is this disease? What are its symptoms, and how is it diagnosed? What are the treatment strategies? These questions are discussed along with long-term care, services for Alzheimer patients and their families, support groups, and how and when to place a family member in a nursing home. Also covers financial and legal matters concerning patients who are afflicted with this debilitating disease.

This book serves as a guide for the patient's family. A checklist is provided for evaluating nursing homes. Additionally, there are many suggestions for helping a family cope with this crisis.

[3-53] *What Is Periodontal Disease?* Joel M. Berns. Chicago: Quintessence Publishing Co., 1982.

Concentrates on the cause, signs, and prevention of periodontal disease. Using colorful drawings, the author illustrates the nature of this disease and how it impacts on the gums and teeth. Some explanation is given about the treatment for periodontal disease.

[3-54] *Why Replace A Missing Back Tooth?* Joel M. Berns. Chicago: Quintessence Publishing Co., 1984.

Using straightforward explanations and illustrations, the author explains the necessity for replacing a back tooth that has been extracted. He discusses the problems that may develop if the area of the missing tooth is not filled with a false tooth.

[3-55] *Why Root Canal Therapy?* Joel M. Berns. Chicago: Quintessence Publishing Co., 1986.

Root canal therapy is a complex procedure that may be used to save a decaying tooth. In this book the author explains why this therapy is needed and how it is performed. Replete with colorful drawings, it shows the anatomy of a tooth, the effect of the decaying process which creates the need for root canal therapy, and the step-by-step procedure of this therapy.

DICTIONARIES

[3-56] *Acronyms, Initialisms, and Abbreviations Dictionary.* 16th edition. Edited by Jennifer Mossman. Detroit: Gale Research Company, 1992. Published annually.

Serves as a guide to the interpretation of acronyms, abbreviations, contractions, initialisms, and alphabetic symbols in a wide array of fields, including medicine, physiology, pharmacy, and other related health areas and non-health fields. In addition to the abbreviation or acronym, entries may include the meaning, English translation (for non-English entries), designation of the foreign language to which the term belongs, location or country of origin, subject area, sponsor, and source code.

[3-57] *Dictionary of Food Ingredients.* Robert S. Igoe. New York: Van Nostrand Reinhold, 1983.

Briefly describes almost one thousand food ingredients, including each ingredient's functions, properties, and applications. Serves as a guide for food professionals and consumers. When applicable, provides chemical formulations and usage levels.

[3-58] *Dorland's Illustrated Medical Dictionary.* 27th edition. Philadelphia: W. B. Saunders, 1988.

A dictionary of medical terms with illustrations of the muscles, nerves, skeleton, skin, blood vessels, and other features of the human anatomy. Also illustrated are medical instruments and types of surgical sutures and knots. Provides a variety of technical tables that are intended mainly for use by the medical professional.

[3-59] *Folk Name and Trade Diseases.* E. R. Plunkett, Stamford, CT: Barrett Book Co., 1978.

For centuries, common names have been used to describe a myriad of occupational diseases and disorders. Often they have described the associated occupation and the ailment. For example, "drummer's thumb" is the "rupture of the long extensor tendon from drumming," and "quick draw leg" is a "bullet wound of the leg sustained while practicing a fast draw from a gun-belt holster." These terms range from the hilarious to the serious. All of us have heard some of these names, but we may not always know their meaning or origin. *Folk Name and Trade Diseases* will part the veil of the mystery because it is a dictionary of these terms, as illustrated by the definitions cited above. Whenever possible, the author has disclosed the first authoritative reference to the name, including the year of use. With almost 1,500 ailments cited, the reader is in for an enjoyable and educational trip through this lexicon of trade-disease and trade-disorder names.

[3-60] *Illustrated Dictionary of Dentistry.* Stanley Jablonski. Philadelphia: W. B. Saunders, 1982.

Provides definitions and explanations of dental terms, concepts, instruments, materials, diseases, and disorders. Encompasses all specialties of dentistry and allied fields, including peripheral terms that are important to dental practitioners. The scope also includes selected medical, physiological, and chemical terms. A guide to the nomenclature of dentistry.

[3-61] *Medical Acronyms and Abbreviations.* Marilyn F. Delong. Oradell, NJ: Medical Economics Books, 1989.

A dictionary of acronyms and abbreviations used in the health care field. For each acronym and abbreviation, there is provided a brief definition. Includes all medical and surgical specialties in addition to nursing, pharmacology, dietetics, and administration.

[3-62] *Medical Sign Language: Easily Understood Definitions of Commonly Used Medical, Dental, and First Aid Terms.* W. Joseph Garcia. Springfield, IL: Charles C. Thomas, 1983.

A unique dictionary of medical and dental terms that not only defines each term but also translates these terms into the American Sign Language (ASL) for the deaf. Supplementing the definitions are drawings that depict the appropriate ASL signs and explanations of how to make each sign. Coverage encompasses diseases, symptoms, drugs, medical procedures, body parts, etc. A separate section contains anatomical drawings.

[3-63] *Melloni's Illustrated Medical Dictionary.* 2nd edition. Ida Dox, Biagio J. Melloni, and Gilbert M. Eisner. Baltimore: Williams and Wilkins, 1985.

The distinguishing feature of this medical dictionary is its extensive use of illustrations to enhance the definitions of medical terms. Using more than 2,500 colored drawings that clarify textual statements, it provides clear explanations. Also useful are the tables of arteries, bones, muscles, nerves, and veins. These tables list each member of an anatomical class and describe its location, function, and other related information. The scope includes dental features, organs, skin, medical instruments, and a large assortment of other types of medical information.

[3-64] *Stedman's Medical Dictionary.* 25th edition. Baltimore: Williams and Wilkins, 1990.

A dictionary of medical terms, procedures, human anatomical features, and other expressions related to medicine. Contains color plates that illustrate the skeleton, muscles, nerves, veins, arteries, and other anatomical components of the body.

DIRECTORIES

[3-65] *9479 Questionable Doctors: Disciplined by States or the Federal Government.* Ingrid VanTuinen, Phyllis McCarthy, and Sidney Wolfe. Washington, DC: Public Citizen's Health Research Group, 1991.

Based on a national study conducted by Public Citizen's Health Research Group, this list cites 9,479 names of physicians and other health professionals who have been disciplined for reasons associated with their medical or dental practices. It reports the doctor's name, hometown and state, the state or agency that took the disciplinary action, the date of the action, the specific action taken, the nature of the offense, and explanatory notes. Also includes the findings of the national study on the quality control system for controlling doctors. Although this publication does not contain the names of all disciplined doctors, it is an informative report.

[3-66] *ABMS Compendium of Certified Medical Specialists.* 3rd edition. 7 volumes. Evanston, IL: American Board of Medical Specialties, 1990. Published every two years.

Contains biographical sketches of physicians who are certified in one or more of the twenty-four medical specialties that are recognized by the American Board of Medical Specialties (ABMS). The medical specialists are arranged alphabetically by specialty. Also presented is a geographical categorization which enables the reader to identify a specialist by the city in which his/her practice is located. Profiles include the physician's address, telephone number, year certified in the specialty or subspecialty, medical school education, type of professional practice, and other related information.

This directory also lists the individual medical specialty boards with their addresses, telephone numbers, and certification requirements.

[3-67] *AIDS Information Sourcebook.* 3rd edition. Edited by H. Robert Malinowsky and Gerald J. Perry. Phoenix: Oryx Press, 1991.

A comprehensive guide to information sources on acquired immunodeficiency syndrome (AIDS). This book is both a directory of organizations, programs, and facilities in the United States, Puerto Rico, and Canada, and an annotated bibliography of a wide variety of publications on AIDS. Among these publications are books, articles, brochures, pamphlets, periodicals, directories, education programs, film/video/audio resources, and online databases.

The *Sourcebook* contains a chronology of the history of AIDS which includes dates and events that have had a significant impact on AIDS awareness and research. The directory section presents descriptive profiles of organizations, facilities, and programs (arranged by state and city) that provide services related to AIDS. Provides a glossary of AIDS terms.

[3-68] *American Chiropractic Association, Membership Directory.* Arlington, VA: American Chiropractic Association, 1990. Published annually.

An alphabetical listing of chiropractors who are members of the American Chiropractic Association, including their addresses and telephone numbers. Arranged by city within state.

[3-69] *American Dental Directory.* Chicago: American Dental Association, 1990. Published annually.

A comprehensive guide to licensed dentists in the United States and its territorial possessions. Also includes foreign affiliates of the American Dental Association. Lists dentists by state, territorial possession, and federal service. For each dentist, it reports the address, year of birth, dental specialty, dental school, year of graduation, and other related information.

In a separate section dentists are listed according to specialty. Within this publication is a listing of the state dental examining boards for licensure.

[3-70] *American Medical Directory: Directory of Physicians in the United States, Puerto Rico, Virgin Islands, Certain Pacific Islands, and U.S. Physicians Temporarily Located in Foreign Countries.* 32nd edition. 4 volumes. Chicago: American Medical Association, 1990. Recently, published biennially.

A directory of physicians arranged by a consolidated alphabetization of their names and an alphabetization by city within state. For each physician there is reported the professional address, medical school from which he/she was graduated, year of license in present state, primary and secondary medical specialty fields, type of practice (e.g., patient care, research, teaching, administration), certified specialty, and if he/she has earned the Physician's Recognition Award for completing the continuing medical education program that is recognized by the American Medical Association. Osteopathic physicians who are members of the AMA are also listed and designated.

[3-71] *The Best Hospitals in America.* Linda Sunshine and John W. Wright. New York: Henry Holt, 1987.

An informative guide to what the authors describe as the best hospitals in America. Arranged by state, this list has a description of each medical center that includes the areas of specialization, names of well-known specialists on staff, significant medical achievements that have occurred at the hospital, admission policy, per diem room charges and average cost per patient stay (approximate, since the charges have been subject to change since the date of this book's publication), and sundry statistical data (e.g., staff size, number of beds, average length of patient stay, and information on emergency room/trauma center visits). The index enables the reader to identify which hospitals and clinics specialize in the treatment and/or research of specific diseases and disorders.

[3-72] *The Blue Book of Optometrists.* 41st edition. Stoneham, MA: Butterworth-Heinemann Publishers, 1991. Published biennially.

A directory of optometrists in the United States, Puerto Rico, and Canada that reports the office address, telephone number, education, specialty, and other descriptive information for each optometrist. Also provides a directory of state examining boards for optometrists and a listing of state optometric associations. Publishes a directory of optometric educational programs, a summary of state laws on optometry, and a directory of miscellaneous associations and organizations related to the field.

[3-73] *Consumer Sourcebook.* 5th edition. Edited by Kay Gill and Robert Wilson. Detroit: Gale Research Company, 1988.

A directory of private organizations and governmental agencies at all levels of government that either advocate and protect consumer rights or provide information, usually free of charge, that assists consumers with their rights. Cites addresses and telephone numbers, and, in some cases, names of contact persons. Lists more than 6,200 consumer information sources that have been organized in twenty-six subject categories that include health care, food and drug safety, insurance, aging, child services, product safety, and other consumer interests. Also offers guidelines for protection in selected areas of consumer activity.

[3-74] *Directory of Alzheimer's Disease Treatment Facilities and Home Health Care Programs.* Phoenix: Oryx Press, 1989.

A national directory of facilities and programs that serve Alzheimer patients and their families. These services include diagnosis and treatment, long-term residential care, adult day care, respite care, home health care, and family support groups. Each entry's profile usually includes the address, telephone number, and names of the administrative and medical directors in addition to the names of the principal medical practitioners. The description of each facility often includes its type, date founded, accreditation, ownership, name of parent organization or system affiliation, physical setting and features, and the training and research services provided.

A program profile cites the referral and admission policies, programs and services provided by program type, financial coverages that are accepted, and other related information. The entries are arranged alphabetically by city within state. A "program type index" facilitates identifying an agency that offers a specific type of program.

[3-75] *Directory of Medical Rehabilitation Programs.* Phoenix: Oryx Press, 1990.

Encompassing the entire United States, this directory presents the names and descriptions of agencies, programs, and facilities that provide medical rehabilitation services. Each description may include the address, telephone number, names of key personnel, accreditation, affiliations, number of beds, levels of training that are offered, admission policies, diagnostic services, medical conditions for which rehabilitation is provided, types of financial coverage that are accepted, and other information.

Among the medical diagnoses served by the listed centers are paraplegia/quadriplegia, traumas, stroke, neuromuscular disorders, language disorders, chronic pain, and cardiovascular disease. These centers are listed by city within state. Includes an "Organization Name Index" and a "Diagnosis Treated Index."

[3-76] *Directory of Medical Specialists.* 25th edition. 3 volumes. Wilmette, IL: Marquis Who's Who, Macmillan Directory Division, 1991. Published annually.

A directory of certified medical specialists arranged by specialty and geograhic location. It provides a biographical profile of each physician, including certification(s), type of practice, education, postgraduate training, career history, address, telephone number, and other related information. All those listed have been certified by one or more of the individual boards of the American Board of Medical Specialties. Contains an explanation of each specialty board's purpose and function, certification requirements, and examination procedures.

[3-77] *Directory of Nursing Homes.* 3rd edition. Phoenix: Oryx Press, 1988.

This guide to the nursing homes in the United States and some of its territorial possessions provides for each facility its address, telephone number, administrator's name, level of health care for which it is licensed, size of staff by type of professional, admission requirements, description of activities offered to residents, and other related information. The nursing homes are listed alphabetically by city within state. There also is a listing of homes by their affiliation (religious denomination, fraternal organizaztion, etc.). For any nursing home owned by a corporation, the directory reports the address and telephone number of the corporate headquarters.

[3-78] *Directory of Pain Treatment Centers in the U.S. and Canada.* Phoenix: Oryx Press, 1989.

Contains descriptive profiles of centers in the United States and Canada that treat chronic pain. Organized alphabetically by state and city within state (by province and city in Canada), these profiles report the name, address, telephone number, medical director's name, administrator's name, and principal practitioners at each center. The program profile describes the types of pain treated, methods used, referral policy, evaluation and screening procedures, and diagnostic services.

The facility profile reports the kinds of financial coverage that are accepted, type of facility, and number of beds available. Also comments on the operating philosophy and goals, physical setting, and unique features of the center.

Three indexes are provided; namely, an alphabetical center-name index, a symptom index, and a treatment procedure index. Also lists chapters of the National Chronic Pain Outreach Association.

[3-79] *Directory of Residential Facilities for Emotionally Handicapped Children and Youth.* 2nd edition. Edited by Barbara S. Sherman. Phoenix: Oryx Press, 1988.

A national directory of residential treatment facilities for children who have emotional handicaps and behavior disorders. Including public and private facilities, this directory publishes the names and descriptive profiles of facilities arranged alphabetically within state. The descriptive information includes the name of the facility, address, telephone number, name of contact person, how referrals are made, funding sources, average length of stay, age range of clients, characteristics exhibited by clients (including IQ range), tuition and fees, professional staff, social and rehabilitative services offered, etc.

Guidelines are presented for finding and applying to one of these residential facilities for children.

[3-80] *Directory of Special Libraries and Information Centers.* 14th edition. Edited by Janice A. DeMaggio. Detroit: Gale Research Company, 1991. Published annually.

A guide to U.S., Canadian, and other large foreign special information collections that are maintained by special and general libraries, research libraries, company libraries, university libraries, archives, information centers, government agencies, nonprofit organizations, and others.

Each of these special collections is profiled alphabetically, reporting the name of the parent or sponsoring organization, name of the library or information center, principal subject or kind of material in the collection, address, telephone number, name of the person in charge, special collections in the holdings, special services provided, etc. Individual profiles also indicate whether outsiders may use the special collection.

Subject, geographic, and personnel indexes are provided to access these centers.

Augmenting this directory is the *Subject Directory of Special Libraries and Information Centers,* in which the profiles are presented in subject order.

[3-81] *Drug, Alcohol, and Other Addictions: A Directory of Treatment Centers and Prevention Programs Nationwide.* Phoenix: Oryx Press, 1989.

Encompassing the United States and its territorial possessions, this directory lists by city within state the treatment centers and prevention programs for alcohol, drugs, and other behavioral addictive disorders. Profiles of the centers and programs disclose address, name of contact person and his/her telephone number, types of addictions treated, methods of treatment, hotline number, specialty groups served (age, ethnic group, sex, etc.), program setting, client services provided, and other related information.

[3-82] *Encyclopedia of Associations. Volume One. National Organizations of the U.S.* Edited by Deborah M. Burek. Detroit: Gale Research Company, 1992. Published annually.

A directory of national and international organizations headquartered in the United States that have voluntary memberships. Includes health and medical organizations in addition to those in other fields. Encompasses organizations concerned with AIDS, birth defects, cancer, medical and health accreditation, board certification, dentistry, pediatrics, disabilities, and many other sectors of health care. The organization profiles disclose the organization's name, acronym, address, telephone number, name and title of the chief operating official, founding date, membership size, purpose, size of operating budget, computer-based services offered, official publications, date and location of the annual convention, and other descriptive information.

[3-83] *Encyclopedia of Medical Organizations and Agencies.* 3rd edition. Edited by Karen Backus. Detroit: Gale Research Company, 1990.

Organized by health and medical subjects, this is a guide to organizations, agencies, and institutions. For each there is a description that usually includes the address, telephone number, name of chief official, purpose, programs, publications, and other descriptive information. Lists national, regional, and international associations, state government agencies (including medical and dental licensing boards), professional medical and health organizations, medical research centers, foundations, hospital licensure boards, and medical and allied health schools. Subjects under which organizations and agencies appear include aging, alternative medicine, birth defects, child abuse, dentistry, handicap, dermatology, oncology, infectious diseases, mental health, nutrition, obstetrics, osteopathic medicine, substance abuse, surgery, and others.

[3-84] *Guide to Accredited Camps.* Martinsville, IN: American Camping Association, 1991. Published annually.

A directory of camps accredited by the American Camping Association. Organized alphabetically by state, the entries are further classified by day camps and resident camps. Although not restricted to camps for handicapped children, there is one section that is a guide to camps that accommodate this clientele. These camps are categorized by the type of special condition or disability served.

For each camp there is reported its address, summer and off-season telephone numbers, camp director's name, name of organization that operates the camp, type of housing provided, length of camp season, cost, kinds of activities offered, types of disabilities served (if any), and whether special campers are mainstreamed if the camp also serves a broader population. Suggests questions to ask when searching for the right camp.

[3-85] *Health Care U.S.A.* Jean Carper. New York: Prentice-Hall, 1987.

A compendium of consumer health care information. Replete with names of treatment centers, specialists, support groups, health-related government agencies, clinics, and titles of health publications. Contains telephone numbers of organizations, including hotline numbers. This is a national directory of places that provide medical information and care. Included are schools for dyslexic children, heart transplant centers, hospital-based burn centers, headache clinics, and more.

[3-86] *Health Hotlines: 800 Numbers from DIRLINE.* Bethesda, MD: National Library of Medicine, 1989.

A directory of toll-free telephone numbers for health organizations that are listed in DIRLINE, the online database of the National Library of Medicine. These "800" numbers are for organizations that span the health field, including mental health, poison control, AIDS, pediatrics, cancer, drugs and alcohol, learning disabilities, and other areas of disease and medical disorders. This directory is available without charge from the National Library of Medicine.

[3-87] *International Directory of Corporate Affiliations.* Wilmette, IL: National Register Publishing Company, 1991. Published annually.

A directory of foreign parent companies with their domestic and international holdings and of U.S. parent companies with their foreign subsidiaries, affiliates, and divisions. Contains a cross-reference index of parent companies and their divisions, affiliates, and subsidiaries. Company descriptions include address, telephone number, names of officers, line of business, and location and business focus of affiliates, divisions, and subsidiaries. Lists companies by country.

[3-88] *Medical and Health Information Directory. Vol. 1. Organizations, Agencies, and Institutions.* 5th edition. Edited by Karen Backus. Detroit: Gale Research Company, 1990. Updated biennially.

A master guide to health associations, organizations, health-related federal and state government agencies, health-related companies, and consultants who serve the health care industry. Reports the addresses and telephone numbers of medical and dental specialty certifying boards, state licensure agencies, and examining boards for nursing home administrators. Here is a directory of international, national, regional, and state health associations that serve patients and health care professionals regarding specific diseases and medical disorders. The scope of this directory encompasses medicine, dentistry, mental health, aging, osteopathy, vital statistics, and many other areas of health.

[3-89] *Medical and Health Information Directory. Vol. 2. Publications, Libraries, and Other Information Services.* 5th edition. Edited by Karen Backus. Detroit: Gale Research Company, 1990. Updated biennially.

Contains bibliographies of health and medical journals, newsletters, annuals, review serials, abstracting and indexing services, electronic databases, and directories. Provides the names, addresses, and telephone numbers of publishers whose publications are represented in this directory. Descriptive profiles are reported.

The section on directories includes membership directories of professional health and medical associations, lists of companies in the health care industry, and directories in other areas of the health field. Also lists the names of computer-readable databases on medical and health topics, special health and medical libraries, producers of audiovisual products, and publishers of books on health. A comprehensive guide to information sources.

[3-90] *Medical and Health Information Directory. Vol. 3. Health Services.* 5th edition. Edited by Karen Backus. Detroit: Gale Research Company, 1991. Updated biennially.

Diagnostic and treatment centers, clinics, support groups, home health care agencies, shelters, special libraries, and academic programs are reported in this directory. Listed are addresses, telephone numbers, and other special information so the reader can identify health service programs and centers that address AIDS, arthritis, burns, cancer, cystic fibrosis, family planning, hemophilia, kidney dialysis and transplantation, mental health, multiple sclerosis, muscular dystrophy, pain, sickle cell anemia, sleep disorders, spinal cord injuries, substance abuse, and Sudden Infant Death Syndrome. This volume also lists agencies that provide hospice services, home health care, sports medicine, and other types of health services.

[3-91] *Medical Device Register.* 2 volumes. Montvale, NJ: Medical Economics Data, 1992. Published annually.

Guide to medical products and their manufacturers and exclusive distributors in the United States. Volume 1 contains a directory of products and the suppliers of each, reporting the supplier's name, address, telephone number, list prices, and product specifications (when available). In Volume 2 are profiles of individual medical suppliers that provide address, telephone number, method of distribution, names of key executives, listing of all medical products sold, and other descriptive information.

The Trade Name Index in Volume 2 allows the reader to identify the medical supplier when only the product's trade name is known. Other information contained in these volumes are medical trade show information, an index of medical suppliers organized by geographic region, and a directory of local dealers for each manufacturer. These two volumes are a complement to *Medical Device Register: International Volume* [3-92].

[3-92] *Medical Device Register: International Volume.* Montvale, NJ: Medical Economics Data, 1992. Published annually.

A directory of every manufacturer and exclusive distributor of medical devices outside of the United States. For each supplier there is reported the address, telephone number, list prices, and product specifications (when available). Also reports the supplier's method of distribution, names of key executives, all medical products offered, subsidiaries, and other descriptive information. Contains a directory of each foreign nation's distributors of medical products. This volume is a complement to *Medical Device Register* [3-91].

[3-93] *National Continuing Care Directory: Retirement Communities With Nursing Care.* 2nd edition. Edited by Ann Trueblood Raper and Anne C. Kalicki. Glenview, IL: Scott, Foresman, 1988. Co-published by the American Association of Retired Persons, Washington, DC.

Continuing care retirement communities are a relatively recent development in the array of housing options for retirees. This is a directory of some of these communities that are available to those who are interested in this lifestyle. Within this directory are profiles of individual communities that describe facilities and services, waiting-list time, accreditation, certification of nursing care beds by Medicare and Medicaid, special features, address, telephone number, and other helpful information.

Checklists are provided that help with the analysis of individual retirement communities and comparisons between them.

[3-94] *National Health Directory.* 14th edition. John T. Grupenhoff. Rockville, MD: Aspen Publishers, 1990.

A guide to key health officials at the federal, state, city, and county levels. Also provides names of members of legislative committees that address health issues. Information includes addresses and telephone numbers.

[3-95] *Principal International Businesses.* Parsippany, NJ: Dun's Marketing Services, 1991. Published annually.

A directory of the most prominent and largest businesses in countries around the world (according to Dun and Bradstreet International). Lists firms alphabetically within country and in a composite list for all countries. Also organizes them by line of business (SIC code). Entry profiles include address, SIC code, name of parent company, name of senior operating officer, and other information.

[3-96] *REHAB: A Comprehensive Guide to Recommended Drug-Alcohol Treatment Centers in the United States.* Stan Hart. New York: Harper & Row, 1988.

Based on personal visitations to alcoholism and drug treatment centers in the United States, this publication provides extensive descriptive information about each center plus evaluative comments and a rating. Included are the center's address, telephone number, general description, average length of treatment, cost, insurance accepted, residential accommodations, brief description of the detoxification unit, age limitations for admitting patients, policy regarding leaving the premises, treatment philosophy and procedure, size and qualifications of the staff, explanation of therapy, visitations, the author's evaluation, etc.

[3-97] *Research Centers Directory.* 2 volumes. 15th edition. Edited by Karen Hill. Detroit: Gale Research Company, 1990. Published annually.

A directory of permanently established research centers, institutes, bureaus, and other similar nonprofit research organizations in the medical and health sciences and other fields. Descriptions of individual entries include address, telephone number, director's name, sources of support, fields of research, specialized collections and databases, publications, and other related information. Indexes by names of research centers, acronyms of the centers, names of sponsoring institution, subjects, and special capabilities.

[3-98] *State Administrative Officials Classified by Function.* Lexington, KY: The Council of State Governments, 1992. Published biennially.

A directory of state government officials, both elected and appointed. Information is arranged by state within function. Cites names of officials, addresses, and telephone numbers. Includes all states, the District of Columbia, and U.S. possessions and territories. Among the officials listed are those responsible for the state departments of health, bureaus of vital statistics and records, and agencies for professional licensing.

[3-99] *State Executive Directory Annual.* Edited by Rosalie Ruane. Washington, DC: Carroll Publishing Co., 1992.

This directory lists the elected officials and administrative officers of the individual states. These persons are identified by their functional areas, and it reports their addresses and telephone numbers. The arrangement by area of responsibility is by state and by composite for all states. Includes state health departments, licensure boards, and bureaus of vital statistics and records. Also provides a section that serves as a national telephone directory for state government officials and administrative officers.

[3-100] *Substance Abuse and Kids: A Directory of Education, Information, Prevention, and Early Intervention Programs.* Phoenix: Oryx Press, 1989.

Focusing on children up to the age of 18 years, this is a national directory of 1,500 programs that provide services for the prevention, education, and early intervention of substance abuse. Profiles of programs include the name of the program, address, telephone number, name of contact person, hotline number, ages/grades that are being served, addictions or disorders targeted, prevention programs and services offered, fees, and other descriptive information.

[3-101] *Substance Abuse Residential Treatment Centers for Teens.* Phoenix: Oryx Press, 1990.

Arranged by cities within states, this is a national directory of residential and inpatient treatment programs for alcohol, drug, and behavioral disorders among preteens and teenagers. Profiling more than 1,000 programs, these descriptions include the program's name, address, telephone number, contact person, hotline number, accreditation, licensure, facility evaluation, the addictions or disorders that are treated, treatment methods, staffing, fees, and other information.

There are three useful indexes, namely, by organization name, by addiction or disorder, and by treatment method. The last two are arranged with the treatment centers classified first by state under the addiction/disorder and then by state under the method of treatment. This provides for the geographical identification of centers according to two principal criteria.

[3-102] *Yearbook and Directory of Osteopathic Physicians.* Chicago: American Osteopathic Association. Published annually.

This annual directory and yearbook of the osteopathic profession contains the names of osteopathic physicians arranged by city within state. A similar listing is made of Canadian osteopathic physicians. Profiles of individual physicians include name, osteopathic education, year of birth, area of certification, specialty, address, and other professional information. Also includes the licensing requirements of each state, the requirements for each of the osteopathic specialty certification boards, and osteopathic predoctoral and postdoctoral education. As a yearbook of the osteopathic profession, it contains a variety of business matters of the American Osteopathic Association.

ENCYCLOPEDIAS AND HANDBOOKS

[3-103] *The Allergy Encyclopedia.* Edited by Craig T. Norback. New York: New American Library, 1981.

This handbook on allergies answers many of the common questions that are asked about allergens and related matters. It explains the allergen characteristics of the regions and states within the United States; provides a pollen calendar for each state; discusses the causes, symptoms, diagnosis, and treatments for different allergies; and provides guidelines on how to manage an allergy emergency. Suggestions are given for allergen-free cooking. Contains a directory of hospital-affiliated allergy centers and clinics. Parents will find useful the listing and description of summer camps for allergic and asthmatic children.

[3-104] *Allergy in the World: A Guide for Physicians and Travelers.* Edited by Alexander Roth. Honolulu: The University Press of Hawaii, 1978.

The traveler's guide to allergens in fifty countries and areas of the world. Especially valuable for international travelers who suffer from pollens, molds, and other allergens. For each country, there is a brief description of geographic and climatic conditions and a listing of the sources of airborne allergens. Whenever possible, mold and pollen calendars are provided. Clinical observations for each country offer helpful information for the allergy-prone traveler. Also includes related reference materials for each nation.

[3-105] *Alternatives in Healing.* Simon Mills and Steven J. Finando. New York: New American Library, 1988.

Today's patient has the opportunity to choose treatment from a number of alternative medical systems. Each has its distinctive philosophy and approach to healing. In this handbook the reader is introduced to acupuncture, chiropractic, homeopathy, medical herbalism, osteopathy, and traditional medicine. Each system is explained, and a comparison of diagnostic and treatment approaches is presented for each system germane to selected medical conditions. This apprises the reader of what contribution, if any, a single medical system can make to the treatment of an individual disease or medical disorder.

[3-106] *The American Cancer Society Cookbook.* Anne Lindsay. New York: Hearst Books, 1988.

This is a guide to healthy eating. It provides nutritional instruction and more than 200 recipes for healthy diets that may reduce the risk of cancer. Each recipe reports the number of calories and grams of fat per serving. It also discloses the vitamin, mineral, and fiber ratings. Categories include appetizers, soups, salads, poultry, meat, fish, sauces, breads, vegetables, desserts, and others. Discloses how the foods we eat impact on the risk of cancer.

[3-107] *The American Medical Association Encyclopedia of Medicine.* Charles B. Clayman, Medical Editor. New York: Random House, 1989.

The layperson's ready-reference encyclopedia for medical information. Its comprehensive introductory coverage of diseases and medical disorders and their causes, symptoms, and treatments makes it a valuable sourcebook for answering health-related questions. Includes definitions of terms, descriptions of procedures, and explanations of anatomical features and physiological functions. Its scope also encompasses dentistry, mental health, and first aid. Contains a glossary of generic and brand-name drugs.

[3-108] *Anatomy of the Human Body.* Henry Gray. 30th American edition. Edited by Carmine D. Clemente. Philadelphia: Lea & Febiger, 1985.

This is the widely recognized textbook on gross human anatomy. Its perpetuation through successive editions has spanned more than 125 years. Originated by Henry Gray, this publication contains detailed descriptions and drawings of the different anatomical components of the human body. It covers cytology, muscles, joints, skin, heart, blood vessels, lymphatic system, central nervous system, respiratory system, digestive system, and other anatomical features.

[3-109] *Atlas of Human Anatomy.* Frank H. Netter. West Caldwell, NJ: CIBA-GEIGY Corporation, 1989.

This is a collection of clear, crisp, colorful, and understandable illustrations of the different components of the human anatomy. The layperson, student, and health professional are introduced to drawings that depict with unusual clarity the details of human gross anatomy. Coverage includes the bones, muscles, organs, nerves, blood vessels, glands, etc.

[3-110] *The Calorie Factor: The Dieter's Companion.* Margo Feiden. New York: Simon & Schuster, 1989.

This is a calorie counter. Its comprehensive coverage of many types of foods, their methods of preparation, and the number of calories in each portion make this an informative guide. Calories and carbohydrates are reported for fast foods (by vendor), breakfast foods, vegetables, meats and poultry, frozen dinners, pizzas, pot pies, stews, pasta dinners, beverages, candies, infant formulas and baby foods, and others. Calories are also reported for vending machine foods, camper's dry mix foods, meals and snacks that are served by selected airlines, and alcoholic beverages. Also, the author reports the calories contained in various pharmaceuticals: namely, vitamins and dietary supplements, syrups, lozenges and cough drops, tablets and capsules, etc. There is a caloric analysis of special weight-loss and weight-gain products. This is a one-stop calorie reference source.

[3-111] *Change Your Smile.* 2nd edition. Ronald E. Goldstein. Chicago: Quintessence Publishing Co., 1988.

Contains answers to many of the questions that are often asked about dental appearance. Whether it be a bad bite, crooked teeth, stained teeth, gaps between teeth, gum disease, or other cosmetic dental problems, this book explains the different treatments available and lists the advantages and disadvantages of different remedies.

[3-112] *Columbia University College of Physicians and Surgeons Complete Guide to Early Child Care.* Genell J. Subak-Sharpe, editorial director. New York: Crown, 1990.

This is a comprehensive handbook on pediatric care. Its scope covers the physical, psychological, and dental development of children during their first five years of life. Written as an aid to parents, it responds to many of their questions. Includes matters pertaining to preparation for a child's birth, events and issues germane to the different stages of growth and development, behavioral concerns, nutritional matters, diseases and disorders, ensuring a child's safety at different ages, first aid procedures, and many other health topics. Contains special charts, tables, and highlighted features that address key questions about pediatric care.

[3-113] *Columbia University College of Physicians and Surgeons Complete Guide to Pregnancy.* Genell J. Subak-Sharpe, editorial director. New York: Crown, 1988.

A handbook for parents-to-be. This guide answers many of the questions frequently asked about pregnancy. It includes everything from planning the pregnancy to how to get back in shape after childbirth. There are discussions of infertility, the developing fetus, medical care and nutritional practices during pregnancy, complications that may occur, labor and delivery, and other related topics. A glossary of terms associated with pregnancy is provided.

[3-114] *Columbia University College of Physicians and Surgeons Complete Home Medical Guide.* Revised edition. Genell J. Subak-Sharpe, editorial director. New York: Crown, 1989.

Although no single volume can be all-inclusive in the field of health, this comprehensive medical information compendium is exceptionally useful to the layperson. Its scope encompasses an explanation of the American medical system; basic first aid procedures; how the human body works; diseases and medical disorders, including their causes, symptoms, and treatments; the proper use of drugs and their interactions; a directory of poison control centers; and other valuable medical information. Coverage extends from the fetus to the aged. It addresses medical, dental, and mental health.

[3-115] *The Complete Book of Cosmetic Surgery: A Candid Guide for Men, Women, and Teens.* Elizabeth Morgan. New York: Warner Books, 1988.

This is a guide for the prospective patient of cosmetic surgery. It provides the essential information for making the decision whether to undergo this form of surgery. Guidelines are given for how to evaluate the prospective surgeon. For each type of cosmetic surgery the author explains what the operation will and will not accomplish, what the surgeon will do during surgery, what the healing process involves, the length of the operation and recovery, side effects and complications, costs, insurance coverage, and other related topics.

[3-116] *The Complete Book of Medical Tests.* Mark A. Moskowitz and Michael E. Osband. New York: W. W. Norton, 1984.

Answers many questions patients have regarding medical diagnostic tests. Responds to fifty of the common general questions patients have concerning medical tests. Also discusses specific medical tests by explaining their purpose, procedure, patient preparation, risks and discomforts, symptoms and diseases for which each test is performed, and how the results are expressed. Costs are reported; however, most are now obsolete.

Includes an explanation of tests commonly administered during pregnancies. Also discloses those tests that are used to diagnose each of various common diseases and symptoms. Explains the effects of exercise on the results of medical tests.

[3-117] *The Complete Book of Natural Medicines.* David Carroll. New York: Summit Books, 1980.

Explains some of the different healing systems collectively known as natural medicine. Discusses the techniques used by natural medicine to maintain or achieve wellness. Presents specific ailments and one or more natural medical procedures followed to treat each ailment. The emphasis is on schools of natural cure, i.e., remedies that involve neither synthetic chemicals nor surgery.

Included among the natural healing approaches are herbal medicine, acupressure, nutrition therapy, fasting, clay therapy, breathing exercises, homeopathy, and others. Healing programs are presented for arthritis, bronchitis, colds, constipation, depression, headaches, hiccups, high blood pressure, menstrual irregularities, anxiety, and more.

[3-118] *Complete Guide to Early Child Care.*

For full title and description, see [3-112].

[3-119] *Complete Guide to Medical Tests.* H. Winter Griffith. Tucson, AZ: Fisher Books, 1988.

This is a compendium of medical diagnostic tests and procedures with an explanation of each. Descriptive profiles feature the purpose of the test, what procedures are performed during the test, pretest preparation, posttest consequences and care, time required for patient involvement, equipment used during the test, who performs the procedure and where, reliability of the test, and the estimated average cost. For each test, there is also an explanation of the risks and precautions. Information is presented that helps the patient interpret the test results, including what constitutes normal values and an explanation of abnormal values. There is a listing of drugs that may affect test results.

[3-120] *Complete Guide to Pregnancy.*

For full title and description, see [3-113].

[3-121] *Complete Guide to Prescription and Non-Prescription Drugs.* 9th edition. H. Winter Griffith. New York: Putnam Publishing Group, 1992. Published annually.

Contains profile charts of prescription and nonprescription drugs. These charts report the brand name(s) for the generic drug name(s), whether a drug is habit forming, its uses, dosage, how to take it, possible adverse reactions or side effects, warnings and precautions, information regarding its use during pregnancy and breast-feeding, special instructions for persons over age 60, and possible interactions with other drugs and substances.

[3-122] *Complete Guide to Sports Injuries.* H. Winter Griffith. Los Angeles: The Body Press, 1986.

A guide to sports-related injuries, diseases, and other medical disorders. With the use of illustrated and clearly presented charts, the reader is provided standard-format profiles of injuries, diseases, and disorders that explain causes, signs and symptoms, prevention, diagnostic measures, possible complications, treatment, probable outcome, and other matters pertaining to the sports-related medical problem. Provides appendixes on special topics, such as caring for a cast and the patient in the cast, the safe use of crutches, injuries commonly associated with individual sports, drugs in sports, and physical therapy techniques.

[3-123] *Complete Guide to Symptoms, Illness and Surgery.* 2nd edition. H. Winter Griffith. Los Angeles: The Body Press, 1989.

Employing easy-to-read charts of symptoms, illnesses, and surgical procedures, the reader is informed about a disease or medical disorder. The first principal section contains a separate chart for each major symptom with information suggesting the disease or disorder that may be indicated. The reader is then told what to do. In another section are charts for different diseases and disorders. These profiles report the signs and symptoms, body parts involved, causes, risks, diagnostic measures, treatment, possible complications, probable outcome, and other types of information.

A third portion of this handbook profiles different surgical procedures, explaining reasons for the surgery, parts of the body involved, risks, description of the operation, anesthesia used, average length of hospital stay, postoperative care, etc.

[3-124] *Complete Home Medical Guide.*

For full title and description, see [3-114].

[3-125] *The Complete Parent's Guide to Telephone Medicine.* Jeffrey L. Brown. New York: Putnam Publishing Group, 1988.

Here is a guide for parents of infants and young children. It assists the parent with diagnosing the child's illness or injury. Uniquely, it instructs the parent whether a call to the pediatrician is needed, and, if it is, when it should be made. The author tells the parent the types of information that should be assembled before calling a doctor or going to a physician's office. The emphasis is on when to call the doctor and how to prepare for this call so that maximum value can be derived from the conversation.

Using an easy-to-read format, the reader can find the appropriate health situation and receive a capsule summary, including what the doctor needs to know, when to call the doctor, and information about the treatment.

[3-126] *Countries of the World and Their Leaders, Yearbook.* Edited by Frank E. Bair. 2 volumes. Detroit: Gale Research Company, 1990.

A comprehensive guide to the nations of the world, with national profiles that provide descriptions of the people, geography, government, economy, health conditions, political conditions, culture, appropriate clothing, customs, telecommunications, and transportation. It discloses information and regulations about matters of health in the different countries as they relate to the traveler. Provides guidance concerning passports, visas, duty, and travel warnings.

Covers the vaccination requirements of individual countries, recommendations on various diseases worldwide, the potential health risk to travelers to different countries, the recommended immunization schedule for both infants and children prior to age seven and those who were not immunized by that age, and other health information for international travel.

[3-127] *Current Pediatric Therapy.* 13th edition. Sydney S. Gellis and Benjamin M. Kagan. Philadelphia: W. B. Saunders, 1990. Published biennially.

A collection of articles written by physicians on the treatment of childhood diseases and medical disorders. Because it is intended for medical practitioners, *Current Pediatric Therapy* will be beyond the comprehension of some lay readers. Coverage addresses medical conditions of the fetus through those of the teenager. These conditions and their treatments include the areas of nutrition, mental and emotional disturbances, the nervous system, respiratory problems, digestive disorders, diseases, orthopedic disorders, skin problems, allergies, poisoning, HIV-1 infection, SIDS, sexual abuse, and genetic diseases. The discussion of treatment involves dosages, prescriptions, special regimens, rehabilitation, and immunization schedules.

[3-128] *Diagnostic and Statistical Manual of Mental Disorders (DSM-111-R).* 3rd edition. Revised. Washington, DC: American Psychiatric Association, 1987.

Written primarily for mental health professionals, *DSM-111-R* classifies mental disorders and provides information that assists with the diagnosis of these disorders. Profiles of mental disorders include essential and associated features, diagnostic criteria, age at onset, course of the disorder, impairment, predisposing factors, prevalence, sex ratio, differential diagnosis, complications, and familial pattern. Due to the complexity of the process for conducting a diagnosis of mental disorder, laypersons should not attempt to use this book for this purpose.

[3-129] *Drug Evaluations Annual.* Chicago: American Medical Association, 1992. Published annually. A continuation of the former title, *AMA Drug Evaluations.*

This is the health care professional's guide to the clinical use of drugs. It provides an analytical description of each medicine, including comparative evaluations between drugs. Generally, the drug profiles cover actions, uses, adverse reactions and precautions, drug interactions, pharmacokinetics, dosage, and preparations. Evaluations are based on a distillation of current scientific research literature and the experience of expert clinicians.

The drugs are arranged by therapeutic classification. Includes extensive bibliographies of drug research references.

[3-130] *Drug Interactions Guide Book.* Richard Harkness. Englewood Cliffs, NJ: Prentice-Hall, 1991.

A guide to clinically significant adverse drug interactions. Whether the interaction is between two medications or between a medication and food or alcohol, *Drug Interactions Guide Book* will reveal the probability of an interaction, the effect in terms of which drug's action will be increased or decreased, potential consequences of the interaction, and what to do to prevent or reduce the interaction. The author cautions laypersons not to attempt to manage chemical interactions themselves, but instead, to leave this task to the physician. Also listed are common diseases and medical disorders and the drugs used to treat them.

[3-131] *Drugs Available Abroad: A Guide to Therapeutic Drugs Available and Approved Outside the U.S.* Edited by Jerry L. Schlesser. Detroit: Gale Research Company, 1991. Published annually.

Many therapeutic drugs are available in foreign countries but not in the United States. Depending on the regulations of a given nation, some of these medicines require a prescription, while others are obtainable over the counter. *Drugs Available Abroad* is a guide to therapeutic drugs that have been approved by various foreign regulatory agencies and that are in use abroad but are not generally accessible to persons in the United States.

Descriptive monographs of more than 1,000 drugs are contained in this book. Within each profile is the generic name of the drug, names of the countries in which the drug is available, uses and actions of the drug, forms of the drug (tablets, capsules, etc.), recommended dosage, precautions, adverse effects, brand name(s), the manufacturer, an indication if the drug is being readied for U.S. FDA approval, and other descriptive information. Nations reported include Australia, Canada, the Caribbean, Central America, Mexico, Scandinavia, South Africa, and Western Europe.

Contains five indexes; namely, Drug Name, Drug Action, Clinical Indications, Manufacturing Company, and Country in Use. The Directory of Regulatory Authorities presents an overview of drug approval requirements and protocols of individual foreign regulatory authorities.

[3-132] *The Essential Guide to Prescription Drugs.* James W. Long. New York: Harper-Collins, 1992. Published annually.

A guide for the layman to the use of prescription drugs. It places a major emphasis on how to use medicines and what their various adverse and side effects may be. Includes a discussion of major chronic health disorders and the drugs that are used to treat each condition. Explains how the drug treatment is managed. There are listings of drugs that adversely affect behavior, vision, and sexual function, and drugs that make the skin sensitive to the sun. Also reports those drugs that interact unfavorably with alcohol.

The drug profiles describe each medicinal drug in terms of its use, how it works, the benefits versus the risks, how long the drug has been in use, dosage, precautions, adverse effects, side effects, use during pregnancy and breast feeding, effects on sexual function, and more.

The Extra Pharmacopoeia (Martindale).

See *Martindale, The Extra Pharmacopoeia* [3-142].

[3-133] Family Guide to Dental Health.

For full title and description, see [3-148].

[3-134] First Aid Book.

For full title and description, see [3-141].

[3-135] The Food and Drug Interaction Guide. Brian L. G. Morgan. New York: Simon and Schuster, 1986.

Addresses the interaction between drugs and foods. Focuses on the way foods may reduce or enhance the effect of drugs and on the way medication may lower the value of certain foods. It is this chemical interplay between drugs and nutrients about which the author endeavors to educate the consumer.

For each generic drug that is described the author discusses the use, possible side effects, foods to avoid, and nutritional consequences. The symptoms of nutritional problems are discussed, along with the appropriate treatments. Recommendations are given on how to prevent or counteract nutritional deficiencies.

[3-136] Food Values of Portions Commonly Used. 15th edition. Jean A. T. Pennington. Philadelphia: J. P. Lippincott, 1989.

This guide to the nutrient content of foods includes their calories, protein, fat, cholesterol, carbohydrates, saturated fatty acids, polyunsaturated fatty acids, fiber, vitamins, and minerals. For some foods other ingredients are reported, such as alcohol, biotin, caffeine, gluten, iodine, pectin, salicylates, and sugars. In addition to standard foods, other food categories include beverages, fast foods, infant formulas, and commercial and hospital special dietary formulas.

[3-137] Foreign Travel and Immunization Guide. 13th edition. Kenneth R. Dardick and Hans H. Neumann. Los Angeles: Practice Management Information Corporation, 1990.

Here is the international traveler's guide to health information. Includes immunization requirements of individual nations, information on the different types of immunization, and a potpourri of health guidelines, such as foods to avoid, how to get a

doctor when abroad, swimming in strange places, jet lag, suggested contents of a
medicine kit when traveling in foreign countries, and numerous other vital topics.
Also provides a telephone directory of centers with medical assistance information
in different countries.

[3-138] *Guide to Prescription and Over-the-Counter Drugs.* American Medical Association. Edited by Charles B. Clayman. New York: Random House, 1988.

A comprehensive handbook for the layperson on the use of prescription and non-
prescription drugs. It explains how drugs are classified, how they work in the body,
and how to manage drug treatments.

   There are profiles of many drugs which describe these drugs according to their
purpose, usage, important characteristics, how and when to take the medicine, dosage, precautions, chemical interactions, possible adverse effects, special guidance
for use during pregnancy and breast-feeding, and other important descriptive information. A helpful feature is the explanation of which drugs are prescribed for the
various body systems and for major diseases. Describes how these drugs work and the
effects and associated risks. Includes informative profiles of vitamins, minerals,
drugs of abuse, and food additives. A color identification chart is provided that helps
to recognize individual drugs that come either as tablets or capsules.

[3-139] *Instructions for Patients.* 3rd edition. H. Winter Griffith. Philadelphia: W. B.
Saunders, 1982.

Contains a collection of medical instructions for patients to follow regarding different diseases, medical disorders, and injuries. The pages were designed to be repro-
duced by physicians as handouts to their patients. For each medical condition, there
is a general description followed by an explanation of treatment steps to be taken by
the patient. These steps usually include activities, diet, medications (guidelines, not
specific drugs), and general measures. Each set of instructions concludes with a section titled "Notify our office if any of the following happens." This is a handy reference manual for patients. Even includes basic anatomical illustrations for the physician to complete with diagnostic indications for the patient.

[3-140] *Is Surgery Necessary?* Siegfried J. Kra and Robert S. Boltax. New York: Macmillan, 1981.

Before any decision to undergo surgery, a second opinion is often wanted. Information is needed that will enable the patient to make a wise decision. This handbook
assists with the process of arriving at a plan of medical action. Some of the most
controversial surgical procedures are discussed with the purpose of addressing those
issues that are critical to the decision-making process. A useful guide, but only one
source in the total process.

[3-141] *Johnson & Johnson First Aid Book.* Stephen N. Rosenberg. New York: Warner
Books, 1985.

This is a comprehensive and authoritative handbook on emergency medical first aid
procedures. Explains how to assess an emergency situation. For each type of emergency, this publication provides step-by-step instructions on what to do. Equally important, it tells what not to do. Checklists and illustrations facilitate learning the

proper action to take when confronted with a medical emergency. Coverage includes poisoning, fractures, bleeding, breathing problems, electric shock, back and neck injuries, pregnancy complications, muscle cramps and strains, and other emergency first aid situations.

[3-142] *Martindale, The Extra Pharmacopoeia.* 29th edition. Edited by James E. F. Reynolds. London: The Pharmaceutical Press, 1989. Distributed in the United States by Rittenhouse Book Distributors.

An international guide to prescription and nonprescription clinical drugs throughout the world. Originally published in 1883, this publication has attained international recognition as a significant source of information on the properties, actions, and uses of medicinal drugs.

Chapters are organized around drugs that have similar uses. Usually, there is a chapter introduction that gives background information on the group of drugs being discussed in that chapter. Following this are monographs on individual drugs. The monograph profiles report the chemical and physical properties of clinical drugs along with pharmacological and therapeutic information. The latter includes uses, adverse effects and their treatment, absorption, precautions, and other descriptive information. Includes abstracts of medical and pharmaceutical literature that report on clinical and laboratory research findings.

A separate section describes the composition of over-the-counter drugs. These profiles are not the comprehensive monographs of the prescription drugs. Among the indexes in this handbook are the Index to Clinical Uses, where drugs are listed under the diseases for which they may be administered.

[3-143] *Medical Tests and Diagnostic Procedures: A Patient's Guide to Just What the Doctor Ordered.* Philip Shtasel. New York: Harper & Row, 1990.

Although medical diagnostic procedures and tests are commonly prescribed, they remain a mystery to many patients. When advised to visit a medical specialist, what should one expect? Capsuled within this book are descriptions and explanations of what to expect when going to an allergist, endocrinologist, nephrologist, orthopedic surgeon, rheumatologist, and other specialists. Furthermore, an explanation is given of various laboratory tests so the reader will know what will happen, who will perform the procedure, how long it will take, what the hazard and discomfort ratings are, and more.

[3-144] *Meeting the Needs of People with Disabilities: A Guide for Librarians, Educators, and Other Service Personnel.* Ruth A. Velleman. Phoenix: Oryx Press, 1990.

This is a guide to information sources regarding persons with disabilities and the services that are available to them. It assists both individuals with disabilities and those who endeavor to serve them. The author explains many of the types of disabilities and discusses attitudes toward them. Among the topics that are covered are legal rights of the disabled; living with a disability and related matters such as clothing, telephone services, independent living, travel, use of pets, and recreation; and computer technology for different types of physical impairment. Includes titles of publications and names of organizations that offer information and services about and for the disabled. This book is an encyclopedic handbook of information and a guide to other sources.

A major section is dedicated to special education and rehabilitation. Also, there is a review of major federal legislation that has been enacted since the 1970s regarding persons with disabilities. A section is devoted to services that libraries can provide to this segment of the population.

[3-145] *The Merck Index: An Encyclopedia of Chemicals, Drugs, and Biologicals.* 11th edition. Edited by Susan Budavari. Rahway, NJ: Merck & Co., 1989.

Intended primarily for physicians, pharmacists, and other scientific professionals, this is a compendium of information on drugs, chemicals, and biological substances. Monographs of descriptive information contain the chemical, generic, and trade names; molecular formula and weight; patent and chemical information; literature references; biological, pharmacological, and clinical information; review articles; structural depictions; therapeutic category; toxicity data; and more. The kinds and amount of information varies among the profiles.

There are numerous helpful indexes that include the Therapeutic Category and Biological Activity Index, Formula Index, and the Cross Index of Names.

[3-146] *The Merck Manual of Diagnosis and Therapy.* 16th edition. Robert Berkow, Editor-in-Chief. Rahway, NJ: Merck & Co., 1992.

This is the physician's ready-reference handbook for diagnosis and treatment. Provides information on most diseases, pregnancy, pediatric and adult disorders, psychiatric problems, and dental emergencies. For each disease or disorder a profile is presented that includes etiology, symptoms, signs, diagnosis, and treatment. Drugs and their dosages are indicated.

Describes common clinical procedures and laboratory tests for diagnostic purposes. The current therapy is described for medical ailments. Contains a section on clinical pharmacology. Reference guides are provided for normal values, calculating dosages, and making conversions to metric equivalents.

[3-147] *Modern Nutrition in Health and Disease.* 7th edition. Edited by Maurice E. Shils and Vernon R. Young. Philadelphia: Lea & Febiger, 1988.

A basic and comprehensive text on nutrition. Explores all areas, including the nature and characteristics of all the vitamins and minerals, physiologic and metabolic interrelations, the assessment and therapeutic treatment of malnutrition, and the management of diet and nutrition in the prevention and treatment of disease. These and other topics are addressed with a collection of papers (chapters) written by experts in the field of nutrition. An extensive appendix provides a large array of technical and statistical data on nutrition.

[3-148] *The Mount Sinai Medical Center Family Guide to Dental Health.* Jack Klatell, Andrew Kaplan, and Gray Williams, Jr. New York: Macmillan, 1991.

A sourcebook on dental health that answers a broad range of questions varying from basic dental care to advanced professional care and oral pathology. Encompasses cleaning of teeth, repair of cavities, periodontics, endodontics, prosthodontics, implants, dental pain control, oral and maxillofacial surgery, orthodontics, and temporomandibular disorders (TMDs). Also addresses pediatric dentistry and gerodontic dental health care. Explains how certain common medical problems affect dental treatment.

[3-149] *New Family Medical Guide.* Better Homes and Gardens. Edited by Edwin Kiester, Jr. Des Moines: Meredith Corporation, 1989.

A survey of the human body and its health. Using an abbreviated approach, this encyclopedia of health explains the purpose and function of the different body parts and discusses the diseases and disorders that can develop. Encompasses the circulatory, nervous, and immune systems; genetics; pain; infectious diseases; arthritis; cancer; pregnancy; and other areas of health. Contains colorful illustrations. A chapter explains selected operations and is useful for the person who is contemplating surgery.

[3-150] *Nutrition Almanac.* 3rd edition. Lavon J. Dunne. New York: McGraw-Hill, 1990.

This is a handbook on nutrition. It is not only complete with descriptive and analytical information on nutrients, the author provides an explanation of more than 130 common ailments which includes those nutrients that have been found to be helpful with their treatment. The reader is informed which vitamins and minerals, when taken together, have an improved effectiveness on the body. Conversely, there are listed those vitamins and minerals that, when taken together, counteract the effectiveness of each substance. Thus the reader can learn how to maximize the benefit of vitamins and minerals.

The complete nutrient analysis of more than 600 foods appears in a Table of Food Composition. This facilitates a comparison of food values for individual items in different food groups. The analysis of specific foods includes vitamins, minerals, lipids, amino acids, calories, proteins, carbohydrates, and fiber. Sample recipes are presented that demonstrate how to prepare nutritious foods. Finally, there is a section that explains the medicinal use of individual herbs.

[3-151] *The Patient's Guide to Medical Tests.* 3rd edition. Cathey Pinckney and Edward R. Pinckney. New York: Facts On file, 1986.

Explains the purpose and use of more than 1,000 medical tests. Contained in the description of each test is an explanation of what is done, when the test is performed, the risk factors, the amount of pain or discomfort that may be experienced, and the accuracy and significance of the test. For each test there is a discussion of normal reference values and an interpretation of abnormal values. The estimated average cost of each test is presented; however, allowance must be made for inflation since the date of publication.

[3-152] *The People's Book of Medical Tests.* David S. Sobel and Tom Ferguson. New York: Summit Books, 1985.

Contains descriptive profiles of medical diagnostic tests with explanations of the purpose, preparation, procedure, risks, results, and cost (allow for inflation since the publication date). In the discussion of results are general explanations of abnormalities that may occur and guidelines for understanding the outcome. Based on hundreds of interviews, the authors describe how the patient feels during each procedure.

[3-153] ***Physicians' Desk Reference (PDR).*** 46th edition. Montvale, NJ: Medical Economics Data, 1992. Published annually and updated within the year by the *PDR Supplement.*

Although written primarily for physicians, the *PDR* contains drug-related information often sought by the layperson. It is a compendium of major pharmaceuticals and diagnostic products with a description of each. The profiles include ingredients, usage, dosage, precautions, adverse reactions, drug interactions, safety rating for use during pregnancy, potential for substance abuse, and other descriptive material. Also includes a listing of certified poison control centers with their emergency telephone numbers.

[3-154] ***Physicians' Desk Reference for Nonprescription Drugs.*** 13th edition. Montvale, NJ: Medical Economics Data, 1992. Published annually.

A guide to the description and explanation of over-the-counter (nonprescription) drugs. Drug profiles include ingredients, usage, dosage, precautions, chemical interactions, warnings, how supplied, and other important information about these drugs. Similar profiles are provided for home-use medical diagnostic products. Contains a listing of poison control centers and other selected health associations and organizations. Features a color identification chart for over-the-counter drugs.

[3-155] ***Sports Health: The Complete Book of Athletic Injuries.*** William Southmayd and Marshall Hoffman. New York: Putnam Publishing Group, 1981.

A comprehensive book on sports medicine. Describes the different parts of the human body in terms of their functions as related to sports. Explains various sports injuries, what happens, the symptoms, and how each is treated. Answers many of the questions that are asked about sports and health. Discusses conditioning exercises and nutritional guidelines for athletes. Addresses the issue of the growing child and his/her involvement in sports, with attention to injuries that are common to children in sports.

[3-156] ***Surgery: A Layman's Guide to Common Operations.*** Edward L. Stern. Tarzana, CA: Lawman Press, 1988.

For the layperson who is contemplating surgery, this book explains what is involved in some of the most common operations. Medical conditions are explained and both surgical and, if available, non-surgical alternatives are covered.

[3-157] ***Surgery: Yes or No?*** Natalie Rogers. New York: Arco, 1980.

Provides the information needed when deciding whether or not to undergo an operation. Focusing on fifteen medical disorders, the author explains what is involved so the reader can make an informed decision. Dispels many myths about individual surgical procedures.

[3-158] *United States Pharmacopeia Drug Information for the Consumer.* United States Pharmacopeial Convention, Inc. New York: Consumers Union of the U.S., 1990.

A guide to prescription and over-the-counter drugs. Each drug is listed alphabetically according to its generic name, and there is a listing of its brand name(s). Profiles of the individual drugs include purpose, usage, steps to follow before taking the medicine, precautions, and side effects. Explains how to administer the drug. Special instructions are given regarding use of individual drugs during pregnancy and breast-feeding.

[3-159] *Warning Symptoms.* Joan N. Larson. American Family Health Institute. Springhouse, PA: Springhouse Corporation, 1986.

Cites common medical warning symptoms and explains their cause(s) and what steps to take in response to each symptom. Contains many illustrations that clarify the narrative. Among the symptoms covered are the general ones of fever, headaches, dizziness, and others. Also includes symptoms pertaining to the eyes and ears, heart, lungs, digestive tract, urinary system, muscles, joints, and other parts of the body. A handy book for helping the reader learn how to respond to a medical situation.

GOVERNMENT DOCUMENTS

[3-160] *Code of Federal Regulations.* Office of the Federal Register. Washington, DC: U. S. Government Printing Office, 1992. Revised at least once each calendar year, with the component titles issued on a quarterly schedule. Supplemented five days weekly by the *Federal Register.*

Often cited as *CFR*, the *Code of Federal Regulations* consists of 50 titles that are a compilation of the general and permanent regulations in force by executive departments and agencies of the federal government. Most of these rules were first published in the *Federal Register*. To determine the latest version of a rule, refer to the *CFR* and then to subsequent issues of the *Federal Register,* because the latter updates the *CFR*. Each of the 50 titles specializes on specific subjects. The titles are divided into chapters, parts, and sections.

LOOSE-LEAF MATERIALS

[3-161] *Surgery On File: Eye, Ear, Nose and Throat Surgery.* The Diagram Group. New York: Facts On File, 1989.

Within this loose-leaf publication is patient information on individual medical and surgical procedures that are performed to relieve or correct conditions of the eyes, ears, nose, and throat. Coverage includes diagnostic procedures, operations, and support therapies. A common format is used to profile the different surgical operations and medical procedures. The descriptive profiles explain each procedure: why it is performed; the risks and benefits associated with it; how the surgical procedure is performed, including what is done to prepare for surgery, what preoperative steps will be undertaken the day of the surgery, and what the surgeon will do during the operation; what is to be expected afterward, including postoperative procedures, possible complications, and what to do during convalescence.

Focusing on invasive procedures, this publication is easy to read, uses language that is understandable to the typical patient, and contains helpful illustrations. It is copyright-free, and it is designed for the patient to photocopy the selected surgical profile.

[3-162] *Surgery On File: General Surgery.* The Diagram Group. New York: Facts On File, 1988.

A loose-leaf publication designed for the patient contemplating surgery. Explains fifty medical and surgical procedures. A common format is used to profile the different surgical operations and medical procedures. The descriptive profiles explain each procedure: why it is performed; the risks and benefits associated with it; how the surgical procedure is performed, including what is done to prepare for surgery, what preoperative steps will be undertaken the day of the surgery, and what the surgeon will do during the operation; what is to be expected afterward, including postoperative procedures, possible complications, and what to do during convalescence.

Focusing on invasive procedures, this publication is easy to read, uses language that is understandable to the typical patient, and contains helpful illustrations. It is copyright-free, and it is designed for the patient to photocopy the selected surgical profile.

[3-163] *Surgery On File: Obstetrics and Gynecology.* The Diagram Group. New York: Facts On File, 1988.

Provides patient information on key obstetrical and gynecological medical and surgical procedures. Includes diagnostic procedures, operations, and support therapies. A common format is used to profile the different surgical operations and medical procedures. The descriptive profiles explain each procedure: why it is performed; the risks and benefits associated with it; how the surgical procedure is performed, including what is done to prepare for surgery, what preoperative steps will be undertaken the day of the surgery, and what the surgeon will do during the operation; what is to be expected afterward, including postoperative procedures, possible complications, and what to do during convalescence.

Focusing on invasive procedures, this publication is easy to read, uses language that is understandable to the typical patient, and contains helpful illustrations. It is copyright-free, and it is designed for the patient to photocopy the selected surgical profile.

[3-164] *Surgery On File: Orthopedics and Trauma Surgery.* The Diagram Group. New York: Facts On File, 1988.

Information is provided for patients concerning medical and surgical procedures that are followed regarding orthopedics and trauma surgery. Addresses diagnostic procedures, operations, and support therapies. A common format is used to profile the different surgical operations and medical procedures. The descriptive profiles explain each procedure: why it is performed; the risks and benefits associated with it; how the surgical procedure is performed, including what is done to prepare for surgery, what preoperative steps will be undertaken the day of the surgery, and what the surgeon will do during the operation; what is to be expected afterward, including postoperative procedures, possible complications, and what to do during conva-lescence.

Focusing on invasive procedures, this publication is easy to read, uses language that is understandable to the typical patient, and contains helpful illustrations. It is copyright-free, and it is designed for the patient to photocopy the selected surgical profile.

[3-165] *Surgery On File: Pediatrics.* The Diagram Group. New York: Facts On File, 1988.

Medical and surgical procedures for the pediatric patient are explained in this loose-leaf publication. It includes diagnostic procedures, operations, and support thera-pies. A common format is used to profile the different surgical operations and med-ical procedures. The descriptive profiles explain each procedure: why it is performed; the risks and benefits associated with it; how the surgical procedure is performed, including what is done to prepare for surgery, what preoperative steps will be undertaken the day of the surgery, and what the surgeon will do during the operation; what is to be expected afterward, including postoperative procedures, possible complications, and what to do during convalescence.

Focusing on invasive procedures, this publication is easy to read, uses language that is understandable and contains helpful illustrations. It is copyright-free, and it is designed for photocopying the selected surgical profile.

NEWSLETTERS

Newsletters have become a medium for communicating medical and health infor-mation. They are usually only a few pages long and specialized, and although some are published on a regular schedule, others are issued irregularly. Due to the volu-minous number of newsletters, it was not feasible to profile the majority of them in this edition; consequently, a few have been selected in different health areas to in-troduce to the reader what is available. For extensive bibliographies that profile newsletters, the reader is referred to *Medical and Health Information Directory,* Volume 2 [3-89], *Newsletters in Print* [3-12], and the *Oxbridge Directory of Newsletters* [3-13].

[NOTE: The information contained in this *Newsletters* section is based on material found in *Medical and Health Information Directory.* Volume 2. 5th edition. Detroit: Gale Research Company, 1990, and printed with permission.]

[3-166] *AARP Bulletin.* Washington, DC: American Association of Retired Persons. Published monthly except in August.

Reports on events and issues of interest to persons aged fifty and older. These in-clude legislative affairs that impact on senior citizens, medical research, Medicare, Medicaid, pension benefits, social security, housing, and other issues pertaining to the welfare of older Americans.

[3-167] *Adolescent Medicine—Newsletter.* Washington, DC: Adolescent Medicine, Inc. Published monthly.

Disseminates research and development information about the health of teenagers that has been derived from physicians and psychiatrists in private practice and from public and private organizations that care for adolescents. Topics covered include diseases, drugs, accidents, sports injuries, pregnancy, and other health issues concerning teenagers.

[3-168] *Aging Action Alert.* Silver Spring, MD: CD Publications. Published monthly.

Keeps its readers abreast of issues regarding the elderly. Focuses on housing, medical care, drugs, nutrition, and education.

[3-169] *AHPA Newsletter.* Atlanta: Arthritis Health Professions Association. Published quarterly.

For persons either suffering from or interested in rheumatic disease, this newsletter reports practices, trends, and research findings on this class of diseases which includes arthritis. Provides information on the cause and treatment of arthritis.

[3-170] *The AIDS Letter.* New York: Royal Society of Medicine. Published bimonthly.

For persons interested in staying current on research and other developments regarding AIDS and the HIV virus, this newsletter provides timely information. Its coverage monitors the progress of research and immunization, reports recent actions of governments worldwide concerning AIDS, and focuses on the different social issues surrounding this disease.

[3-171] *AIDS Policy and Law.* Washington, DC: Buraff Publications. Published biweekly.

Provides news about legislation, regulations, and litigation at the federal, state, and local levels concerning AIDS. Contains information on fair employment practices regarding AIDS. This is a means for learning about political developments, laws, and legal actions stemming from matters pertaining to AIDS.

[3-172] *Alternatives.* Ingram, TX: Mountain Home Publishing. Published monthly.

Directed to new discoveries in natural health care. Addresses natural alternatives to drugs and surgery. Analyzes the use of nutritional and health food products in the prevention and treatment of diseases and medical disorders.

[3-173] *Alzheimer's Research Review.* Rockville, MD: American Health Assistance Foundation. Published quarterly.

Helps families which have a member who is afflicted with Alzheimer's disease by offering them useful information. Discloses advances in the study of this disease by covering the progress of research.

[3-174] *AROCC Newsletter.* Buffalo, NY: Association for Research of Childhood Cancer, Inc. Published bimonthly.

Discloses pediatric cancer research news. Reports on fund-raising projects and community activities for children with cancer.

[3-175] *Association of Birth Defect Children—Newsletter.* Orlando, FL: Association of Birth Defect Children. Published quarterly.

A source of current information on the prevention and treatment of birth defects. Coverage spans prosthesis devices, rehabilitation surgery, and services for the disabled. Reports judicial decisions, and recommends articles and books on birth defects.

[3-176] *Asthma and Allergy Advocate.* Milwaukee: American Academy of Allergy and Immunology. Published quarterly.

Offers a potpourri of information on allergies, including controversial allergy treatments, tips for children with allergies, research findings, and other allergy-related topics.

[3-177] *Back Pain Monitor.* Atlanta: American Health Consultants. Published monthly.

This newsletter is for persons with back problems. Its scope encompasses the prevention, treatment, rehabilitation, and compensation of these disorders. Includes useful drugs for treating back problems, company-sponsored fitness programs, OSHA rulings, and legal advice pertaining to this type of injury in the workplace.

[3-178] *The Cancer Challenge.* Pittsburgh: Cancer Guidance Institute. Published quarterly.

Written to serve patients with cancer. Its mission is to report on advances in cancer research and to encourage effective medical care, education, and a positive mental attitude for patients and their families.

[3-179] *Cardiac Alert.* Potomac, MD: Phillips Publishing. Published monthly.

Discusses heart disease and its prevention. Presents findings of research that pertain to the heart and offers answers to cardiac questions. Features heart surgery, exercise, diet, drugs used to treat heart disease, and rehabilitation.

[3-180] *Caregivers.* St. Petersburg, FL: Fulfillment Etc. Published monthly.

This newsletter is meant for those persons who give care to the elderly and the handicapped. It offers information that will assist them with their daily efforts. Suggestions are offered on how to render care.

[3-181] *Diabetes.* Alexandria, VA: American Diabetes Association. Published quarterly.

Designed to assist individuals who are coping with diabetes. The articles discuss self-testing, diet, medication, exercise, and other topics related to diabetes.

[3-182] *Drug Abuse Update.* Decatur, GA: Families in Action National Drug Information Center. Published quarterly.

Contains abstracts from various sources, including medical journals, that address the use and effects of drugs that are abused, and trends in the treatment of these drugs. Encompasses all types of drugs, including tobacco, alcohol, heroin, and cocaine.

[3-183] *Living With Allergies.* Menlo Park, CA: American Allergy Association. Published bimonthly.

For sufferers of allergies, this newsletter provides information to help cope with this medical disorder. It covers environmental control methods, diets, recipes, and medications.

[3-184] *Medical Malpractice Litigation Reporter.* Edgemont, PA: Andrews Publications. Published semimonthly.

Written primarily for attorneys, physicians, hospitals, insurers, and medical groups, this newsletter contains summaries and reprints of complete texts of major decisions and pleadings involving medical malpractice litigation. More specifically, its coverage includes errors in diagnosis, mistakes in prescribing medication, surgical complications, birth injuries, resuscitation policies, and other areas germane to the practice of medicine. The emphasis is on the standard of patient care and the patient's consent to receive medical treatment.

[3-185] *Medical Malpractice: Verdicts, Settlements, and Experts.* Nashville: M. Lee Smith, Publishers and Printers. Published monthly.

This newsletter follows current cases and significant new rulings handed down in federal and state courts regarding medical malpractice. Case summaries are categorized by topic. Information for the cases covered include the docket numbers and the names of expert witnesses and legal counsels involved in the cases.

[3-186] *The Melanoma Letter.* New York: Skin Cancer Foundation. Published quarterly.

Publishes articles on the diagnosis and treatment of skin cancer. Keeps readers abreast of developments in melanoma research.

[3-187] *National Foundation for Ileitis and Colitis—Foundation Focus.* New York: National Foundation for Ileitis and Colitis. Published quarterly.

Specializes in reporting on the treatment of ileitis (Crohn's disease) and ulcerative colitis, along with research developments for these medical disorders. Also includes information to help persons cope with these chronic medical conditions. Reports on digestive disease centers.

[3-188] *National Headache Foundation—Newsletter.* Chicago: National Headache Foundation. Published quarterly.

A newsletter that is dedicated to educating its readers on the causes and treatment of headaches. Reports on recent discoveries of headache research.

[3-189] *Occupational Safety and Health Reporter.* Washington, DC: Bureau of National Affairs. Published weekly.

Reports recent developments in federal and state agencies concerning their regulation of occupational health and safety. The focus encompasses legislation, legal decisions, standards, recommendations, enforcement activities, union activities, and state programs. Keeps the reader current on OSHA's regulatory issues.

[3-190] *Occupational Stress.* Oakland, CA: Institute for Labor and Mental Health. Published bimonthly.

Discusses the causes and sources of stress in the workplace. Articles explain ways to combat occupational stress. Presents legal recourses that give workers alternatives when grieving stressful conditions in the work environment.

[3-191] *Parkinson's Disease Foundation—Newsletter.* New York: Parkinson's Disease Foundation. Published quarterly.

Dedicated to serving patients with Parkinson's disease, along with their families and physicians. Reports on drug therapies, support groups, reviews of current medical research, and educational programs that target this disease. Provides helpful tips for patients.

[3-192] *Phobia Society of America—Newsletter.* Rockville, MD: Phobia Society of America. Published quarterly.

Enlightens its readers on the treatment, services, and research on panic and phobic disorders.

[3-193] *Spinal Cord Injury Life.* Woburn, MA: National Spinal Cord Injury Association. Published quarterly.

Published to educate patients, their families, and physicians about spinal cord injuries. Includes articles on treatment and research findings.

[3-194] *Sports Medicine Digest.* Van Nuys, CA: PM. Published monthly.

Designed to serve readers who are interested in the prevention, diagnosis, and treatment of sports-related injuries. Among its varied topics are professional articles on drugs and their effect on athletic performance. This is a useful resource for persons who are interested in sports injuries.

[3-195] *Transplant Action.* Alexandria, VA: American Council on Transplantation. Published bimonthly.

Focuses on the donation of human organs and tissues for transplantation. Covers such issues as ethics, logistics, and finances. Discloses tissue banks and procurement programs. The latter programs are described.

[3-196] *The Workers Bi-Weekly.* Boston: Quinlan Publishing Co. Published biweekly. Formerly titled *OSHA Update.*

Keeps its readers abreast of cases that are before the federal OSHA. Summarizes selected cases, including complaints and citations. Capsules decisions of the review commission.

REPORTS

[3-197] *American National Standard for Buildings and Facilities—Providing Accessibility and Usability for Physically Handicapped People.* New York: American National Standards Institute, 1986.

Within this report are the standards of the American National Standards Institute (ANSI) for creating a barrier-free building or facility that will enable persons with physical handicaps to have access to and use of the structure. They provide architectural specifications. These guidelines are for designing new buildings, for remodeling and rehabilitating existing facilities, and for temporary conditions. The report covers all accessible elements and spaces of construction, including hallways, walkways, ramps, parking spaces, elevators, doors, toilet rooms, bathrooms, auditoriums, and other structural features. It is replete with drawings and dimensions.

4

Where Should I Go to Find Health Information in Computerized Databases?

The past twenty years have seen an astounding growth in the use of computers in all facets of our lives. The information industry embraced this new technology, and the number of databases that can be accessed by computer technology have proliferated. Many of the printed bibliographic indexes are now produced by computer, and the producers of these indexes make their tapes available for purchase. Vendors purchase these tapes, install them in large computers, and provide access to this information via telecommunication networks. With the expansion of computer storage capabilities, the contents of bibliographic databases have expanded to include not only bibliographic citations to the literature, but also abstracts and full text of the documents. The latest technology stores data on compact disc (CD) which can be accessed by a personal computer equipped with a compact disc reader (CD-ROM).

Libraries have been the leaders in using computer technology to gain rapid access to needed information. Many are now equipped with telecommunication links to personal computers, and also with CD-ROM workstations. They offer information from a variety of vendors. Individuals may also gain access to databases from vendors by using their personal computer equipped with a modem.

The professional medical literature was the first to go online with the production of MEDLINE [5-19] by the National Library of Medicine. This early version contained a portion of *Index Medicus* [3-2] MEDLINE has grown through the years to contain the world's major biomedical literature. MEDLINE is included in this chapter because of this wide coverage of all medical problems and technologies, and because it remains the first choice for searching the professional literature. Literature that is appropriate for lay readers can be found in MEDLINE, as well as in some of the other professional databases which are included in this chapter. These databases are also useful sources for locating a specialist for a particular problem, and for identifying research centers treating specific disorders. Because of the complexity of professional databases, readers are encouraged to seek the help of a trained librarian to perform searches for appropriate literature. Many libraries offer online search services, although there may be a charge for this service.

One of the major consumer health information databases, COMBINED HEALTH INFORMATION DATABASE [5-7], is also produced by the federal government. It covers a multitude of patient information materials, mainly on chronic diseases such as arthritis, high blood pressure, and diabetes, as well as information on the prevention of disease, from fourteen of the clearinghouses listed in Chapter 9.

Some of the databases listed in this chapter are quite large, and the coverage of information will overlap, so the same information may be found in more than one database. Contradictory information may also be retrieved from these databases. This contradiction exemplifies the nature of the scientific method. By studying contradictions, researchers are able to advance our understanding of health problems. A patient who is aware of the current status of research in a particular area can make more informed decisions regarding his or her health care. As a rule, computer databases are updated more frequently than printed indexes, thus allowing for retrieval of more recent information.

This chapter contains examples of the information that can be found in the various health related databases, whether it is actual data, or citations to articles which discuss particular problems. The question are arranged by topics similar to those found in Chapter 2. Often more than one database may provide answers to a question, and these are listed in capital letters, followed by a number in brackets. For more information about the contents of a database, use the number in brackets to locate the database in Chapter 5. A listing of the producers and vendors of the databases can be found in Appendix II.

WHERE SHOULD I GO TO FIND . . .	*TRY*

Alternative Medical Care

journal articles that discuss alternative health care, such as chiropractic and homeopathic medicine?	HEALTH PERIODICALS DATABASE [5-15] MEDLINE [5-19]

Associations and Organizations

the address and telephone number for a voluntary organization that provides information related to a specific disease?	DIRLINE [5-10] ENCYCLOPEDIA OF ASSOCIATIONS [5-12]
the address and telephone number for a specific organization of health professionals?	DIRLINE [5-10] ENCYCLOPEDIA OF ASSOCIATIONS [5-12]

WHERE SHOULD I GO TO FIND. . .	*TRY*
fact sheets and pamphlets published by a voluntary health organization or a government agency?	COMBINED HEALTH INFORMATION DATABASE [5-7] HEALTH REFERENCE CENTER [5-17]
the address and telephone number for a support group for a specific disease or disorder?	DIRLINE [5-10]

The Body's Structure and Functions

descriptions from a medical textbook of the normal anatomy and physiology of the human body?	COMPREHENSIVE CORE MEDICAL LIBRARY [5-8] SCIENTIFIC AMERICAN MEDICINE [5-27]
studies about blood autotransfusions for elective surgery?	EMBASE [5-11] HEALTH PLANNING AND ADMINISTRATION [5-16] MEDLINE [5-19] NURSING AND ALLIED HEALTH [5-21]
articles from the professional journal literature regarding the safety of the blood supply?	EMBASE [5-11] HEALTH PLANNING AND ADMINISTRATION [5-16] MEDLINE [5-19] NURSING AND ALLIED HEALTH [5-21]

Definitions

definitions of medical terms and concepts expressed in lay language?	AIDS KNOWLEDGE BASE [5-2] COMBINED HEALTH INFORMATION DATABASE [5-7] CONSUMER DRUG INFORMATION [5-9] HEALTH REFERENCE CENTER [5-17] PDQ: PATIENT INFORMATION FILE [5-23]

Dental Health

articles on the latest research for the prevention of dental caries or cavities?	HEALTH PERIODICAL DATABASE [5-15] HEALTH REFERENCE CENTER [5-17]

(answer continues)

WHERE SHOULD I GO TO FIND. . .	*TRY*
articles on the latest research for the prevention of dental caries or cavities?	MAGAZINE INDEX [5-18] MEDLINE [5-19]
articles that describe orthodontic treatment for adult patients?	HEALTH PERIODICALS DATABASE [5-15] HEALTH REFERENCE CENTER [5-17] MAGAZINE INDEX [5-18] MEDLINE [5-19]
guidelines for dental care for AIDS patients?	AIDS KNOWLEDGE BASE [5-2] AIDSLINE [5-3] HEALTH PLANNING AND ADMINISTRATION [5-16] MEDLINE [5-19]

The Disabled

articles about special nursing care for the disabled?	MEDLINE [5-19] NURSING AND ALLIED HEALTH [5-21]
articles about physical therapy for the disabled?	MEDLINE [5-19] NURSING AND ALLIED HEALTH [5-21] REHABDATA [5-26]
patient education materials concerning disabilities?	COMBINED HEALTH INFORMATION DATABASE [5-7] HEALTH REFERENCE CENTER [5-17]
articles on sports for the disabled?	REHABDATA [5-26] SPORT [5-29]

Diseases

Diseases in General

information from a medical textbook on a specific disease or disorder?	COMPREHENSIVE CORE MEDICAL LIBRARY [5-8] SCIENTIFIC AMERICAN MEDICINE [5-27]
articles from the professional literature related to adult diseases and disorders?	EMBASE [5-11] MEDLINE [5-19] MENTAL HEALTH ABSTRACTS [5-20] NURSING AND ALLIED HEALTH [5-21]

WHERE SHOULD I GO TO FIND. . .	*TRY*

Diseases in General

summaries, in lay language, of professional articles on a disease or disorder?	HEALTH PERIODICALS DATABASE [5-15] HEALTH REFERENCE CENTER [5-17]
a description, in lay language, of a disease or disorder?	COMBINED HEALTH INFORMATION DATABASE [5-7] HEALTH REFERENCE CENTER [5-17]
access to patient education materials for many chronic diseases and disorders?	AGELINE [5-1] ALCOHOL AND ALCOHOL PROBLEMS SCIENCE DATABASE [5-4] COMBINED HEALTH INFORMATION DATABASE [5-7] HEALTH PERIODICALS DATABASE [5-15] HEALTH REFERENCE CENTER [5-17] MAGAZINE INDEX [5-18] SMOKING AND HEALTH [5-28]
descriptions of tests that are performed to diagnose a specific disease or disorder?	HEALTH REFERENCE CENTER [5-17]
articles from the professional literature about nursing care for a specific disease or disorder?	MEDLINE [5-19] NURSING AND ALLIED HEALTH [5-21]

Selected Health Problems

educational materials on the prevention of AIDS?	AIDS KNOWLEDGE BASE [5-2] AIDLINE [5-3] COMBINED HEALTH INFORMATION DATABASE [5-7]
research studies on the treatment of alcoholism?	ALCOHOL AND ALCOHOL PROBLEMS SCIENCE DATABASE [5-4] EMBASE [5-11] MEDLINE [5-19] PSYCINFO [5-25]
research studies for the treatment of cancer?	CANCERLIT [5-6] EMBASE [5-11] MEDLINE [5-19] PDQ: PATIENT INFORMATION FILE [5-23] PDQ PROTOCOL FILE [5-24]

WHERE SHOULD I GO TO FIND. . .   *TRY*

Selected Health Problems

statistics on health problems associated
with smoking?

COMBINED HEALTH INFORMATION
DATABASE [5-7]
MEDLINE [5-19]
SMOKING AND HEALTH [5-28]

| Drugs: Use and Abuse |

information about the generic form of a
proprietary drug?

CONSUMER DRUG INFORMATION [5-9]
HEALTH REFERENCE CENTER [5-17]

information about the possible adverse
effects of a certain drug?

CONSUMER DRUG INFORMATION [5-9]
EMBASE [5-11]
HEALTH REFERENCE CENTER [5-17]
MEDLINE [5-19]

articles about drug dosage levels for the
elderly?

AGELINE [5-1]
CONSUMER DRUG INFORMATION [5-9]
EMBASE [5-11]
HEALTH REFERENCE CENTER [5-17]
MEDLINE [5-19]

articles about the safety of administering
drugs during pregnancy?

CONSUMER DRUG INFORMATION [5-9]
EMBASE [5-11]
HEALTH REFERENCE CENTER [5-17]
MEDLINE [5-19]

research studies on drug therapies for
AIDS?

AIDS KNOWLEDGE BASE [5-2]
AIDSLINE [5-3]
MEDLINE [5-19]

articles on drug therapy for alcoholism?

ALCOHOL AND ALCOHOL PROBLEMS
SCIENCE DATABASE [5-4]
EMBASE [5-11]
MEDLINE [5-19]
MENTAL HEALTH ABSTRACTS [5-20]

information on admission to a research
drug treatment protocol for cancer therapy?

PDQ PROTOCOL FILE [5-24]

articles about drug abuse treatment
programs?

HEALTH PERIODICALS DATABASE [5-15]
HEALTH REFERENCE CENTER [5-17]
MEDLINE [5-19]

WHERE SHOULD I GO TO FIND. . .	***TRY***
articles about drug abuse treatment programs?	MENTAL HEALTH ABSTRACTS [5-20] PSYCINFO [5-25]
information about the interactions of drugs?	CONSUMER DRUG INFORMATION [5-9] HEALTH REFERENCE CENTER [5-17]

Food Facts

information about the interactions of foods with drugs?	CONSUMER DRUG INFORMATION [5-9] HEALTH REFERENCE CENTER [5-17]
articles from the popular literature on a specific diet plan?	HEALTH PERIODICALS DATABASE [5-15] HEALTH REFERENCE CENTER [5-17] MAGAZINE INDEX [5-18]
articles on nutritional requirements for supporting therapy for certain diseases or disorders?	MEDLINE [5-19] NURSING AND ALLIED HEALTH [5-21]
research reports on food contamination caused by pesticides?	TOXLINE [5-30]

Geriatrics

articles about the economic and psychological adjustment to retirement?	AGELINE [5-1] MAGAZINE INDEX [5-18] PSYCINFO [5-25]
educational materials about the diagnosis and treatment for Alzheimer's disease?	COMBINED HEALTH INFORMATION DATABASE [5-7] HEALTH REFERENCE CENTER [5-17]
articles about the special nursing needs of the elderly?	MEDLINE [5-19] NURSING AND ALLIED HEALTH [5-21]
articles about drug dosage levels for the elderly?	AGELINE [5-1] CONSUMER DRUG INFORMATION [5-9] EMBASE [5-11]

(answer continues)

WHERE SHOULD I GO TO FIND. . .	*TRY*
articles about drug dosage levels for the elderly?	HEALTH REFERENCE CENTER [5-17] MEDLINE [5-19]

Health Care Centers and Services

the address for a health research institution?	DIRLINE [5-10]
articles on the economics of health care for the aged?	AGELINE [5-1] HEALTH PLANNING AND ADMINISTRATION [5-16] MEDLINE [5-19]
information about evaluating hospice facilities for AIDS patients?	AIDS KNOWLEDGE BASE [5-2] AIDSLINE [5-3] HEALTH PLANNING AND ADMINISTRATION [5-16]
articles on standards for health care facilities?	HEALTH PLANNING AND ADMINISTRATION [5-16] MEDLINE [5-19] NURSING AND ALLIED HEALTH [5-21]
information about health care services for Alzheimer patients?	AGELINE [5-1] COMBINED HEALTH INFORMATION DATABASE [5-7] HEALTH REFERENCE CENTER [5-7]

Health Care Equipment and Prostheses

research reports that evaluate a prosthesis?	EMBASE [5-11] MEDLINE [5-19]
the addresses and telephone numbers of trade associations whose members produce health equipment or devices?	ENCYCLOPEDIA OF ASSOCIATIONS [5-12]
information about reported problems or recall of medical equipment or devices?	HEALTH DEVICES ALERTS [5-13]

WHERE SHOULD I GO TO FIND...	*TRY*
the address, telephone number, and marketing information for the manufacturer of medical equipment and devices?	HEALTH DEVICES SOURCEBOOK [5-14]
articles about diagnostic equipment used in health care facilities?	HEALTH PLANNING AND ADMINISTRATION [5-16] MEDLINE [5-19] NURSING AND ALLIED HEALTH [5-21]
articles, in lay language, about new prostheses?	HEALTH PERIODICALS DATABASE [5-15] HEALTH REFERENCE CENTER [5-17]

Health Care Professionals

examples in the literature for codes of professional ethics?	BIOETHICSLINE [5-5] MEDLINE [5-19] NURSING AND ALLIED HEALTH [5-21]
the address and telephone number for a professional society?	DIRLINE [5-10]
articles about the education of personnel working in health care facilities?	HEALTH PLANNING AND ADMINISTRATION [5-16] MEDLINE [5-19] NURSING AND ALLIED HEALTH [5-21]

Health and Matters of Law

policy issues related to AIDS testing?	AIDSLINE [5-3] BIOETHICSLINE [5-5] MEDLINE [5-19] HEALTH PLANNING AND ADMINISTRATION [5-16]
information on legal issues related to drug testing in the workplace?	BIOETHICSLINE [5-5] HEALTH PERIODICALS INDEX [5-15] MAGAZINE INDEX [5-18] MEDLINE [5-19] PSYCINFO [5-25]

WHERE SHOULD I GO TO FIND. . .	*TRY*
articles that discuss patients' rights?	BIOETHICSLINE [5-5] HEALTH PLANNING AND ADMINISTRATION [5-16] HEALTH REFERENCE CENTER [5-17] MEDLINE [5-19] NURSING AND ALLIED HEALTH [5-21]
the legal implications of an unsafe workplace?	MEDLINE [5-19] OCCUPATIONAL SAFETY AND HEALTH [5-22]
articles on legal cases that relate to smoking and disease?	CANCERLIT [5-6] MEDLINE [5-19] SMOKING AND HEALTH [5-28]

Mental Health

articles on family stress caused by caregiving for an elderly family member?	AGELINE [5-1] MENTAL HEALTH ABSTRACTS [5-20] PSYCINFO [5-25]
literature on the psychological aspects of AIDS?	AIDS KNOWLEDGE BASE [5-2] AIDSLINE [5-3] MEDLINE [5-19] MENTAL HEALTH ABSTRACTS [5-20]
information on the psychological aspects of the treatment and prevention of alcoholism?	ALCOHOL AND ALCOHOL PROBLEMS SCIENCE DATABASE [5-4] HEALTH REFERENCE CENTER [5-17] MEDLINE [5-19] MENTAL HEALTH ABSTRACTS [5-20] PSYCINFO [5-25]
discussion in the literature of the ethical considerations of certain mental health therapies?	BIOETHICSLINE [5-5] MENTAL HEALTH ABSTRACTS [5-20] MEDLINE [5-19] PSYCINFO [5-25]
descriptions of social programs for mental retardation?	HEALTH PERIODICALS DATABASE [5-15] HEALTH REFERENCE CENTER [5-17]

WHERE SHOULD I GO TO FIND...	*TRY*
descriptions of social programs for mental retardation?	MENTAL HEALTH ABSTRACTS [5-20] PSYCINFO [5-25]
case studies on drug treatment for mental illness?	MEDLINE [5-19] MENTAL HEALTH ABSTRACTS [5-20] PSYCINFO [5-25]

Occupational Health and Safety

literature on the proper procedure for removal of hazardous substances?	OCCUPATIONAL SAFETY AND HEALTH [5-22] TOXLINE [5-30]
what constitutes an unsafe workplace?	OCCUPATIONAL SAFETY AND HEALTH [5-22]

Pediatric and Adolescent Diseases

information about the proper pediatric dosage level of a drug?	CONSUMER DRUG INFORMATION [5-9] HEALTH REFERENCE CENTER [5-17] MEDLINE [5-19]
articles from the popular literature on infant growth and development?	HEALTH PERIODICALS DATABASE [5-15] HEALTH REFERENCE CENTER [5-17] MAGAZINE INDEX [5-18]
articles from the professional literature related to child psychology?	MEDLINE [5-19] MENTAL HEALTH ABSTRACTS [5-20] PSYCINFO [5-25]
articles on the diagnosis and treatment for a specific childhood disease?	EMBASE [5-11] HEALTH PERIODICALS DATABASE [5-15] HEALTH REFERENCE CENTER [5-17] MEDLINE [5-19]
information on the treatment, staging, and prognosis for childhood cancer?	PDQ: PATIENT INFORMATION FILE [5-23]

WHERE SHOULD I GO TO FIND. . .	*TRY*
the location of and entry criteria for a research pediatric cancer treatment protocol?	PDQ PROTOCOL FILE [5-24]
articles on the adverse effects of second-hand smoke upon children?	EMBASE [5-11] HEALTH PERIODICALS DATABASE [5-15] HEALTH REFERENCE CENTER [5-17] MEDLINE [5-19] SMOKING AND HEALTH [5-28]

Physical Fitness

measurements for physical fitness in children?	SPORT [5-29]
articles from the popular literature about physical fitness of adolescents?	HEALTH PERIODICALS DATABASE [5-15] HEALTH REFERENCE CENTER [5-17] MAGAZINE INDEX [5-18]
articles from the professional literature about physical fitness programs for the frail elderly?	AGELINE [5-1] HEALTH REFERENCE CENTER [5-17] MEDLINE [5-19] NURSING AND ALLIED HEALTH [5-21]

Rehabilitation

descriptions of nursing care for rehabilitation programs?	MEDLINE [5-19] NURSING AND ALLIED HEALTH [5-21]
current research for the treatment of physical or mental disabilities?	EMBASE [5-11] MEDLINE [5-19] MENTAL HEALTH ABSTRACTS [5-20] PSYCINFO [5-25] REHABDATA [5-26]
articles on the functional evaluation of physical disabilities?	REHABDATA [5-26]
articles on sports for the handicapped?	REHABDATA [5-26] SPORT [5-29]

WHERE SHOULD I GO TO FIND. . .   *TRY*

Sex and Reproduction

articles from the professional literature on the ethical considerations of reproductive technology and genetic intervention?

BIOETHICSLINE [5-5]
MEDLINE [5-19]

information about the safety of taking a certain drug during pregnancy and breast feeding?

CONSUMER DRUG INFORMATION [5-9]
HEALTH REFERENCE CENTER [5-17]

research studies on treatment for sexual dysfunction?

EMBASE [5-11]
MEDLINE [5-19]
MENTAL HEALTH ABSTRACTS [5-20]
PSYCINFO [5-25]

Sports Medicine

research on medical treatment for specific sports injuries?

EMBASE [5-11]
MEDLINE [5-19]

articles from the popular literature on therapies for sports injuries?

HEALTH PERIODICALS DATABASE [5-15]
HEALTH REFERENCE CENTER [5-17]
MAGAZINE INDEX [5-18]

articles from the professional literature about exercise physiology?

MEDLINE [5-19]
NURSING AND ALLIED HEALTH [5-21]
SPORT [5-29]

information about the age at which children can participate in contact sports?

SPORT [5-29]

Surgery

information from a medical textbook about a specific surgical procedure?

COMPREHENSIVE CORE MEDICAL LIBRARY [5-8]

(answer continues)

WHERE SHOULD I GO TO FIND. . .	*TRY*
information from a medical textbook about a specific surgical procedure?	SCIENTIFIC AMERICAN MEDICINE [5-27]
citations to articles about a specific surgical procedure?	EMBASE [5-11] MEDLINE [5-19]
research on the newest surgical techniques used in cancer treatment?	CANCERLIT [5-6] MEDLINE [5-19] PDQ: PATIENT INFORMATION FILE [5-23] PDQ PROTOCOL FILE [5-24]
articles discussing the ethical issues of organ transplantation?	BIOETHICSLINE [5-5] MEDLINE [5-19]

Toxicology

information about certain chemicals causing cancer?	CANCERLIT [5-6] MEDLINE [5-19] OCCUPATIONAL SAFETY AND HEALTH [5-22] TOXLINE [5-30]
patient information about the possible toxicity of a drug?	CONSUMER DRUG INFORMATION [5-9] HEALTH REFERENCE CENTER [5-17]
case studies on the toxicity of a chemical, drug, or pesticide?	EMBASE [5-11] MEDLINE [5-19] TOXLINE [5-30]

5

Descriptive Profiles of Computerized Databases

Descriptions are provided on the following pages for the databases cited in Chapter 4. The alphabetical listing of entries by the file name provides information on database contents, including the type of information that can be retrieved (bibliographic citations, abstracts, or full-text), the sources that are included (magazines, journals, books, etc.), the level of the information in the database (i.e., whether it is for lay readers or health professionals), the general health topics that are covered, and the producers and vendors for each database. Item entry numbers correspond to those used in Chapter 4.

Some of the databases that are produced specifically for health professionals have been included because they often provide access to information which is appropriate for lay readers. In addition, they are also useful for locating specialists and research centers for specific health problems by identifying authors of recent research studies. Librarians have more experience searching these professional databases and finding materials which are appropriate for the layperson. Many libraries provide search services for patrons. Check with your local library to learn if these search services are available, and whether there will be a charge for the search services. Librarians can also offer advice on how to locate the materials that have been identified in a database search.

The major vendors for health databases are BRS, DIALOG, and the National Library of Medicine. Addresses and telephone numbers for these vendors, and also for the producers of the various databases, can be found in Appendix II.

[5–1] AGELINE. A bibliographic database produced by the American Association of Retired Persons, providing citations and abstracts which focus on middle age and aging. Major areas of coverage include economics, demographics, family relationships, health and health care services, leisure, psychological factors, and retirement. The database covers English-language literature from 1978 to the present, from journal articles, reports, monographs, book chapters, conference papers, dissertations, and summaries of selected federally funded research projects in aging. AGELINE is available from BRS and DIALOG.

[5–2] AIDS KNOWLEDGE BASE. From the San Francisco General Hospital, this database is produced by Maxwell Electronic Publishing to provide current comprehensive information about all aspects of acquired immune deficiency syndrome (AIDS). Topics covered include epidemiology, diagnosis, prevention, treatment, patient education, and social and psychological aspects of AIDS. This full-text database, which covers the time period from 1986 to the present, is designed for clinicians, nurses, researchers, and public health educators, and includes documents which support patient education. AIDS KNOWLEDGE BASE is available from BRS.

[5–3] AIDSLINE. Produced by the National Library of Medicine, AIDSLINE provides access to the world's scientific literature on acquired immune deficiency syndrome (AIDS). This bibliographic database covers the clinical and research aspects of AIDS, such as diagnosis and treatment, as well as epidemiology and health policy issues. Included are citations and selected abstracts to articles in journals published from 1980 to the present, in over 70 countries, with 84% of the articles in English. AIDSLINE is available from BRS, DIALOG, and the National Library of Medicine.

[5–4] ALCOHOL AND ALCOHOL PROBLEMS SCIENCE DATABASE. Produced by CRI, Inc., under a contract with the National Institute on Alcohol Abuse and Alcoholism, the ALCOHOL AND ALCOHOL PROBLEMS SCIENCE DATABASE, is a comprehensive alcoholism resource. Included are bibliographic records with abstracts from the U.S. and foreign literature covering clinical and professional journals, books, reports, and conference proceedings from 1972 to the present. Topics cover all aspects of alcoholism research, including psychology, physiology, biochemistry, epidemiology, treatment, prevention, education, employment, legislation, and public policy. ALCOHOL AND ALCOHOL PROBLEMS SCIENCE DATABASE is available from BRS.

[5–5] BIOETHICSLINE. This database is produced by the Bioethics Information Retrieval Project of the Kennedy Institute of Ethics at Georgetown University. BIOETHICSLINE covers ethics and related public policy issues in health care and biomedical research. The database includes bibliographic citations from journal articles, monographs, newspaper articles, court decisions, bills, laws, and unpublished documents. These citations cover such topics as euthanasia, organ donation and transplantation, the allocation of health care resources, patients' rights, codes of professional ethics, reproductive technologies, genetic intervention, abortion, mental health therapies, AIDS, human experimentation, and animal experimentation. BIOETHICSLINE in available from the National Library of Medicine.

[5–6] CANCERLIT. CANCERLIT, produced by the National Cancer Institute in cooperation with the National Library of Medicine, contains bibliographic records, with abstracts, for cancer-related literature published from 1963 to the present. Included are articles from journals, abstracts of papers from professional meetings, reports, dissertations, and monographs. Topics cover all aspects of experimental and clinical cancer therapy, mechanisms of carcinogenesis, and chemical, viral and other agents that cause cancer. CANCERLIT is available from BRS, DIALOG, and the National Library of Medicine, and in CD-ROM format.

[5–7] COMBINED HEALTH INFORMATION DATABASE. The COMBINED HEALTH INFORMATION DATABASE, produced by the cooperative efforts of 14 government agencies and clearinghouses, provides access to health information for both health professionals, their patients, educators, and the general public. Included in the database are patient and professional educational materials, health promotion and health education programs, journal articles, brochures, fact sheets, books, government documents, product descriptions, and audiovisual materials. Some online documents are full-text. Topics covered include arthritis and musculoskeletal and skin diseases, cholesterol, high blood pressure and smoking education, Alzheimer's disease, diabetes, digestive diseases, disease prevention, AIDS education, kidney and urologic diseases, and patient education programs from the Veterans Administration. The COMBINED HEALTH INFORMATION DATABASE is available from BRS.

[5–8] COMPREHENSIVE CORE MEDICAL LIBRARY. Produced by BRS Information Technology, COMPREHENSIVE CORE MEDICAL LIBRARY is a full-text database, designed as a ready-reference tool for practicing physicians, covering literature from the fields of emergency, internal, and critical care medicine. Included are current and retrospective issues of 72 professional medical journals, and current editions of 24 medical textbooks and reference works. COMPREHENSIVE CORE MEDICAL LIBRARY is available from BRS.

[5–9] CONSUMER DRUG INFORMATION. CONSUMER DRUG INFORMATION is a full-text database of the *Consumer Drug Digest* published by the American Society of Hospital Pharmacists. It is designed to provide consumers, pharmacists, physicians, and nurses with general drug information, and guidelines for use of the most commonly prescribed drugs. It describes 270 drugs marketed in the United States, and includes over 5,000 brand names representing over 90% of the prescriptions written. Each record includes trade and generic names for the drug, as well as information on use, dosage, precautions, storage, methods of administration, and undesired effects. Information is also given for food and drug interactions, pediatric dosage, and pregnancy and breast feeding cautions. CONSUMER DRUG INFORMATION is available from BRS and DIALOG.

[5–10] DIRLINE. Directory of Information Resources Online (DIRLINE), produced by the National Library of Medicine, is an online interactive database containing information about health and biomedical organizations that are considered to be information resource centers. These organizations include federal, state, and local government agencies; information and referral centers; professional societies; self-help, support groups, and voluntary associations; academic and research institutions; hospitals; libraries; and museums. Each record contains location and descriptive information about the organization which may include publications, holdings, and services provided. DIRLINE is available from the National Library of Medicine.

[5–11] EMBASE. EMBASE corresponds to the 46 specialty abstract journals and two literature indexes which comprise the print *Excerpta Medica* published in the Netherlands. International in scope, EMBASE provides comprehensive coverage of the professional biomedical journal literature covering over 4,000 journals. The major topics covered include drug literature, clinical medicine, adverse drug reactions, bioengineering, cancer, environmental health, geriatrics, and public health. EMBASE is available from BRS and DIALOG.

[5–12] ENCYCLOPEDIA OF ASSOCIATIONS. The ENCYCLOPEDIA OF ASSOCIATIONS database corresponds to the print *Encyclopedia of Associations* [3–82] family of publications published by Gale Research Inc., containing information on over 90,000 non-profit membership organizations worldwide. Each record provides name, address, telephone number, executive officer, and descriptions of the professional societies, trade associations, cultural, religious and health-related organizations covered by the database. The ENCYCLOPEDIA OF ASSOCIATIONS is available from DIALOG.

[5–13] HEALTH DEVICES ALERTS. Produced by ECRI, HEALTH DEVICES ALERTS is a comprehensive database of reported medical device problems, hazards, recalls, evaluations, and updates compiled from medical, legal and technical literature, national reporting networks, and government sources. Reports cover problems with diagnostic and therapeutic medical equipment, including implanted devices, disposable medical products, and clinical laboratory reagents. HEALTH DEVICES ALERTS is available from DIALOG.

[5–14] HEALTH DEVICES SOURCEBOOK. HEALTH DEVICES SOURCEBOOK, produced by ECRI, and a companion file to HEALTH DEVICES ALERTS, is a directory containing the address and marketing information of the manufacturers and distributors of 4,000 classes of medical devices. The file contains product records, manufacturer records, and service records for diagnostic and therapeutic medical devices and materials, and clinical laboratory equipment and reagents. HEALTH DEVICES SOURCEBOOK is available from DIALOG.

[5–15] HEALTH PERIODICALS DATABASE. HEALTH PERIODICALS DATABASE, produced by Information Access, provides in-depth coverage on a wide range of health subjects. Included are medical journals; health, fitness, and nutrition publications; and selected health-related articles from many popular publications. Summaries that are written for the layperson are included for the professional medical journal articles, and full text is provided for many of the articles from popular publications. Subjects covered include prenatal care, dieting, drug abuse, AIDS, biotechnology, cardiovascular diseases, public health, safety, sports medicine, and toxicology. HEALTH PERIODICALS DATABASE is available from DIALOG and in CD-ROM format.

[5–16] HEALTH PLANNING AND ADMINISTRATION. The HEALTH PLANNING AND ADMINISTRATION database is produced cooperatively by the National Library of Medicine and the American Hospital Association. International in scope, it includes professional articles from health administration and planning journals, technical reports, monographs, and theses covering such topics as health care planning, organization, financing, management, manpower, and related subjects. HEALTH PLANNING AND ADMINISTRATION is available from BRS, DIALOG, and the National Library of Medicine, and in CD-ROM format.

[5–17] HEALTH REFERENCE CENTER. A CD-ROM system produced by Information Access HEALTH REFERENCE CENTER provides comprehensive coverage of consumer health information. The database includes full-text coverage of consumer magazines and newsletters, and summaries in lay language for articles from professional journals. Also included are medical education pamphlets published by medical associations, foundations, and government agencies, as well as the full text of five medical reference books namely, *Mosby's Medical and Nursing Dictionary*, *Columbia University College of Physicians and Surgeons Complete Home Medical Guide* [3–114], *The People's Book of Medical Tests* [3–152], *USP-DI Advice for the Patient* [3–158], *and Consumer Health Information Source Book* [3–8]. Available only in CD-ROM format.

[5–18] MAGAZINE INDEX. Produced by Information Access, MAGAZINE INDEX provides bibliographic information for articles published in over 500 popular magazines, with full-text records from more than 100 of these general interest magazines. It offers extensive coverage of health related topics, including consumer information, health care, leisure activities, nutrition, and science. MAGAZINE INDEX is available from BRS, and DIALOG, and in CD-ROM format.

[5–19] MEDLINE. Produced by the National Library of Medicine, MEDLINE is one of the major sources for comprehensive biomedical information. This bibliographic database corresponds to three printed indexes: *Index Medicus* [3–2], *Index to Dental Literature* [3–3], and the *International Nursing Index*. International in scope, it includes over 3,500 professional journals covering all aspects of clinical and experimental medicine and the allied health fields. Also included are biological and physical sciences, social sciences, humanities, and information sciences as they relate to health care. MEDLINE is available from BRS, DIALOG, and the National Library of Medicine, and in CD-ROM format.

[5–20] MENTAL HEALTH ABSTRACTS. MENTAL HEALTH ABSTRACTS, produced until 1982 by the National Institute of Mental Health, and now produced by IFI/Plenum, covers world-wide information relating to all aspects of mental health. Included are abstracts from articles in 1,200 journals from 41 countries, books, monographs, technical reports, conference proceedings, and symposia. Topics covered include aging and geriatrics, alcoholism and drug abuse, child psychology, ethics, family, mental health services, mental retardation, personality, psychopharmacology, schizophrenia, sexology, sleep, stress, suicide, treatment and therapy, and violence. MENTAL HEALTH ABSTRACTS is available from DIALOG.

[5–21] NURSING AND ALLIED HEALTH. The NURSING AND ALLIED HEALTH database corresponds to the print *Cululative Index to Nursing and Allied Health Literature*. It provides access to more than 300 nursing journals, publications of the American Nurses' Association and the National League for Nursing, primary journals in the allied health disciplines, and new books in all related areas. Selected articles from the biomedical, psychological, and popular literature are also indexed. NURSING AND ALLIED HEALTH is available from BRS and DIALOG, and in CD-ROM format.

[5–22] OCCUPATIONAL SAFETY AND HEALTH. OCCUPATIONAL SAFETY AND HEALTH is produced by the Clearinghouse at the National Institute for Occupational Safety and Health (NIOSH), covering more than 400 journals and 70,000 monographs and technical reports. Topics cover all aspects of occupational safety and health, including hazardous agents, unsafe workplace environment, and toxicology. OCCUPATIONAL SAFETY AND HEALTH is available from DIALOG.

[5–23] PDQ: PATIENT INFORMATION FILE. Produced by the National Cancer Institute, PDQ: PATIENT INFORMATION FILE is designed especially for patients and other laypersons. An editorial board, composed of leading oncologists from the National Cancer Institute and from throughout the United States, reviews each summary on a monthly basis to maintain both currency and accuracy of the information. Each summary in this full-text database contains information on general prognosis, stage explanations, treatment overview, and treatment options for nearly 80 types of adult and childhood cancer. PDQ: PATIENT INFORMATION FILE is available from BRS and National Library of Medicine, and in CD-ROM format.

[5–24] PDQ PROTOCOL FILE. The Physician Data Query (PDQ) PROTOCOL FILE is a full-text database produced by the National Cancer Institute for trained oncologists. It contains clinical summaries of over 1,000 ongoing cancer treatment protocols directly supported by the National Cancer Institute (NCI), as well as new treatment protocols submitted voluntarily to NCI by other investigators. Each protocol document contains a title, unique protocol identification number, chairman of the protocol, study objectives, patient entry criteria, details of the treatment regimen, and a listing of the participating organizations. Detailed information is provided for ongoing clinical trials, and this database can be used to retrieve information relevant to specific kinds of cancers, locating protocols being used in a specific geographic area, determining entry criteria for patients enrolled in a study, and retrieving information about specific drugs and technologies used for treatment. PDQ PROTOCOL FILE is available from BRS and the National Library of Medicine, and in CD-ROM format.

[5–25] PSYCINFO. PSYCINFO, the online version of the printed *Psychological Abstracts*, produced by the American Psychological Association, covers the international literature in psychology and related disciplines. These disciplines include psychiatry, sociology, anthropology, education, pharmacology, physiology, and linguistics. The bibliographic references and abstracts are obtained from more than 1,300 sources including professional journals, technical reports, dissertations, conference reports, and monographs. PSYCINFO is available from BRS and DIALOG, and in CD-ROM format.

[5–26] REHABDATA. The REHABDATA database, produced by the National Rehabilitation Information Center, covers research and literature related to the rehabilitation of persons with physical or mental disabilities. Topics covered include applied therapy and research, such as disability management, functional evaluation, independent living, placement, and evaluation. The scope of coverage ranges from technical research reports to consumer-oriented periodicals and monographs. REHABDATA is available from BRS.

[5–27] SCIENTIFIC AMERICAN MEDICINE. Produced by Scientific American Inc., SCIENTIFIC AMERICAN MEDICINE is a full-text database designed as a ready-reference tool for practicing physicians and medical information professionals. Chapters are divided among the fifteen subspecialties of internal medicine providing information on patient management, diagnostic techniques, basic medical science, and drug regimens, plus summary articles on current medical topics. SCIENTIFIC AMERICAN MEDICINE is available from BRS.

[5–28] SMOKING AND HEALTH. SMOKING AND HEALTH, produced by the Office on Smoking and Health, corresponds to the print *Smoking and Health Bulletin,* providing bibliographic citations to journal articles and other literature related to the effects of smoking on health. Topics covered include mortality and morbidity, neoplastic diseases, non-neoplastic respiratory diseases, cardiovascular diseases, pregnancy and infant health, behavioral and psychological aspects, smoking prevention and cessation methods, tobacco economics, and legislation. SMOKING AND HEALTH is available from DIALOG.

[5–29] SPORT. Produced by the Sport Information Resource Center, SPORT is a bibliographic database, international in scope, corresponding to the print *Sport Bibliography,* covering all aspects of sports, fitness, and recreation. Articles from more than 2,000 sports-related journals and monographs are included, with the audience level indicated for each document. SPORT includes material in the areas of individual and team sports, recreation, coaching and administration, physical fitness, physical education, biomechanics, sports medicine, exercise physiology, the history, psychology and sociology of sport, and sports for the disabled. SPORT is available from BRS and DIALOG, and in CD-ROM format.

[5–30] TOXLINE. TOXLINE, produced by the National Library of Medicine, is a collection of bibliographic files covering the pharmacologic, biomedical, physiological, and toxicological effects of drugs and other chemicals on our health and on the environment. The database, 75% of which is derived from MEDLINE [5–19], contains bibliographic records, as well as research in progress. Topics covered include adverse drug reactions, air pollution, animal venom antidotes, carcinogenesis via chemicals, chemically induced diseases, drug toxicity, food contamination, environmental pollution, occupational hazards, pesticides and herbicides, and waste disposal and water treatment. TOXLINE is available from BRS, DIALOG, and the National Library of Medicine, and in CD-ROM format.

6

Where Should I Go to Find Health Information in Organizations?

Organizations, both professional and voluntary, are valuable sources of health information. These organizations provide answers to questions about health problems, health professionals, and health centers and services, as well as other health related issues. Many of these groups are listed on the following pages. However, this chapter is a selective list, giving answers to frequently asked health related questions. For a more extensive listing of organizations, consult the health directories found in Chapter 3.

The entries in this chapter provide the national or main office for an organization. In many cases, these organizations also have local branches or offices. By writing or calling the national headquarters, one may find a local affiliate. Readers are reminded also to check the telephone directory or public library for local listings.

All organizations listed on the following pages provide information upon request in the form of referrals, expert information, or printed materials. They are listed under the following broad categories: Information about Health Centers; Information about Health Professionals; Information about Health Problems; Information about Health Procedures; and Other Health Related Information.

The item numbers that accompany each answer refer to the numbers and additional information that appear in Chapter 7.

WHERE SHOULD I GO TO FIND . . .   *TRY*

Information About Health Centers

the services that are provided at the   American Hospital Association [7-4]
hospital near my home?

WHERE SHOULD I GO TO FIND. . .	*TRY*
information about whether the hospital near my home is accredited?	American Hospital Association [7-4] Joint Commission on Accreditation of Healthcare Organizations [7-2]
how to report a complaint about incorrect charges on my hospital bill?	American Hospital Association [7-4]
if my hospital is affiliated with a medical school?	American Hospital Association [7-4] Council on Teaching Hospitals [7-6]
tips on how to choose a hospital?	Council of Better Business Bureaus [7-5]
if a nursing home is accredited?	Joint Commission on Accreditation of Healthcare Organizations [7-2] American Association of Homes for the Aging [7-8]
if a hospice is accredited?	Joint Commission on Accreditation of Healthcare Organizations [7-2]
information about the accreditation of a surgicenter near my home?	Joint Commission on Accreditation of Healthcare Organizations [7-2]
if a plastic surgery clinic is accredited?	American Association for Accreditation of Ambulatory Plastic Surgery Facilities [7-1]
information about the services provided at a vein clinic?	Society for Vascular Surgery [7-3]
the name and address of the medical school nearest to me?	Association of American Medical Colleges [7-7]

Information About Health Professionals

Physician Licensure and Certification

biographical information about my physician, such as when my physician was licensed and where my physician went to medical school?	American Medical Association [7-9]
the name of a local practicing physician in a specified medical field?	Medical Society/Association for Alabama [7-31] Alaska [7-32]

WHERE SHOULD I GO TO FIND. . .   *TRY*

Physician Licensure and Certification

the name of a local practicing physician in   Medical Society/Association for
a specified medical field?   Arizona [7-33]
                                                     Arkansas [7-34]
                                                     California [7-35]
                                                     Colorado [7-36]
                                                     Connecticut [7-37]
                                                     Delaware [7-38]
                                                     District of Columbia [7-39]
                                                     Florida [7-40]
                                                     Georgia [7-41]
                                                     Hawaii [7-42]
                                                     Idaho [7-43]
                                                     Illinois [7-44]
                                                     Indiana [7-45]
                                                     Iowa [7-46]
                                                     Kansas [7-47]
                                                     Kentucky [7-48]
                                                     Louisiana [7-49]
                                                     Maine [7-50]
                                                     Maryland [7-51]
                                                     Massachusetts [7-52]
                                                     Michigan [7-53]
                                                     Minnesota [7-54]
                                                     Mississippi [7-55]
                                                     Missouri [7-56]
                                                     Montana [7-57]
                                                     Nebraska [7-58]
                                                     Nevada [7-59]
                                                     New Hampshire [7-60]
                                                     New Jersey [7-61]
                                                     New Mexico [7-62]
                                                     New York [7-63]
                                                     North Carolina [7-64]
                                                     North Dakota [7-65]
                                                     Ohio [7-66]
                                                     Oklahoma [7-67]
                                                     Oregon [7-68]
                                                     Pennsylvania [7-69]
                                                     Rhode Island [7-70]
                                                     South Carolina [7-71]
                                                     South Dakota [7-72]
                                                     Tennessee [7-73]
                                                     Texas [7-74]
                                                     Utah [7-75]

                                                     (*answer continues*)

WHERE SHOULD I GO TO FIND. . .	*TRY*

Physician Licensure and Certification

the name of a local practicing physician in a specified medical field?	Medical Society/Association for Vermont [7-76] Virginia [7-77] Washington [7-78] West Virginia [7-79] Wisconsin [7-80] Wyoming [7-81] Guam [7-82] Puerto Rico [7-83] Virgin Islands [7-84]
where to file a complaint against a physician?	See State Medical Societies/Associations listed above See also State Licensing Boards in Chapter 10
if my physician is board certified in a medical specialty, and what that means?	American Board of Medical Specialties [7-92] American Medical Association [7-9]
what it means to be board certified in allergy and immunology?	American Board of Allergy and Immunology [7-93]
what it means to be board certified in anesthesiology?	American Board of Anesthesiology [7-94]
what it means to be board certified in colon and rectal surgery?	American Board of Colon and Rectal Surgery [7-95]
what it means to be board certified in dermatology?	American Board of Dermatology [7-96]
what it means to be board certified in emergency medicine?	American Board of Emergency Medicine [7-97]
what it means to be board certified in family practice?	American Board of Family Practice [7-98]
what it means to be board certified in internal medicine?	American Board of Internal Medicine [7-99]
what it means to be board certified in neurological surgery?	American Board of Neurological Surgery [7-100]

WHERE SHOULD I GO TO FIND. . .	*TRY*

Physician Licensure and Certification

what it means to be board certified in neurology?	American Board of Psychiatry and Neurology [7-111]
what it means to be board certified in nuclear medicine?	American Board of Nuclear Medicine [7-101]
what it means to be board certified in obstetrics and gynecology?	American Board of Obstetrics and Gynecology [7-102]
what it means to be board certified in ophthalmology?	American Board of Ophthalmology [7-103]
what it means to be board certified in orthopedic surgery?	American Board of Orthopedic Surgery [7-104]
what it means to be board certified in otolaryngology?	American Board of Otolaryngology [7-105]
what it means to be board certified in pathology?	American Board of Pathology [7-106]
what it means to be board certified in pediatrics?	American Board of Pediatrics [7-107]
what it means to be board certified in physical medicine and rehabilitation?	American Board of Physical Medicine and Rehabilitation [7-108]
what it means to be board certified in plastic surgery?	American Board of Plastic Surgery [7-109]
what it means to be board certified in preventive medicine?	American Board of Preventive Medicine [7-110]
what it means to be board certified in psychiatry?	American Board of Psychiatry and Neurology [7-111]
what it means to be board certified in radiology?	American Board of Radiology [7-112]
what it means to be board certified in surgery?	American Board of Surgery [7-113]
what it means to be board certified in thoracic surgery?	American Board of Thoracic Surgery [7-114]
what it means to be board certified in urology?	American Board of Urology [7-115]

WHERE SHOULD I GO TO FIND. . .   *TRY*

Physicians in Specific Practices

a physician who performs disability evaluations?	American Academy of Disability Evaluating Physicians [7-123] National Association of Disability Examiners [7-124]
a practitioner of holistic medicine?	American Holistic Medical Association [7-133]
a physician who specializes in occupational medicine?	American College of Occupational Medicine [7-135]
a physician who practices in the field of physical medicine and rehabilitation?	American Academy of Physical Medicine and Rehabilitation [7-150] American Congress of Rehabilitation Medicine [7-151]
information on the education and training requirements for psychiatrists?	American Academy of Child & Adolescent Psychiatry [7-142] American Academy of Clinical Psychiatrists [7-143] American Psychiatric Association [7-144]
information about the education and training requirements for a psychoanalyst?	American Psychoanalytic Association [7-146] American Academy of Psychoanalysis [7-145]
a physician who practices psychosomatic medicine?	Academy of Psychosomatic Medicine [7-147]

Physicians in Foreign Countries

the address and medical training of a physician practicing in Canada?	Canadian Medical Association [7-85]
the address and medical training of a physician practicing in England?	British Medical Association [7-88] Royal College of Physicians [7-89] Royal College of Surgeons [7-90]
the address and medical training of a physician practicing in Mexico?	Mexican Medical Association [7-91]
an English-speaking physician practicing in a specified foreign country?	Internal Association for Medical Assistance to Travelers [7-86]

WHERE SHOULD I GO TO FIND...	*TRY*
Physicians in Foreign Countries	
an English-speaking physician practicing in a specified foreign country?	Travel Health Information [7-87]
the address of a U.S. physician temporarily located in a foreign country?	American Medical Association [7-9]
information about U.S. physicians serving as volunteer physicians in foreign countries?	National Council for International Health [7-25] Care Medico [7-26]
Other Health Professionals	
educational requirements for one of the allied health professions?	American Society of Allied Health Professions [7-10] American Medical Association [7-9] National Health Council [7-11]
the requirements for becoming a licensed chiropractor?	American Chiropractic Association [7-12]
the location and telephone number of my local dental society, for referral to a dentist?	American Dental Association [7-13]
information on the accreditation of home health care providers?	Joint Commission on the Accreditation of Healthcare Organizations [7-2]
a listing of qualified medical illustrators?	Association of Medical Illustrators [7-14]
educational requirements for a medical records administrator?	American Medical Record Association [7-15]
the location and telephone number of a medical writer in my area?	American Medical Writers Association [7-16]
information about the practice of midwifery?	American College of Nurse-Midwives [7-17] American College of Obstetricians and Gynecologists [7-18] Planned Parenthood [7-19]
information about the nursing profession?	American Nurses Association [7-21] National League of Nursing [7-22]

WHERE SHOULD I GO TO FIND. . .	*TRY*

Other Health Professionals

information about nursing education?	American Association of Colleges of Nursing [7-20]
the education and training requirements for an optometrist?	American Optometric Association [7-23]
the education and training requirements for an osteopath?	American Osteopathic Association [7-24]
information about overseas jobs for health professionals?	National Council for International Health [7-25]
the educational requirements for pharmacists?	American Pharmaceutical Association [7-27]
the education and training requirements for physical therapists?	American Physical Therapy Association [7-28]
the education and training requirements for podiatrists?	American Podiatric Medical Association [7-29]
the location and telephone number of a psychologist in my area?	American Psychological Association [7-30]

Information About Health Problems

the current treatments for acne?	American Academy of Dermatology [7-121] American Society for Dermatologic Surgery [7-172]
information about acoustic neuroma?	Acoustic Neuroma Association [7-173]
the definition of and treatment for agoraphobia?	Anxiety Disorders Association of American [7-174] PASS Group (Panic Attack Sufferers' Support Group) [7-175]
educational materials about AIDS?	American Alliance for Health, Physical Education, Recreation and Dance [7-176] American Council on Life Insurance [7-180] National Center for Homecare Education and Research [7-177]

WHERE SHOULD I GO TO FIND...   *TRY*

WHERE SHOULD I GO TO FIND...	*TRY*
educational materials about AIDS?	National Parent-Teachers Association [7-178] SIECUS (Sex Information and Education Council of the U.S.) [7-179] See also additional questions for AIDS in Chapter 8
information about the prevention and treatment of alcoholism?	AL-ANON Family Group Headquarters [7-181] Alcoholics Anonymous World Services [7-183] National Council on Alcoholism [7-184] Alcohol Education for Youth [7-182]
current diagnostic methods for allergies?	American Academy of Allergy and Immunology [7-116] American Academy of Otolaryngic Allergy [7-117] Asthma and Allergy Foundation of American [7-185]
current research on Alzheimer's disease?	Alzheimer's Disease and Related Disorders Association [7-187] Alzheimer's Disease Education and Referral Center [7-186] American Academy of Neurology [7-134]
information about amyotrophic lateral sclerosis (ALS)?	Amyotrophic Lateral Sclerosis Association [7-188]
a support group for anorexia nervosa and bulimia?	National Association of Anorexia Nervosa and Associated Disorders [7-189] Anorexia and Related Eating Disorders [7-190] BASH (Bulimia Anorexia Self-Help) [7-191]
a support group for anxiety disorders?	Anxiety Disorders Association of America [7-174] PASS Group (Panic Attack Sufferers' Support Group) [7-175]
water therapy and water exercises for arthritis?	Arthritis Foundation [7-192] American College of Rheumatology [7-152]

WHERE SHOULD I GO TO FIND. . .	*TRY*
a support group for asbestosis?	Asbestos Information Association [7-193] Asbestos Victims of America [7-194]
current therapy for asthma?	Asthma and Allergy Foundation of America [7-185] American Academy of Allergy and Immunology [7-116] American College of Allergy and Immunology [7-118] National Asthma Center [7-195]
information about autism?	National Society for Children and Adults with Autism [7-196]
current therapy for back problems?	American Back Society [7-197]
current therapy for Bell's palsy?	American Academy of Otolaryngology-Head & Neck Surgery [7-164]
current research on birth defects?	Association of Birth Defect Children [7-198] March of Dimes Birth Defects Foundation [7-199] National Easter Seal Society [7-200]
support groups for blindness?	American Council of the Blind [7-201] American Council of Blind Parents [7-202] Eye Bank Association of America [7-203] Guide Dog Foundation for the Blind Training Center [7-204] Helen Keller National Center for Deaf-Blind Youth and Adults [7-205] Lions Clubs International [7-206] National Alliance of Blind Students [7-207] National Society to Prevent Blindness [7-208]
current diet and exercise therapy for high blood pressure?	American Heart Association [7-209] Citizens for the Treatment of High Blood Pressure [7-210]
support groups for pediatric brain disorders?	National Brain Research Association [7-211]

WHERE SHOULD I GO TO FIND. . .	*TRY*
research information about brain tumors?	National Brain Tumor Foundation [7-212]
support groups for breast cancer?	National Alliance of Breast Cancer Organizations [7-213] Y-Me Breast Cancer Support Program [7-214]
the latest treatment for burns?	American Burn Association [7-215]
information about survival rates for cancer?	American Cancer Society [7-216] Candelighters Childhood Cancer Foundation [7-217]
information about diet therapy for candidiasis?	The Candida Research and Information Foundation [7-218]
information about the diagnosis of celiac sprue?	Celiac Sprue Society [7-219]
current research and therapy for cerebral palsy?	American Academy for Cerebral Palsy and Developmental Medicine [7-220] United Cerebral Palsy Association [7-221]
current diagnostic procedures for chronic fatigue syndrome?	Chronic Fatigue Immune Dysfunction Syndrome Association [7-222] Chronic Fatigue Immune Dysfunction Syndrome Society [7-223]
treatment and rehabilitation methods for cleft palate?	American Cleft Palate-Craniofacial Association [7-224] American Cleft Palate Foundation [7-225]
current therapy for colitis?	American College of Gastroenterology [7-129] National Foundation for Ileitis and Colitis [7-226]
information about Cooley's anemia?	AHEPA Cooley's Anemia Foundation [7-227]
information about Cornelia De Lange syndrome?	Cornelia De Lange Syndrome Foundation [7-228]
symptoms of Cri du Chat syndrome?	Cri du Chat Syndrome Society [7-229]

WHERE SHOULD I GO TO FIND. . .	*TRY*
current therapy for Crohn's disease?	American College of Gastroenterology [7-129] National Foundation for Ileitis and Colitis [7-226]
information about genetic screening for cystic fibrosis?	Cystic Fibrosis Foundation [7-231]
information about deafness and other hearing disorders?	American Deafness & Rehabilitation Association [7-232] American Otological Society [7-139] Deafness Research Foundation [7-233] International Hearing Dog Association [7-234] National Captioning Institute [7-235] National Hearing Aid Society [7-236] SHH (Self Help for Hard of Hearing People) [7-237]
current information about the diagnosis and treatment for depression?	American Academy of Child and Adolescent Psychiatry [7-142] American Academy of Clinical Psychiatrists [7-143] American Academy of Psychoanalysis [7-145] American Psychoanalytic Association [7-146] American Psychiatric Association [7-144] American Psychological Association [7-30] National Depressive and Manic Depressive Association [7-238]
the latest research findings on diabetes?	American Diabetes Association [7-239] Endocrine Society [7-127] Juvenile Diabetes Foundation [7-240]
diagnostic information for Down's syndrome?	American College of Obstetricians and Gynecologists [7-18] National Down's Syndrome Society [7-241]
educational materials on drug abuse that are suitable for young children?	American Council for Drug Education [7-242] Narcotics Educational Foundation [7-244] National Federation of Parents for Drug-Free Youth [7-245]

WHERE SHOULD I GO TO FIND. . .	*TRY*
educational materials on drug abuse that are suitable for young children?	See also questions for Drug Abuse in Chapter 8
information about the adverse effects of marijuana?	Potsmokers Anonymous [7-246]
the latest treatment for dwarfism?	Human Growth Foundation [7-247]
about the diagnosis of dyslexia?	Orton Dyslexia Society [7-248]
the latest treatment for endometriosis?	American College of Obstetricians and Gynecologists [7-18] Endometriosis Association [7-249]
support groups for epilepsy?	American Epilepsy Society [7-250] Epilepsy Foundation of America [7-251]
information about Epstein-Barr syndrome?	Chronic Fatigue Immune Dysfunction Syndrome Association [7-222] Chronic Fatigue Immune Dysfunction Syndrome Society [7-223]
the latest research on eye disorders?	American Academy of Ophthalmology [7-136] National Eye Research Foundation [7-252]
information about the inheritance of familial polyposis?	Familial Polyposis Registry [7-253]
the latest research related to fertility disorders?	American College of Obstetricians and Gynecologists [7-18] American Fertility Society [7-254] Fertility Research Foundation [7-255] Resolve [7-256]
brochures about fibrocystic breast disease?	College of American Pathologists [7-257]
information about Fragile X syndrome?	Fragile X Foundation [7-258]
a support group for Friedreich's ataxia?	Friedreich's Ataxia Group in American [7-259]

WHERE SHOULD I GO TO FIND. . .	*TRY*
the diagnosis and treatment for Gaucher disease?	National Gaucher Foundation [7-260]
the latest research on hair loss?	American Academy of Dermatology [7-121] American Hair Loss Council [7-261] American Society for Dermatologic Surgery [7-172] National Alopecia Areata Foundation [7-262]
the latest treatment for head injuries?	National Head Injury Foundation [7-263] See also question related to head injuries in Chapter 8
the latest research on headaches?	American Association for the Study of the Headache [7-264] National Headache Foundation [7-265]
rehabilitation programs for heart disease?	American College of Cardiology [7-119] American Heart Association [7-209]
information about hemochromatosis?	Hemochromatosis Research Foundation [7-266]
the latest research findings on the treatment of hemophilia?	American Society of Hematology [7-132] National Hemophilia Foundation [7-267]
information about the prevention of hepatitis?	American Association for the Study of Liver Disease [7-268] American Hepatitis Association [7-269] American Liver Foundation [7-270] National Foundation for Infectious Diseases [7-271]
information about the diagnosis of Huntington's disease?	Huntington's Disease Society of American [7-272]
current diet and exercise therapy for hypertension?	American Heart Association [7-209] Citizens for the Treatment of High Blood Pressure [7-210]
diet information for hypoglycemia?	National Hypoglycemia Association [7-273]
the latest treatment for ileitis?	National Foundation for Ileitis and Colitis [7-226]

WHERE SHOULD I GO TO FIND. . .	**TRY**
the latest therapy for impotence?	American Urological Association [7-171]
information about iron overload disease?	Iron Overload Diseases Association [7-274]
the latest research on kidney disease?	American Association of Kidney Patients [7-275] American Kidney Fund [7-276] National Kidney Foundation [7-277]
information about the diagnosis and treatment of leprosy?	American Leprosy Foundation [7-278] American Leprosy Missions [7-279]
survival statistics for leukemia?	American Cancer Society [7-216] American Society of Hematology [7-132] Leukemia Society of America [7-280]
genetic information about lipid diseases?	National Lipid Disease Foundation [7-282]
the latest research findings on the treatment of liver disease?	American Association for the Study of Liver Disease [7-268] American Liver Foundation [7-270]
information about Lou Gehrig's disease?	Amyotrophic Lateral Sclerosis Association [7-188]
the causes and prevention of lung diseases?	American College of Chest Physicians [7-120] American Lung Association [7-230]
about the diagnosis and treatment for lupus?	Lupus Foundation of America [7-283] National Lupus Erythematosus Foundation [7-284]
the incidence of Lyme disease?	The Lyme Borreliosis Foundation [7-285]
about the diagnosis of macular disease?	American Academy of Ophthalmology [7-136] Association for Macular Diseases [7-286]
about the diagnosis of Marfan syndrome?	National Marfan Foundation [7-287]
information on the treatment of Ménière's disease?	American Otological Society [7-139] EAR Foundation [7-288]

(answer continues)

WHERE SHOULD I GO TO FIND. . .	*TRY*
information on the treatment of Ménière's disease?	International Ménière's Disease Research Institute [7-289]
latest research on multiple sclerosis?	National Multiple Sclerosis Society [7-290]
support groups for muscular dystrophy?	Muscular Dystrophy Association [7-291]
symptoms of myasthenia gravis?	Myasthenia Gravis Foundation [7-292]
the latest research on narcolepsy?	American Narcolepsy Association [7-293] Narcolepsy and Cataplexy Foundation of America [7-294]
information about genetic testing for neurofibromatosis?	National Neurofibromatosis Foundation [7-295]
support groups for obesity?	Gastroplasty Support Group [7-296] National Association to Aid Fat Americans [7-297]
information for the diagnosis of obsessive-compulsive disorder?	American Academy of Clinical Psychiatrists [7-143] American Psychoanalytic Association [7-146] American Psychiatric Association [7-144] American Psychological Association [7-30] The OCD Foundation [7-298]
information about osteogenesis imperfecta?	Osteogenesis Imperfecta Foundation [7-299]
how to prevent osteoporosis?	American Brittle Bone Society [7-300] National Osteoporosis Foundation [7-301]
tests for the diagnosis of Paget's disease?	Paget's Disease Foundation [7-302]
recent research related to pain?	American Academy of Pain Medicine [7-303] American Pain Society [7-304] International Association for the Study of Pain [7-305] National Chronic Pain Outreach Association [7-306]

WHERE SHOULD I GO TO FIND. . .	*TRY*
recent research on the treatment of Parkinson's disease?	American Parkinson Disease Association [7-307] National Parkinson Association [7-308] Parkinson Support Group of America [7-309]
a support group for PMS (Premenstrual Syndrome)?	Premenstrual Syndrome Action [7-310]
information on the prevalence of post–polio symptoms?	Polio Survivors Association [7-311] Post-Polio League for Information [7-312]
about the early diagnosis of porphyria?	American Porphyria Foundation [7-313]
about safe exercise during pregnancy?	American College of Obstetricians and Gynecologists [7-18]
current therapies for rare diseases?	National Information Center for Orphan Drugs and Rare Diseases [7-314] National Organization for Rare Disorders [7-315]
information about the causes and prevention of respiratory diseases?	American College of Chest Physicians [7-120] American Lung Association [7-230] Cystic Fibrosis Foundation [7-231]
a support group for retinitis pigmentosa?	National Retinitis Pigmentosa Foundation [7-316]
information about the causes of Reye's syndrome?	American Reye's Syndrome Association [7-317] National Reye's Syndrome Foundation [7-318]
therapy programs for rheumatism?	American College for Rheumatology [7-152]
a support group for sarcoidosis?	Sarcoidosis Family Aid and Research Foundation [7-319]
new drug therapies for schizophrenia?	American Academy of Clinical Psychiatrists [7-143]

(answer continues)

WHERE SHOULD I GO TO FIND. . .   *TRY*

new drug therapies for schizophrenia?

American Psychiatric Association [7-144]
National Alliance for the Mentally Ill
[7-320]

about the diagnosis and treatment for
scleroderma?

United Scleroderma Foundation [7-321]

latest research information about scoliosis?

National Scoliosis Foundation [7-322]
The Scoliosis Association [7-323]

educational materials about the prevention
of sexually transmitted diseases?

American Foundation for the Prevention of
Venereal Disease [7-324]
American Public Health Association [7-325]
American Social Health Association [7-326]
Planned Parenthood [7-19]
SIECUS (Sex Information and Education
Council of the U.S.) [7-179]

latest research on the treatment of sickle
cell disease?

Center for Sickle Cell Disease [7-327]
National Association for Sickle Cell Disease
[7-328]

the latest therapy for sinusitis?

American Rhinological Society [7-153]
American Laryngological, Rhinological and
Otological Society [7-140]

a support group for Sjögren's syndrome?

Sjögren's Syndrome Foundation [7-329]

guidelines for the prevention of skin
cancer?

American Academy of Dermatology
[7-121]
American Cancer Society [7-216]
Skin Cancer Foundation [7-330]

information about rare skin disorders?

American Academy of Dermatology
[7-121]
D.E.B.R.A. (Dystrophic Epidermolysis
Bullosa Research Association of America)
[7-331]
National Foundation for Ectodermal
Dysplasia [7-332]
Xeroderma Pigmentosum Registry
[7-333]

the latest research on sleep disorders?

American Sleep Disorders Association
[7-334]

WHERE SHOULD I GO TO FIND. . .	*TRY*
rehabilitation for speech disorders?	American Speech-Language-Hearing Association [7-335] National Council on Stuttering [7-336] Stuttering Resource Foundation [7-337]
a support group for spina bifida?	Spina Bifida Association of American [7-338]
about the drug therapy for spinal cord injuries?	American Academy of Neurology [7-134] National Spinal Cord Injury Association [7-339] Spinal Cord Society [7-340]
recent research on sports injuries?	American College of Sports Medicine [7-341] American Orthopaedic Society for Sports Medicine [7-138] Women's Sports Foundation [7-342]
information about the diagnosis and treatment for sprue?	Celiac Sprue Society [7-219]
information about the prevention of stroke?	American Heart Association [7-209] National Stroke Association [7-343] The Stroke Foundation [7-344]
a support group for sudden infant death syndrome (SIDS)?	American Sudden Infant Death Syndrome Institute [7-345] National Sudden Infant Death Syndrome Foundation [7-346] Sudden Infant Death Syndrome Clearinghouse [7-347]
about the prevalence of Tay-Sachs Disease?	National Tay-Sachs and Allied Diseases Association [7-348]
about the latest research on temporomandibular joint (TMJ) syndrome?	American Dental Association [7-13]
a support group for tinnitus?	American Tinnitus Association [7-349]
information about the diagnosis and treatment for Tourette's syndrome?	Tourette's Syndrome Association [7-350]

WHERE SHOULD I GO TO FIND. . .	*TRY*
research on the treatment of trauma?	American College of Emergency Physicians [7-125] American Trauma Society [7-351]
a support group for tuberous sclerosis?	National Tuberous Sclerosis Association [7-352]
a support group for urinary incontinence?	HIP (Help for Incontinent People) [7-353] Simon Foundation [7-354]
about the prevention of venereal disease?	American Foundation for the Prevention of Venereal Disease [7-324] American Public Health Association [7-325] American Social Health Association [7-326] SIECUS (Sex Information and Education Council of the U.S.) [7-179]
information on the treatment for vitiligo?	National Vitiligo Foundation [7-355]
a support group for Wegener's granulomatosis?	Wegener's Granulomatosis Support Group [7-356]

Information About Health Procedures

information about a specific abdominal surgery?	American Society of Abdominal Surgeons [7-154]
information about acupuncture?	American Association for Acupuncture and Oriental Medicine [7-357] National Commission for Certification for Acupuncture [7-358]
support groups for amputation?	American Amputee Foundation [7-359] Amputee Services Association [7-360] National Odd Shoe Exchange [7-361]
about success rates for artificial insemination and *in-vitro* fertilization?	American College of Obstetricians and Gynecologists [7-18] American Fertility Society[7-254]
latest research on biofeedback?	Association of Applied Physiology and Biofeedback [7-362]

WHERE SHOULD I GO TO FIND. . .	TRY
about the safety of blood transfusions?	American Association of Blood Banks [7-363] American Red Cross [7-364]
about the benefits of breast feeding?	American Academy of Pediatrics [7-141] American College of Obstetricians and Gynecologists [7-18] La Leche League [7-365]
the latest procedure for cataract surgery?	American Academy of Ophthalmology [7-136] American Society of Cataract and Refractive Surgery [7-366]
guidelines for Cesarean section?	American College of Obstetricians and Gynecologists [7-18]
information about colon surgery?	American Society of Colon and Rectal Surgery [7-155]
the latest research of contact lenses?	American Academy of Ophthalmology [7-136] Contact Lens Association of Ophthalmologists [7-367]
instruction in CPR (cardiopulmonary resuscitation)?	American Heart Association [7-209]
latest research on cryosurgery?	American College of Cryosurgery [7-156]
dental care for the handicapped?	National Foundation of Dentistry for the Handicapped [7-368]
about dialysis for kidney failure?	American Kidney Fund [7-276] National Kidney Foundation [7-277]
guidelines for drug testing in the workplace?	American College of Occupational Medicine [7-135] College of American Pathologists [7-257]
about endoscopy for the diagnosis of gastrointestinal diseases?	American Society for Gastrointestinal Endoscopy [7-131]

WHERE SHOULD I GO TO FIND. . .	*TRY*
about the surgical treatment for epilepsy?	American Association of Neurological Surgeons [7-162] Epilepsy Foundation of America [7-251]
the latest research on hand surgery?	American Association for Hand Surgery [7-159] American Society for Surgery of the Hand [7-160]
latest procedures for heart surgery?	American Association for Thoracic Surgery [7-169] Society of Thoracic Surgeons [7-170]
about the use of hyperbaric therapy?	Undersea and Hyperbaric Medical Society [7-369]
about the use of hypnosis in smoking cessation?	American Society of Clinical Hypnosis [7-370]
information about transcervical balloon tuboplasty for infertility?	American College of Obstetricians and Gynecologists [7-18]
immunization schedules for children?	American Academy of Pediatrics [7-141]
requirements for kidney transplantation?	American Association of Kidney Patients [7-275] American Kidney Fund [7-276] National Kidney Foundation [7-277]
the most recent research on the artificial larynx or voice box?	American Laryngological Association [7-371]
about laser surgery for retinal disorders?	American Academy of Ophthalmology [7-136] American Society for Laser Medicine and Surgery [7-372]
information about liposuction?	American Society of Lipo-Suction Surgery [7-373] American Society of Plastic and Reconstructive Surgeons [7-168]
information about lithotripsy for kidney stones?	National Kidney Foundation [7-277]

WHERE SHOULD I GO TO FIND. . .	*TRY*
recommendations and guidelines for mammography?	American Cancer Society [7-216] American College of Radiology [7-148]
information about surgical treatment for obesity?	American College of Gastroenterology [7-129] American Gastroenterological Association [7-130]
current therapy for sports injuries?	American Academy of Orthopaedic Surgeons [7-163] American Orthopaedic Association [7-137] American Orthopaedic Society for Sports Medicine [7-138]
a support group for ostomies?	United Ostomy Association [7-374]
information on the latest research for pancreatic transplants?	American Diabetes Association [7-239] Juvenile Diabetes Foundation International [7-240] American Pancreatic Association [7-375]
about specific pediatric surgery procedures?	American Pediatric Surgical Association [7-165]
about specific plastic surgery procedures?	American Academy of Facial Plastic & Reconstructive Surgery [7-166] American Association of Plastic Surgeons [7-167] American Society of Plastic and Reconstructive Surgeons [7-168]
current research in therapeutic radiology?	American Society for Therapeutic Radiology and Oncology [7-376]
current surgical procedures for sinusitis?	American Academy of Otolaryngology–Head and Neck Surgery [7-164]
information on general surgical procedures?	American College of Surgeons [7-157] International College of Surgeons [7-158] See also items in this section on specific types of surgery.

WHERE SHOULD I GO TO FIND...	*TRY*
the latest research on ultrasound?	American Institute of Ultrasound in Medicine [7-377]
information on specific vascular surgical procedures?	Society for Vascular Surgery [7-3]
about reversal of a vasectomy?	American Urological Association [7-171]
recommendations on how often x-rays may be safely administered?	American College of Radiology [7-148] Radiological Society of North America [7-149]

Other Health Information

Aging

help for special health problems related to aging?	American Association for International Aging [7-378] American Geriatrics Society [7-379] American Society on Aging [7-381] Asociacíon National por Personas Mayores (National Association for Hispanic Elderly [7-382] CAPS (Children of Aging Parents) [7-383] Gerontological Society of America [7-384] National Center and Caucus on Black Aged [7-385] National Council of Senior Citizens [7-386] National Council on the Aging [7-387] National Indian Council on Aging [7-388] National Pacific/Asian Resource Center on Aging [7-389] Older Women's League [7-390]

Alternative Therapies

about the practice of homeopathy?	National Center for Homeopathy [7-391]
about the practice of naturopathy?	American Association of Naturopathic Physicians [7-392]

WHERE SHOULD I GO TO FIND...	*TRY*

Captioning

information on captioning for the hearing-impaired?

National Captioning Institute [7-235]

Children's Health

the location of a hospice facility for a child?

Children's Hospice International [7-399]

information about prenatal care and health care for children?

National Center for Education in Maternal and Child Health [7-400]
Association for the Care of Children's Health [7-396]
Children's Defense Fund [7-398]

educational materials for small children who must go to the hospital?

Children in Hospitals [7-397]

about the hazards of certain toys?

National Child Safety Council [7-401]

information about health services and health education programs in schools?

American School Health Association [7-395]

about the diagnosis and reporting procedures for child abuse?

Clearinghouse on Child Abuse and Neglect [7-393]
National Committee for Prevention of Child Abuse [7-394]

about the proper use of car seats and transporting children with special needs?

American Academy of Pediatrics [7-141]

Consumer Health

if a certain procedure or therapy is fraudulent?

National Council Against Health Fraud [7-402]

information about specific health problems or specific health and safety issues?

American Council on Science and Health [7-403]
American Health Foundation [7-404]
Center for Science in the Public Interest [7-405]
National Center for Health Education [7-406]
National Council on Patient Information and Education [7-407]

(answer continues)

WHERE SHOULD I GO TO FIND. . .	TRY

Consumer Health

information about specific health problems or specific health and safety issues?	Public Citizen Health Research Group [7-408]
my rights as a hospital patient as described in the *Patient Bill of Rights?*	American Hospital Association [7-4] American Medical Association [7-9]
the name and location of a self-help group for a specific disorder?	National Self-Help Clearinghouse [7-411]
the adverse health effects of a certain pesticide?	National Coalition Against the Misuse of Pesticides [7-409] Rachel Carson Council [7-410]

Drugs

the adverse effects of a certain drug?	Drug Information Association [7-412]
written instructions on how to take medications (Patient Medication Instruction Sheets)?	U.S.P.C. (United States Pharmacopeial Convention) [7-413]
about the availability of an orphan drug?	National Information Center for Orphan Drugs and Rare Diseases [7-314] National Organization for Rare Disorders [7-315]

Dying

an example of a living will?	Choice in Dying [7-416]
the requirements for providing for durable powers of attorney?	Choice in Dying [7-416]
a self-help group for the grieving?	Compassionate Friends [7-415] Grief Education Institute [7-417]
information on the right to die?	Choice in Dying [7-416] Hemlock Society [7-418]
the latest statistics on teenage suicide?	American Association of Suicidology [7-414]

Emergencies

information about disaster medical care?	American College of Emergency Physicians [7-125]

WHERE SHOULD I GO TO FIND. . .	*TRY*

Emergencies

information about disaster medical care?	American Red Cross [7-364] Wilderness Medical Society [7-126]
how to obtain a medical identification card or a medical identification bracelet?	Medic Alert Foundation [7-419]

Exercise and Fitness

exercise programs for older persons?	Aerobics and Fitness Association of America [7-420] Aquatic Exercise Association [7-421] American Heart Association [7-209]
tests for determining the fitness of young children?	National Fitness Foundation [7-422] President's Council on Physical Fitness and Sports [7-423]

Health Insurance

advice when I believe an insurance claim has been unfairly rejected?	Health Insurance Association of America [7-424] National Association of Insurance Commissioners [7-425] National Insurance Consumer Organization [7-427]
how to report a fraudulent claim filed for payment from my health insurance?	National Healthcare Anti-Fraud Association [7-426]

Medical Records

the procedure for obtaining my medical record?	American Medical Association [7-9] See previous listing for specific state Medical Society/Association
information about locating my medical record in the event of my physician's death or retirement?	American Medical Association [7-9]

Nutrition

information about special diets for specific disorders?	American Dietetic Association [7-428]

WHERE SHOULD I GO TO FIND. . .   TRY

Nutrition

information about improving my daily
nutrition?

Center for Science in the Public Interest
[7-405]
Community Nutrition Institute [7-429]
Public Voice for Food and Health Policy
[7-430]

Rehabilitation

information about rehabilitation programs
for the handicapped?

American Coalition of Citizens with
Disabilities [7-431]
American Congress of Rehabilitation
Medicine [7-151]
American Physical Therapy Association
[7-28]
Federation of the Handicapped [7-432]
National Rehabilitation Association [7-433]
Rehabilitation International [7-434]

about sports activities for the handicapped?

American Alliance for Health, Physical
Education, Recreation and Dance [7-176]
Center for Dance Medicine [7-435]
National Wheelchair Athletic Association
[7-436]
National Wheelchair Basketball Association
[7-437]
North American Riding for the
Handicapped Association [7-438]

special travel assistance for the
handicapped?

Flying Wheels Travel [7-439]
Mobility International [7-440]
Society for the Advancement of Travel for
the Handicapped [7-441]

Reproduction

the latest research on birth control and
contraception?

American College of Obstetricians and
Gynecologists [7-18]
Planned Parenthood [7-19]

educational materials related to childbirth?

American Society for Psychoprophylaxis in
Obstetrics (ASPO-Lamaze) [7-442]
International Childbirth Education
Association (ICEA) [7-444]

WHERE SHOULD I GO TO FIND...	*TRY*

Reproduction

a self-help group for parents of multiple births?	National Organization of Mothers of Twins Clubs [7-445] Twinline [7-447]
statistics on multiple births?	Center for Study of Multiple Birth [7-443]
the location of a sperm bank in my area?	American Fertility Society [7-254] Fertility Research Foundation [7-255]
the legal aspects of surrogate parenthood?	Surrogate Parent Foundation [7-446]
the risks of working near video-display terminals during pregnancy?	American College of Obstetricians and Gynecologists [7-18]

Sick Building

information about Sick Building syndrome?	National Safe Workplace Institute [7-448]

Transplantation

the procedures for planning and documenting intentions to make organ donations?	American Council on Transplantation [7-452] Lion's Club International (Eye Donor Registry) [7-206] Living Bank [7-449] Medic Alert Organ Donor Program Foundation [7-450] National Kidney Foundation [7-277] National Society to Prevent Blindness [7-208]
about the experimental status of bone marrow transplantation?	American Medical Association [7-9]
the latest research about tissue or organ transplantation?	American Association of Tissue Banks [7-451] American Council on Transplantation [7-452] American Diabetes Association [7-239] American Society of Transplant Surgeons [7-453] Children's Transplant Association [7-454] National Kidney Foundation [7-277]

WHERE SHOULD I GO TO FIND. . .	*TRY*

Travel and Health

the procedure for obtaining a medical passport?	Medical Passport Foundation [7-456]
information on the health aspects of travel?	Healthcare Abroad [7-455] International Association for Medical Assistance to Travelers [7-86] Travel Health Information Service [7-87]

7

Health Organizations Listed According to the Type of Medical Question

This chapter contains additional information about the health organizations cited in Chapter 6. Entries contain the names, addresses, and telephone numbers for the national office of each organization. Readers can learn about the nearest local chapter or branch office by checking with the national office.

Information provided by these organizations will vary with the nature of the organization. Those that supply information about health centers or health professionals will answer questions related to licensure and certification, and they may provide referrals, while those organizations related to specific health problems or procedures may provide direct answers to questions, referral to an expert in the area, referral to a self-help group, or printed educational materials.

Entries in this chapter are listed alphabetically under the following broad categories: Organizations According to Information about Health Centers, Organizations According to Information about Health Professionals, Organizations According to Information about Specific Health Problems, Organizations According to Information about Specific Health Procedures, and Organizations According to Other Health Information.

The item entry numbers for organizations correspond to those used in Chapter 6. Some of these organizations have been placed in several categories; however, the identification number appears only with the first entry. When searching for a number, ignore the gaps and pursue the numerical sequence until your number is found.

For an alphabetical listing of non-governmental organizations, see Appendix III.

ORGANIZATIONS ACCORDING TO INFORMATION ABOUT HEALTH CENTERS

Clinics

[7-1] American Association for the Accreditation of Ambulatory
Plastic Surgery Facilities
1202 Allanson Road
Mundelein, IL 60060
(708)949-6058

[7-2] Joint Commission on Accreditation of Health Care
Organizations (JCAHO)
One Renaissance Boulevard
Oakbrook Terrace, IL 60181
(708)916-5600

[7-3] Society for Vascular Surgery
13 Elm Street
Manchester, MA 01944
(508)526-8330

Hospice

Joint Commission on Accreditation of Health Care Organizations (JCAHO)
One Renaissance Boulevard
Oakbrook Terrace, IL 60181
(708)916-5600

Hospitals

[7-4] American Hospital Association
840 North Lake Shore Drive
Chicago, IL 60611
(312)280-6000

[7-5] Council of Better Business Bureaus
4200 Wilson Boulevard
Arlington, VA 22203
(703)276-0100

[7-6] Council on Teaching Hospitals
One DuPont Circle NW
Washington, DC 20036
(202)828-0490

Joint Commission on Accreditation of Health Care Organizations (JCAHO)
One Renaissance Boulevard
Oakbrook Terrace, IL 60181
(708)916-5600

Medical Schools
[7-7] Association of American Medical Colleges
Suite 200
One DuPont Circle NW
Washington, DC 20036
(202)828–0400

Nursing Homes
[7-8] American Association of Homes for the Aging
Suite 400
1129 20th Street NW
Washington, DC 20036
(202)296–5960

Joint Commission on Accreditation of Health Care Organizations (JCAHO)
One Renaissance Boulevard
Oakbrook Terrace, IL 60181
(708)916–5600

ORGANIZATIONS ACCORDING TO INFORMATION ABOUT HEALTH PROFESSIONALS

Allied Health Professions
[7-9] American Medical Association
515 North State Street
Chicago, IL 60610
(312)464–4818

[7-10] American Society of Allied Health Professions
Suite 700
1101 Connecticut Avenue NW
Washington, DC 20036
(202)857–1150

[7-11] National Health Council
Suite 1118
350 Fifth Avenue
New York, NY 10018
(212)268–8900

Chiropractors
[7-12] American Chiropractic Association
1701 Clarendon Boulevard
Arlington, VA 22201
(703)276–8800

Dentists

[7-13] American Dental Association
211 East Chicago Avenue
Chicago, IL 60611
(312)440–2500

Home Health-Care Providers

Joint Commission on Accreditation of Health Care Organizations (JCAHO)
One Renaissance Boulevard
Oakbrook Terrace, IL 60181
(708)916–5600

Medical Illustrators

[7-14] Association of Medical Illustrators
2692 Huguenot Springs Road
Midlothian, VA 23113
(804)794–2908

Medical Records Administrators

[7-15] American Medical Records Association
Suite 1400
919 North Michigan Avenue
Chicago, IL 60611
(312)787–2672

Medical Writers

[7-16] American Medical Writers Association
Suite 410
5282 River Road
Bethesda, MD 20816
(301)493–0003

Midwives

[7-17] American College of Nurse-Midwives
Suite 1000
1522 K Street NW
Washington, DC 20005
(202)289–0171

[7-18] American College of Obstetricians and Gynecologists
409 12th Street SW
Washington, DC 20024
(202)638–5577

[7-19] Planned Parenthood Federation of America
810 Seventh Avenue
New York, NY 10019
(212)541–7800

Nurses

[7-20] American Association of Colleges of Nursing
Suite 530
One Dupont Circle NW
Washington, DC 20036
(202)463–6930

[7-21] American Nurses Association
2420 Pershing Road
Kansas City, MO 64108
(816)474–5720

[7-22] National League of Nursing
10 Columbus Circle
New York, NY 10019
(212)582–1022

Optometrists

[7-23] American Optometric Association
243 N. Lindbergh Boulevard
St. Louis, MO 63141
(314)991–4100

Osteopaths

[7-24] American Osteopathic Association
142 East Ontario
Chicago, IL 60611
(312)280–5800

Overseas Health Professionals

[7-25] National Council for International Health
Suite 600
1701 K Street NW
Washington, DC 20006
(202)833–5900

[7-26] Care Medico
660 First Avenue
New York, NY 10016
(212)686–3110

Pharmacists

[7-27] American Pharmaceutical Association
2215 Constitution Avenue NW
Washington, DC 20037
(202)628–4410

Physical Therapists

[7-28] American Physical Therapy Association
111 North Fairfax Street
Alexandria, VA 22314
(703)684–2784

Podiatrists
[7-29] American Podiatric Medical Association
9312 Old Georgetown Road
Bethesda, MD 20814
(301)571–9200

Psychologists
[7-30] American Psychological Association
1200 17th Street NW
Washington, DC 20036
(202)955–7600

Physicians—Complaints, Licensure, and Referrals
American Medical Association
515 North State Street
Chicago, IL 60610
(312)464–4818

[7-31] Medical Association of the State of Alabama
19 South Jackson Street
PO Box 1900
Montgomery, AL 36102
(205)263–6441

[7-32] Alaska State Medical Association
4107 Laurel Street
Anchorage, AK 99508
(907)562–2662

[7-33] Arizona Medical Association
810 West Bethany Home Road
Phoenix, AZ 85013
(602)246–8901

[7-34] Arkansas Medical Society
Suite 300
10 Corporate Hill
PO Box 5776
Little Rock, AR 72215
(501)224–8967

[7-35] California Medical Association
221 Main Street
PO Box 7690
San Francisco, CA 94120
(415)541–0900

[7-36] Colorado Medical Society
PO Box 17550
Denver, CO 80217
(303)779–5455

[7-37] Connecticut State Medical Society
160 St. Ronan Street
New Haven, CT 06511
(203)865–0587

[7-38] Medical Society of Delaware
1925 Lovering Avenue
Wilmington, DE 19806
(302)658–7596

[7-39] Medical Society of the District of Columbia
Suite 400
1707 L Street NW
Washington, DC 20036
(202)466–1800

[7-40] Florida Medical Association
760 Riverside Avenue
PO Box 2411
Jacksonville, FL 32203
(904)356–1571

[7-41] Medical Association of Georgia
938 Peachtree Street NE
Atlanta, GA 30309
(404)876–7535

[7-42] Hawaii Medical Association
1360 South Beretania Street
Honolulu, HI 96814
(808)536–7702

[7-43] Idaho Medical Association
PO Box 2668
Boise, ID 83701
(208)344–7888

[7-44] Illinois State Medical Society
Suite 700
20 North Michigan Avenue
Chicago, IL 60602
(312)782–1654

[7-45] Indiana State Medical Association
3935 North Meridian Street
Indianapolis, IN 46208
(317)925–7545

[7-46] Iowa Medical Society
1001 Grand Avenue
West Des Moines, IA 50265
(515)223–1401

[7-47] Kansas Medical Society
1300 Topeka Avenue
Topeka, KS 66612
(913)235–2383

[7-48] Kentucky Medical Association
3532 Ephraim McDowell Drive
Louisville, KY 40205
(502)459–9790

[7-49] Louisiana State Medical Society
1700 Josephine Street
New Orleans, LA 70113
(504)561–1033

[7-50] Maine Medical Association
PO Box 190
Manchester, ME 04351
(207)622–3374

[7-51] Medical & Chirurgical Faculty of the State of Maryland
1211 Cathedral Street
Baltimore, MD 21201
(301)539–0872

[7-52] Massachusetts Medical Society
1440 Main Street
Waltham, MA 02154
(617)893–4610

[7-53] Michigan Medical Society
120 West Saginaw
East Lansing, MI 48823
(517)337–1351

[7-54] Minnesota Medical Association
Suite 400
2221 University Avenue SE
Minneapolis, MN 55414
(612)378–1875

[7-55] Mississippi State Medical Association
735 Riverside Drive
Jackson, MS 39202
(601)354–5433

[7-56] Missouri State Medical Association
113 Madison Street
PO Box 1028
Jefferson City, MO 65102
(314)636–5151

[7-57] Montana Medical Association
2021 11th Avenue
Helena, MT 59601
(406)443–4000

[7-58] Nebraska Medical Association
1512 FirsTier Bank Building
Lincoln, NE 68508
(402) 474–4472

[7-59] Nevada State Medical Association
Suite 101
3660 Baker Lane
Reno, NV 89509
(702)825–6788

[7-60] New Hampshire Medical Society
4 Park Street
Concord, NH 03301
(603)224–1909

[7-61] Medical Society of New Jersey
2 Princess Road
Lawrenceville, NJ 08648
(609)896–1766

[7-62] New Mexico Medical Society
Suite 400
7770 Jefferson Street NE
Albuquerque, NM 87109
(505)828–0237

[7-63] Medical Society of the State of New York
420 Lakeville Road
Lake Success, NY 11042
(516)488–6100

[7-64] North Carolina Medical Society
222 North Person Street
PO Box 27167
Raleigh, NC 27611
(919)833–3836

[7-65] North Dakota Medical Association
PO Box 1198
Bismarck, ND 58502
(701)223–9475

[7-66] Ohio State Medical Association
1500 Lake Shore Drive
Columbus, OH 43204
(614)486–2401

[7-67] Oklahoma State Medical Association
601 NW Expressway
Oklahoma City, OK 73118
(405)843–9571

[7-68] Oregon Medical Association
5210 SW Corbett Street
Portland, OR 97201
(503)226–1555

[7-69] Pennsylvania Medical Society
777 East Park Drive
PO Box 8820
Harrisburg, PA 17105
(717)558–7750

[7-70] Rhode Island Medical Society
106 Francis Street
Providence, RI 02903
(401)331–3207

[7-71] South Carolina Medical Association
PO Box 11188
Columbia, SC 29211
(803)798–6207

[7-72] South Dakota State Medical Association
1323 South Minnesota Avenue
Sioux Falls, SD 57105
(605)336–1965

[7-73] Tennessee Medical Association
112 Louise Avenue
Nashville, TN 37203
(615)327–1451

[7-74] Texas Medical Association
1801 North Lamar Boulevard
Austin, TX 78701
(512)477–6704

[7-75] Utah Medical Association
540 East 500 Street South
Salt Lake City, UT 84102
(801)355–7477

[7-76] Vermont State Medical Society
136 Main Street, Box H
Montpelier, VT 05601
(802)223–7898

[7-77] Medical Society of Virginia
4205 Dover Road
Richmond, VA 23221
(804)353–2721

[7-78] Washington State Medical Association
Suite 900
2033 Sixth Avenue
Seattle, WA 98121
(206)441–9762

[7-79] West Virginia State Medical Association
PO Box 4106
Charleston, WV 25364
(304)925–0342

[7-80] State Medical Society of Wisconsin
PO Box 1109
Madison, WI 53701
(608)257–6781

[7-81] Wyoming Medical Society
PO Drawer 4009
Cheyenne, WY 82003
(307)635–2424

[7-82] Guam Medical Society
PO Box 8718
Tamuning, GU 96911
(671)646–5824

[7-83] Puerto Rico Medical Association
Box 9387
Santurce, PR 00908
(809)721–6969

[7-84] Virgin Islands Medical Society
PO Box 5986
St. Croix, VI 00823
(809)778–5305

Physicians—Foreign Countries
Canada
[7-85] Canadian Medical Association
1867 Alta Vista Drive
PO Box 8650
Ottawa, Ontario K16 OG8
(613)731–9331

English-Speaking
[7-86] International Association for Medical Assistance to Travelers
417 Center Street
Lewiston, NY 14092
(716)754–4883

[7-87] Travel Health Information
5827 West Washington Boulevard
Milwaukee, WI 53208
(414)774–4600
(800)433–5256

Great Britain
[7-88] British Medical Association
BMA House, Tavistock Square
London WC1H 9JP, England
(01)387–4499

[7-89] Royal College of Physicians
11 St. Andrew's Place
London NW1 4LE, England
(01)935–1174

[7-90] Royal College of Surgeons
35 - 43 Lincoln's Inn Fields
London WC2A 3PN, England
(01)405–3474

Mexico
[7-91] Asociación de Médicos Mexicanos
Santiago Papasquiaro
140 Sur Zona Industrial
Gomez Palacio, DGO, Mexico

Physicians—Specialty Board Certification
[7-92] American Board of Medical Specialties
Suite 805
One Rotary Center
Evanston, IL 60201
(708)491–9091

[7-93] American Board of Allergy and Immunology
University City Science Center
3624 Market Street
Philadelphia, PA 19104
(215)349–9466

[7-94] American Board of Anesthesiology
100 Constitution Plaza
Hartford, CT 06103
(203)522–9857

[7-95] American Board of Colon and Rectal Surgery
Suite 410
875 Telegraph Road
Taylor, MI 48180
(313)295–1740

[7-96] American Board of Dermatology
Henry Ford Hospital
Detroit, MI 48202
(313)871–8739

[7-97] American Board of Emergency Medicine
Suite D
200 Woodland Pass
East Lansing, MI 48823
(517)332–4800

[7-98] American Board of Family Practice
2228 Young Drive
Lexington, KY 40505
(606)269–5626

[7-99] American Board of Internal Medicine
University City Science Center
3624 Market Street
Philadelphia, PA 19104
(215)243–1500
(800)441-ABIM
(Includes the subspecialties of Cardiovascular Disease; Critical Care Medicine; Endocrinology and Metabolism; Gastroenterology; Geriatric Medicine; Hematology; Infectious Disease; Medical Oncology; Nephrology; Pulmonary Disease; Rheumatology)

[7-100] American Board of Neurological Surgery
Smith Tower, Suite 2139
6550 Fannin Street
Houston, TX 77030
(713)790–6015

[7-101] American Board of Nuclear Medicine
Room 12–200
900 Veteran Avenue
Los Angeles, CA 90024
(213)825–6787

[7-102] American Board of Obstetrics and Gynecology
Suite 305
4225 Roosevelt Way NE
Seattle, WA 98105
(206)547–4884

[7-103] American Board of Ophthalmology
Suite 241
111 Presidential Boulevard
Bala Cynwyd, PA 19004
(215)664–1175

[7-104] American Board of Orthopedic Surgery
Suite 1150
737 North Michigan Avenue
Chicago, IL 60611
(312)664–9444

[7-105] American Board of Otolaryngology
Suite 936
5615 Kirby Drive
Houston, TX 77005
(713)528–6200

[7-106] American Board of Pathology
PO Box 25915
5401 West Kennedy Boulevard
Tampa, FL 33622
(813)286–2444

[7-107] American Board of Pediatrics
111 Silver Cedar Court
Chapel Hill, NC 27514
(919)929–0461
(Includes Neonatal-Perinatal Medicine; Pediatric Cardiology; Pediatric Critical Care; Pediatric Endocrinology; Pediatric Hematology-Oncology; Pediatric Nephrology; Pediatric Pulmonary)

[7-108] American Board of Physical Medicine and Rehabilitation
Suite 674
Norwest Center
21 First Street SW
Rochester, MN 55902
(507)282–1776

[7-109] American Board of Plastic Surgery
Suite 400, 7 Penn Center
1635 Market Street
Philadelphia, PA 19103
(215)587–9322

[7-110] American Board of Preventive Medicine
Department of Community Medicine
Wright State University School of Medicine
PO Box 927
Dayton, OH 45401
(513)278–6915
(Includes Public Health; Aerospace Medicine; Occupational Medicine)

[7-111] American Board of Psychiatry and Neurology
Suite 335
500 Lake Cook Road
Deerfield, IL 60015
(708)945–7900
(Includes Child Psychiatry; Neurology; Psychiatry)

[7-112] American Board of Radiology
Suite 440
300 Park Street
Birmingham, MI 48009
(313)645–0600

[7-113] American Board of Surgery
Suite 860
1617 John F. Kennedy Boulevard
Philadelphia, PA 19103
(215)568–4000

[7-114] American Board of Thoracic Surgery
Suite 803
1 Rotary Center
Evanston, IL 60201
(708)475–1520

[7-115] American Board of Urology
Suite 150
31700 Telegraph Road
Birmingham, MI 48010
(313)646–9720

Physicians—Specific Practices
Allergists
[7-116] American Academy of Allergy and Immunology
611 East Wells Street
Milwaukee, WI 53202
(414)272–6071
(800)822–2762

[7-117] American Academy of Otolaryngic Allergy
Suite 745
8455 Colesville Road
Silver Spring MD 20910
(301)588–1800

[7-118] American College of Allergy and Immunology
Suite 1080
800 East Northwest Highway
Palatine, IL 60067
(708)359–2800

Cardiologists
[7-119] American College of Cardiology
9111 Old Georgetown Road
Bethesda, MD 20814
(301)897–5400

Chest Physicians
[7-120] American College of Chest Physicians
911 Busse Highway
Park Ridge, IL 60068
(708)698–2200

Dermatologists
[7-121] American Academy of Dermatology
PO Box 3116
Evanston, IL 60201
(708)869–3954

[7-122] Society for Investigative Dermatology
Room 269, Building 100
1001 Potrero Street
San Francisco, CA 94110
(415)647–3992

Disability Examiners
[7-123] American Academy of Disability Evaluating Physicians
PO Box 4313
Arlington Heights, IL 60006
(708)228–6095

[7-124] National Association of Disability Examiners
3299 K Street NW
Washington, DC 20007
(202)965–1544

Emergency Physicians
[7-125] American College of Emergency Physicians
PO Box 619911
Dallas, TX 75261
(214)550–0911

[7-126] Wilderness Medical Society
PO Box 397
Point Reyes Station, CA 94956
(415)663–9107

Endocrinologists
[7-127] Endocrine Society
9650 Rockville Pike
Bethesda, MD 20814
(301)571–1802

[7-128] American Thyroid Association
Mayo Clinic
200 First Street SW
Rochester, MN 55905
(507)284–4738

Gastroenterologists
[7-129] American College of Gastroenterology
4222 King Street
Alexandria, VA 22302
(703)549–4440

[7-130] American Gastroenterological Association
6900 Grove Road
Thorofare, NJ 08086
(609)848–9218

[7-131] American Society for Gastrointestinal Endoscopy
13 Elm Street
Manchester, MA 01944
(508)526–8330

Gynecologists
American College of Obstetricians and Gynecologists
409 12th Street SW
Washington, DC 20024
(202)638–5577

Hematologists
[7-132] American Society of Hematology
6900 Grove Road
Thorofare, NJ 08086
(609)845–0003

Holistic Medicine
[7-133] American Holistic Medical Association
2002 Eastlake Avenue East
Seattle, WA 98102
(206)322–6842

Neurologists
[7-134] American Academy of Neurology
Suite 335
2221 University Avenue SE
Minneapolis, MN 55414
(612)623–8115

Obstetricians
American College of Obstetricians and Gynecologists
409 12th Street SW
Washington, DC 20024
(202)638–5577

Occupational Medicine
[7-135] American College of Occupational Medicine
55 West Seegers
Arlington Heights, IL 60005
(708)228–6850

Ophthalmologists
[7-136] American Academy of Ophthalmology
655 Beach
San Francisco, CA 94120
(415)561–8500

Orthopedists
[7-137] American Orthopaedic Association
222 S. Prospect
Park Ridge, IL 60068
(708)698–1640

[7-138] American Orthopaedic Society for Sports Medicine
70 West Hubbard Street
Chicago, IL 60610
(312)644–2623

Otologists
[7-139] American Otological Society
Loyola University of Chicago Medical Center
Building 105, Room 1870
2160 South First Avenue
Maywood, IL 60153
(708)216–9183

[7-140] American Laryngological, Rhinological and Otological Society
PO Box 155 Bethesda Church Road
East Greenville, PA 18041
(215)679–7180

Pediatricians
[7-141] American Academy of Pediatrics
141 Northwest Point Boulevard
Elk Grove Village, IL 60007
(708)228–5005
(800)433–9016

Psychiatrists
[7-142] American Academy of Child and Adolescent Psychiatry
3615 Wisconsin Avenue NW
Washington, DC 20016
(202)996–7300

[7-143] American Academy of Clinical Psychiatrists
PO Box 3212
San Diego, CA 92103
(619)298–4782

[7-144] American Psychiatric Association
1400 K Street NW
Washington, DC 20005
(202)682–6000

Psychoanalysts
[7-145] American Academy of Psychoanalysis
Suite 206
30 East 40th Street
New York, NY 10016
(212)679–4105

[7-146] American Psychoanalytic Association
309 49th Street
New York, NY 10017
(212)752–0450

Psychosomatic Medicine
[7-147] Academy of Psychosomatic Medicine
5824 Magnolia
Chicago, IL 60660
(312)784–2025

Radiologists
[7-148] American College of Radiology
1891 Preston White Drive
Reston, VA 22091
(703)648–8900

[7-149] Radiological Society of North America
2021 Spring Street
Oakbrook, IL 60521
(708)571–2670

Rehabilitation Medicine
[7-150] American Academy of Physical Medicine and Rehabilitation
Suite 1300
122 S. Michigan Avenue
Chicago, IL 60603
(312)922–9366

[7-151] American Congress of Rehabilitation Medicine
Suite 1310
130 South Michigan Avenue
Chicago, IL 60603
(312)922–9368

Rheumatologists
[7-152] American College of Rheumatology
Suite 480
17 Executive Park Drive NE
Atlanta, GA 30329
(404)633–3777

Rhinologists
[7-153] American Rhinological Society
Suite 105
2929 Baltimore Street
Kansas City, MO 64108
(816)561–4423

American Laryngological, Rhinological, and Otological Society
PO Box 155 Bethesda Church Road
East Greenville, PA 18041
(215)679–7180

Surgeons
Abdominal Surgeons
[7-154] American Society of Abdominal Surgeons
675 Main Street
Melrose, MA 02176
(617)665–6102

Colon and Rectal Surgeons
[7-155] American Society of Colon and Rectal Surgery
800 East NW Highway
Palatine, IL 60067
(708)359–9184

Cryosurgeons
[7-156] American College of Cryosurgery
1567 Maple Avenue
Evanston, IL 60201
(708)869–3954

General Surgeons
[7-157] American College of Surgeons
55 East Erie Street
Chicago, IL 60611
(312)664–4050

[7-158] International College of Surgeons
1516 North Lake Shore Drive
Chicago, IL 60610
(312)787–6274

Hand Surgeons
[7-159] American Association for Hand Surgery
Suite 210
2934 Fish Hatchery Road
Madison, WI 53713
(608)273–8940

[7-160] American Society for Surgery of the Hand
3025 South Parker Road
Aurora, CO 80014
(303)755–4588

Maxillofacial Surgeons
[7-161] American Society of Maxillofacial Surgeons
444 East Algonquin Road
Arlington Heights, IL 60005
(708)228–9900

Neurosurgeons
[7-162] American Association of Neurological Surgeons
22 South Washington
Park Ridge, IL 60068
(708)692–9500

Orthopedic Surgeons
[7-163] American Academy of Orthopaedic Surgeons
222 South Prospect
Park Ridge, IL 60068
(708)823–7186

Otolaryngeal Surgeons
[7-164] American Academy of Otolaryngology—Head and Neck Surgery
1 Prince Street
Alexandria, VA 22314
(703)836–4444

Pediatric Surgeons
[7-165] American Pediatric Surgical Association
Children's Hospital National Medical Center
111 Michigan Avenue NW
Washington, DC 20010
(202)745–2153

Plastic Surgeons
[7-166] American Academy of Facial Plastic and Reconstructive Surgery
Suite 404
1101 Vermont Avenue NW
Washington, DC 20005
(202)842–4500
(800)332-FACE

[7-167] American Association of Plastic Surgeons
811 Harvey, Johns Hopkins Hospitals
600 North Wolfe Street
Baltimore, MD 21205
(301)955–6897

[7-168] American Society of Plastic and Reconstructive Surgeons
444 East Algonquin
Arlington Heights, IL 60005
(708)228–9900
(800)635–0635

Thoracic Surgeons
[7-169] American Association for Thoracic Surgery
13 Elm Street
Manchester, MA 01944
(508)526–8330

[7-170] Society of Thoracic Surgeons
Suite 600
111 East Wacker Drive
Chicago, IL 60601
(312)644–6610

Vascular Surgeons
Society for Vascular Surgery
13 Elm Street
Manchester, MA 01944
(508)526–8330

Urologists
[7-171] American Urological Association
1120 North Charles Street
Baltimore, MD 21201
(301)727–1100

ORGANIZATIONS ACCORDING TO SPECIFIC HEALTH PROBLEMS

Acne
American Academy of Dermatology
PO Box 3116
Evanston, IL 60201
(708)869–3954

[7-172] American Society for Dermatologic Surgery
PO Box 3116
Evanston, IL 60201
(708)869–3954
(800)441-ASDS

Acoustic Neuroma
[7-173] Acoustic Neuroma Association
PO Box 398
Carlisle, PA 17013
(717)249–4783

Agoraphobia
[7-174] Anxiety Disorders Association of America
Suite 513
6000 Executive Boulevard
Rockville, MD 20852
(301)231–9350
(900)737–3400

[7-175] PASS Group (Panic Attack Sufferers' Support Groups)
PO Box 1614
Williamsville, NY 14221
(716)689–4399

AIDS (Acquired Immune Deficiency Syndrome) Education
[7-176] American Alliance for Health, Physical Education, Recreation and Dance
1900 Association Drive
Reston, VA 22091
(703)476–3400

[7-177] National Center for Homecare Education and Research
350 Fifth Avenue
New York, NY 10011
(212)560–3300

[7-178] National Parent-Teachers Association
700 North Rush Street
Chicago, IL 60610
(312)787–0977

[7-179] SIECUS (Sex Information and Education Council of the United States)
32 Washington Place
New York, NY 10003
(212)673–3850

[7-180] American Council of Life Insurance
Department 190
1001 Pennsylvania Avenue NW
Washington, DC 20004
(202)624–2000

For more information, see additional listings in Chapter 8.

Alcoholism
[7-181] AL-ANON Family Group Headquarters
7th Floor
1372 Broadway
New York, NY 10018
(212)302–7240

[7-182] Alcohol Education for Youth
1500 Western Avenue
Albany, NY 12203
(514) 456–3800

[7-183] Alcoholics Anonymous World Services
468 Park Avenue South
New York, NY 10016
(212) 686–1100

[7-184] National Council on Alcoholism
12 West 21st Street
New York, NY 10010
(212) 206–6770
(800) NCA-CALL

Allergies
American Academy of Allergy and Immunology
611 East Wells Street
Milwaukee, WI 53202
(414) 272–6071
(800) 822–2762

American Academy of Otolaryngic Allergy
Suite 745
8455 Colesville Road
Silver Spring, MD 20910
(301) 588–1800

[7-185] Asthma and Allergy Foundation of America
Suite 305
1717 Massachusetts Avenue NW
Washington, DC 20036
(202) 265–0265

Alzheimer's Disease
[7-186] Alzheimer's Disease Education and Referral Center
Suite 304
8737 Colesville Road
Silver Spring, MD 20910
(301) 495–3311

[7-187] Alzheimer's Disease and Related Disorders Association
70 East Lake Street
Chicago, IL 60601
(800) 621–0379

American Academy of Neurology
Suite 335
2221 University Avenue SE
Minneapolis, MN 55414
(612) 623–8115

Amyotrophic Lateral Sclerosis (ALS)
[7-188] Amyotrophic Lateral Sclerosis Association
Suite 321
21021 Ventura Boulevard
Woodland Hills, CA 91364
(818)990–2151

Anorexia Nervosa/Bulimia
[7-190] Anorexia Nervosa and Related Eating Disorders
PO Box 5102
Eugene, OR 97405
(503)344–1144

[7-191] BASH (Bulimia Anorexia Self-Help)
Deaconess Hospital
6150 Oakland Avenue
St. Louis, MO 63139
(314)768–3838
(800)762–3334

[7-189] National Association of Anorexia Nervosa and Associated Disorders
Box 271
Highland Park, IL 60035
(708)831–3438

Anxiety Disorders
Anxiety Disorders Association of America
Suite 513
6000 Executive Boulevard
Rockville, MD 20852
(301)231–9350
(900)737–3400

PASS Group (Panic Attack Sufferers' Support Group)
PO Box 1614
Williamsville, NY 14221
(716)689–4399

Arthritis
[7-192] Arthritis Foundation
1314 Spring Street NW
Atlanta, GA 30309
(404)872–7100

American College of Rheumatology
Suite 480
17 Executive Park Drive NE
Atlanta, GA 30329
(404)633–3777

Asbestosis

[7-193] Asbestos Information Association of North America
Suite 509
1745 Jefferson Davis Highway
Arlington, VA 22202
(703)979–1150

[7-194] Asbestos Victims of America
2715 Porter Street
Soquel, CA 95073
(408)476–3646

Asthma

American Academy of Allergy and Immunology
611 East Wells Street
Milwaukee, WI 53202
(414)272–6071
(800)822–2762

American College of Allergy and Immunology
Suite 1080
800 East Northwest Highway
Palatine, IL 60067
(708)359–2800

Asthma and Allergy Foundation of America
Suite 305
1717 Massachusetts Avenue NW
Washington, DC 20036
(202)265–0265

[7-195] National Asthma Center
National Jewish Center for Immunology and Respiratory Medicine
1400 Jackson Street
Denver, CO 80206
(800)222-LUNG

Autism

[7-196] National Society for Children and Adults with Autism
Suite 1017
1234 Massachusetts Avenue NW
Washington, DC 20005
(202)783–0125

Back Problems

[7-197] American Back Society
Suite 401
2647 East 14th Street
Oakland, CA 94601
(415)536–9929

Bell's Palsy
American Academy of Otolaryngology—Head & Neck Surgery
1 Prince Street
Alexandria, VA 22314
(703)836–4444

Birth Defects
[7-198] Association of Birth Defect Children
Suite 270
5400 Diplomat Circle
Orlando, FL 32810
(407)629–1466

[7-199] March of Dimes Birth Defects Foundation
1275 Mamaroneck Avenue
White Plains, NY 10605
(914)428–7100
(800)533–9255

[7-200] National Easter Seal Society
70 East Lake Street
Chicago, IL 60601
(312)726–6200

Blindness
[7-201] American Council of the Blind
Suite 1100
1010 Vermont Avenue NW
Washington, DC 20005
(202)393–3666
(800)424–8666

[7-202] American Council of Blind Parents
14400 Cedar
University Heights, OH 44121
(216)381–1822

[7-203] Eye Bank Association of America
Suite 308
1725 Eye Street NW
Washington, DC 20006
(202)775–4999

[7-204] Guide Dog Foundation for the Blind Training Center
371 East Jericho Turnpike
Smithtown, NY 11787
(516)265–2121

[7-205] Helen Keller National Center for Deaf-Blind Youths and Adults
111 Middle Neck Road
Sands Point, NY 11050
(516)944–8900

[7-206] Lion's Clubs International
300 22nd Street
Oakbrook, IL 60570
(708)986–1700

[7-207] National Alliance of Blind Students
Suite 1100
1010 Vermont Avenue NW
Washington, DC 20005
(800)424–8666

[7-208] National Society to Prevent Blindness
500 East Remington Road
Schaumberg, IL 60173
(708)843–2020

Blood Pressure
[7-209] American Heart Association
7320 Greenville Avenue
Dallas, TX 75231
(214)750–5300

[7-210] Citizens for the Treatment of High Blood Pressure
Suite 904
888 17th Street NW
Washington, DC 20006
(202)466–4553

Brain Disorders—Pediatric
[7-211] National Brain Research Association
1439 Rhode Island Avenue NW
Washington, DC 20005
(202)483–6272

Brain Tumors
[7-212] National Brain Tumor Foundation
Suite 510
323 Geary Street
San Francisco, CA 94102
(415)296–0404

Breast Cancer
[7-213] National Alliance of Breast Cancer Organizations
1180 Avenue of the Americas
New York, NY 10036
(212)719–0154

[7-214] Y-Me Breast Cancer Support Program
18220 Harwood Avenue
Homewood, IL 60430
(708)799–8228
(800)221–2141

Burns
[7-215] American Burn Association
Suite B10
1130 East McDowell Road
Phoenix, AZ 85006
(602) 239–2391

Cancer
[7-216] American Cancer Society
1599 Clifton Road NE
Atlanta, GA 30329
(404) 320–3333

[7-217] Candelighters Childhood Cancer Foundation
Suite 1001
1901 Pennsylvania Avenue NW
Washington, DC 20006
(202) 659–5136

Candidiasis
[7-218] The Candida Research and Information Foundation
Box 2719
Castro Valley, CA 94546
(415) 582–2179

Celiac Sprue
[7-219] Celiac Sprue Society
PO Box 31700
Omaha, NE 68131
(402) 558–0600

Cerebral Palsy
[7-220] American Academy for Cerebral Palsy and Developmental Medicine
PO Box 11086
1910 Byrd Avenue
Richmond, VA 23230
(804) 282–0036

[7-221] United Cerebral Palsy Association
7 Penn Plaza
New York, NY 10001
(212) 268–6655
(800) USA-5UCP

Chronic Fatigue Syndrome
[7-222] Chronic Fatigue Immune Dysfunction Syndrome Association
PO Box 220398
Charlotte, NC 28222
(704) 362–2343

[7-223] Chronic Fatigue Immune Dysfunction Syndrome Society
PO Box 230108
Portland, OR 97223
(503)684–5261

Cleft Palate
[7-224] American Cleft Palate-Craniofacial Association
1218 Grandview Avenue
Pittsburgh, PA 15211
(412)481–1376

[7-225] American Cleft Palate Foundation
1218 Grandview Avenue
Pittsburgh, PA 15211
(800)242–5338

Colitis
American College of Gastroenterology
4222 King Street
Alexandria, VA 22302
(703)549–4440

[7-226] National Foundation for Ileitis and Colitis
444 Park Avenue South
New York, NY 10016
(212)685–3440

Cooley's Anemia
[7-227] AHEPA Cooley's Anemia Foundation
1707 L Street NW
Washington, DC 20036
(202)628–4974
(800)759–1515

Cornelia De Lange Syndrome
[7-228] Cornelia De Lange Syndrome Foundation
60 Dyer Avenue
Collinsville, CT 06022
(800)223–8355

Cri du Chat Syndrome
[7-229] Cri du Chat Syndrome Society
11609 Oakmont
Overland Park, KS 66210
(913)469–8900

Crohn's Disease
American College of Gastroenterology
4222 King Street
Alexandria, VA 22302
(703)549–4440

National Foundation for Ileitis and Colitis
444 Park Avenue South
New York, NY 10016
(212)685–3440

Cystic Fibrosis
[7-230] American Lung Association
1740 Broadway
New York, NY 10019
(212)315–8700

[7-231] Cystic Fibrosis Foundation
6931 Arlington Road
Bethesda, MD 20814
(301)951–4422

Deafness and Hearing Disorders
[7-232] American Deafness and Rehabilitation Association
PO Box 251554
Little Rock, AR 72225
(501)375–6643

American Otological Society
Loyola University of Chicago Medical Center
Building 105, Room 1870
2160 South First Avenue
Maywood, IL 60153
(708)216–9183

[7-233] Deafness Research Foundation
9 East 38th Street
New York, NY 10016
(212)684–6559 (TDD/TT)
(800)535–3323

[7-234] International Hearing Dog Association
5901 East 89th Avenue
Henderson, CO 80640
(303)287–3277

[7-235] National Captioning Institute
5203 Leesburg Pike
Falls Church, VA 22014
(703)998–2400

[7-236] National Hearing Aid Society
20361 Middlebelt
Livonio, MI 48152
(800)521–5247

[7-237] SHHH (Self Help for Hard of Hearing People)
7800 Wisconsin Avenue
Bethesda, MD 20814
(301)657–2248

Depression
American Academy of Child and Adolescent Psychiatry
3615 Wisconsin Avenue NW
Washington, DC 20016
(202)996–7300

American Academy of Clinical Psychiatrists
PO Box 3212
San Diego, CA 92102
(619)298–4782

American Academy of Psychoanalysis
Suite 206
30 East 40th Street
New York, NY 10016
(212)679–4105

American Psychiatric Association
1400 K Street NW
Washington, DC 20005
(202)682–6000

American Psychoanalytic Association
309 East 49th Street
New York, NY 10017
(212)752–0450

American Psychological Association
1200 17th Street NW
Washington, DC 20036
(202)955–7600

[7-238] National Depressive and Manic Depressive Association
Suite 2812
222 South Riverside Plaza
Chicago, IL 60606
(312)993–0066

Diabetes
[7-239] American Diabetes Association
1660 Duke Street
Alexandria, VA 22314
(703)549–1500
(800)232–3472

Endocrine Society
9650 Rockville Pike
Bethesda, MD 20814
(301)571–1802

[7-240] Juvenile Diabetes Foundation
432 Park Avenue
New York, NY 10016
(212)889–7575
(800)223–1138

Down's Syndrome
[7-241] National Down's Syndrome Society
141 Fifth Avenue
New York, NY 10010
(212)460–9330
(800)221–4602

Drug Abuse
[7-242] American Council for Drug Education
5820 Hubbard Drive
Rockville, MD 20852
(301)984–5700

[7-243] Narcotics Anonymous
PO Box 9999
Van Nuys, CA 91409
(818)780–3951

[7-244] Narcotics Educational Foundation of America
5055 Sunset Boulevard
Los Angeles, CA 90027
(213)663–5171

[7-245] National Federation of Parents for Drug-Free Youth
Suite 200
8730 Georgia Avenue
Silver Spring, MD 20910
(301)585–5437

[7-246] Potsmokers Anonymous
316 East Third Street
New York, NY 10009
(212)254–1777

Dwarfism
[7-247] Human Growth Foundation
4720 Montgomery Lane
Bethesda, MD 20814
(301)656–7540

Dyslexia
[7-248] Orton Dyslexia Society
724 York Road
Baltimore, MD 21204
(301)296–0232
(800)ABCD-123

Endometriosis
American College of Obstetricians and Gynecologists
409 12th Street SW
Washington, DC 20024
(202)638–5577

[7-249] Endometriosis Association
8585 North 76th Place
Milwaukee, WI 53223
(414)355–2200
(800)992-ENDO

Epilepsy
[7-250] American Epilepsy Society
Suite 304
179 Allyn Street
Hartford, CT 06130
(203)246–6566

[7-251] Epilepsy Foundation of America
Suite 406
4351 Garden City Drive
Landover, MD 20785
(301)459–3700

Epstein-Barr Syndrome
Chronic Fatigue Immune Dysfunction Syndrome Association
PO Box 220398
Charlotte, NC 28222
(704)362–2343

Chronic Fatigue Immune Dysfunction Syndrome Society
PO Box 230108
Portland, OR 97223
(503)684–5261

Eye Disorders
American Academy of Ophthalmology
655 Beach Street
San Francisco, CA 94109
(415)561–8500

[7-252] National Eye Research Foundation
Suite 207A
910 Skokie Boulevard
Northbrook, IL 60062
(708)564–4652

Familial Polyposis
[7-253] Familial Polyposis Registry
Department of Colorectal Surgery
Cleveland Clinic Foundation
9500 Euclid Avenue
Cleveland, OH 44195
(216)444–6470

Fertility Disorders
American College of Obstetricians and Gynecologists
409 12th Street SW
Washington, DC 20024
(202)638–5577

[7-254] American Fertility Society
Suite 200
2140 11th Avenue South
Birmingham, AL 35205
(205)933–8494

[7-255] Fertility Research Foundation
Suite 103
1430 Second Avenue
New York, NY 10021
(212)744–5500

[7-256] Resolve
PO Box 474
Belmont, MA 02178
(617)484–2424

Fibrocystic Breast Disease
[7-257] College of American Pathologists
325 Waukegan Road
Northfield, IL 60093
(708)446–8800

Fragile X Syndrome
[7-258] Fragile X Foundation
PO Box 300233
Denver, CO 80220
(800)835–2246

Friedreich's Ataxia
[7-259] Friedreich's Ataxia Group in America
PO Box 11116
Oakland, CA 94611
(415)655–0833

Gaucher Disease
[7-260] National Gaucher Foundation
1424 K Street NW
Washington, DC 20005
(202)393–2777

Hair Loss
American Academy of Dermatology
PO Box 3116
Evanston, IL 60201
(708)869–3954

[7-261] American Hair Loss Council
4500 South Broadway
Tyler, TX 75703
(214)581–8717

American Society for Dermatologic Surgery
PO Box 3116
Evanston, IL 60204
(708) 869–3954
(800)441-ASDS

[7-262] National Alopecia Areata Foundation
Suite 216
714 C Street
San Rafael, CA 94901
(415)456–4644

Head Injuries
[7-263] National Head Injury Foundation
333 Turnpike Road
Southborough, MA 01772
(508)485–9950

Headaches
[7-264] American Association for the Study of Headache
PO Box 5136
San Clemente, CA 92672
(714)498–1846

[7-265] National Headache Foundation
5252 North Western Avenue
Chicago, IL 60625
(312)878–7715
(800)843–2256

Heart Disease
American College of Cardiology
9111 Old Georgetown Road
Bethesda, MD 20814
(301)897–5400

American Heart Association
7320 Greenville Avenue
Dallas, TX 75231
(214)373–6300

Hemochromatosis
[7-266] Hemochromatosis Research Foundation
PO Box 8569
Albany, NY 12208
(518)489–0972

Hemophilia
American Society of Hematology
6900 Grove Road
Thorofare, NJ 08086
(609)845–0003

[7-267] National Hemophilia Foundation
110 Green Street
New York, NY 10012
(212)219–8180

Hepatitis
[7-268] American Association for the Study of Liver Disease
6900 Grove Road
Thorofare, NJ 08086
(609)848–1000

[7-269] American Hepatitis Association
30 East 40th Street
New York, NY 10011
(212)599–5070

[7-270] American Liver Foundation
1425 Pompton Avenue
Cedar Grove, NJ 07009
(201)256–2550
(800)223–0179

[7-271] National Foundation for Infectious Diseases
Suite 750
4733 Bethesda Avenue
Bethesda, MD 20814
(301)656–0003

Huntington's Disease
[7-272] Huntington's Disease Society of America
140 West 22nd Street
New York, NY 10011
(212)242–1968
(800)345–4372

Hypertension
American Heart Association
7320 Greenville Avenue
Dallas, TX 75231
(214)373–6300

Citizens for the Treatment of High Blood Pressure
Suite 904
888 17th Street NW
Washington, DC 20006
(202)466–4553

Hypoglycemia
[7-273] National Hypoglycemia Association
PO Box 120
Ridgewood, NJ 07451
(201)670–1189

Ileitis
American College of Gastroenterology
4222 King Street
Alexandria, VA 22302
(703)549–4440

National Foundation for Ileitis and Colitis
444 Park Avenue South
New York, NY 10016
(212)685–3440

Iron Overload Disease
[7-274] Iron Overload Diseases Association
Suite 911
224 Datura Street
West Palm Beach, FL 33401
(407)659–5616

Kidney Disease
[7-275] American Association of Kidney Patients
Suite LL1
1 Davis Boulevard
Tampa, FL 33606
(813)251–0725

[7-276] American Kidney Fund
Suite 1010
6110 Executive Boulevard
Rockville, MD 20852
(800)638–8299

[7-277] National Kidney Foundation
30 East 33rd Street
New York, NY 10016
(212)889–2210

Leprosy
[7-278] American Leprosy Foundation
Suite 210
11600 Nebel Street
Rockville, MD 20852
(301)984–1336

[7-279] American Leprosy Missions
1 Broadway
Elmwood Park, NJ 07407
(201)794–8650
(800)543–3131

Leukemia
American Cancer Society
1599 Clifton Road NE
Atlanta, GA 30329
(404)320–3333

American Society of Hematology
6900 Grove Road
Thorofare, NJ 08086
(609)845–0003

[7-280] Leukemia Society of America
733 Third Avenue
New York, NY 10017
(212)573–8484

[7-281] National Leukemia Association
Suite 536
585 Stewart Avenue
Garden City, NY 11530
(516)222–1944

Lipid Diseases
[7-282] National Lipid Diseases Foundation
1201 Corbin Street
Elizabeth, NJ 07201
(201)527–8000

Liver Diseases
American Association for the Study of Liver Disease
6900 Grove Road
Thorofare, NJ 08086
(609)848–1000

American Liver Foundation
1425 Pompton Avenue
Cedar Grove, NJ 07009
(201)256–2550
(800)223–0179

Lou Gehrig's Disease
Amyotrophic Lateral Sclerosis Association
Suite 321
21021 Ventura Boulevard
Woodland Hills, CA 91364
(818)990–2151

Lung Diseases
American College of Chest Physicians
911 Busse Highway
Park Ridge, IL 60068
(708)698–2200

American Lung Association
1740 Broadway
New York, NY 10019
(212)315–8700

Lupus
[7-283] Lupus Foundation of America
Suite 203
1717 Massachusetts Avenue NW
Washington, DC 20036
(202)328–4550
(800)558–0121

[7-284] National Lupus Erythematosus Foundation
5430 Van Nuys Boulevard
Van Nuys, CA 91401
(818)885–8787

Lyme Disease
[7-285] Lyme Borreliosis Foundation
PO Box 462
Tolland, CT 06084
(203)871–2900

Macular Diseases
American Academy of Ophthalmology
655 Beach
San Francisco, CA 94120
(415)561–8500

[7-286] Association for Macular Diseases
210 East 64th Street
New York, NY 10021
(212)605–3719

Marfan Syndrome
[7-287] National Marfan Foundation
382 Main Street
Port Washington, NY 11050
(516)883–8712

Ménière's Disease
American Otological Society
Loyola University of Chicago Medical Center
Building 105, Room 1870
2160 South First Avenue
Maywood, IL 60153
(708)216–9183

[7-288] EAR Foundation
2000 Church Street
Nashville, TN 37236
(615)329–7809
(800)545-HEAR

[7-289] International Ménière's Disease Research Institute
Suite 400
300 East Hampden Avenue
Englewood, CO 80110
(800)637–6646

Multiple Sclerosis
[7-290] National Multiple Sclerosis Society
205 East 42nd Street
New York, NY 10017
(212)986–3240
(800)624–8236

Muscular Dystrophy
[7-291] Muscular Dystrophy Association
810 Seventh Avenue
New York, NY 10019
(212)586–0808

Myasthenia Gravis
[7-292] Myasthenia Gravis Foundation
Suite 1352
53 West Jackson
Chicago, IL 60604
(800)541–5454

Narcolepsy
[7-293] American Narcolepsy Association
PO Box 1187
San Carlos, CA 94070
(415)591–7979

[7-294] Narcolepsy and Cataplexy Foundation of America
Suite 2D
1410 New York Avenue
New York, NY 10021
(212)628–6315

Neurofibromatosis
[7-295] National Neurofibromatosis Foundation
Suite 7-S
141 Fifth Avenue
New York, NY 10010
(800)323–7938

Obesity
[7-296] Gastroplasty Support Group
657 Irvington Avenue
Newark, NJ 07106
(201)374–1717

[7-297] National Association to Aid Fat Americans
PO Box 188620
Sacramento, CA 95818
(916)443–0303

Obsessive Compulsive Disorder
American Academy of Clinical Psychiatrists
PO Box 3212
San Diego, CA 92103
(619)298–4782

American Academy of Psychoanalysis
Suite 206
30 East 40th Street
New York, NY 10016
(212)679–4105

American Psychiatric Association
1400 K Street NW
Washington, DC 20005
(202)682–6000

American Psychoanalytic Association
309 49th Street
New York, NY 10017
(212)752–0450

American Psychological Association
1200 17th Street NW
Washington, DC 20036
(202)955–7600

[7-298] The OCD Foundation
PO Box 9573
New Haven, CT 06535
(203)772–0565

Osteogenesis Imperfecta
[7-299] Osteogenesis Imperfecta Foundation
PO Box 14807
Clearwater, FL 34629
(813)855–7077

Osteoporosis
[7-300] American Brittle Bone Society
1256 Merrill Drive
West Chester, PA 19382
(215)692–6248

[7-301] National Osteoporosis Foundation
Suite 822
1625 I Street NW
Washington, DC 20006
(202)223–2226

Paget's Disease
[7-302] Paget's Disease Foundation
165 Cadman Plaza East
Brooklyn, NY 11201
(718)596–1043

Pain
[7-303] American Academy of Pain Medicine
5700 Old Orchard Road
Skokie, IL 60077
(708)966–9510

[7-304] American Pain Society
PO Box 186
Skokie, IL 60076
(708)475–7300

[7-305] International Association for the Study of Pain
Suite 306
909 NE 43rd Street
Seattle, WA 98105
(206) 547–6409

[7-306] National Chronic Pain Outreach Association
8222 Wycliffe Court
Manassas, VA 22110
(703)368–7353

Parkinson's Disease
American Association of Neurological Surgeons
22 South Washington
Park Ridge, IL 60068
(708)692–9500

[7-307] American Parkinson Disease Association
116 John Street
New York, NY 10038
(800)223–2732

[7-308] National Parkinson Association
1501 NW 9th Avenue
Miami, FL 33136
(305)547–6666
(800)327–4545

[7-309] Parkinson Support Group of America
11376 Cherry Hill Road
Beltsville, MD 20705
(301)937–1545

PMS (Premenstrual Syndrome)
[7-310] Premenstrual Syndrome Action
PO Box 16292
Irvine, CA 92716
(714)854–4407

Post–Polio Symptoms
[7-311] Polio Survivors Association
12720 La Reina Avenue
Downey, CA 90242
(213)923–0034

[7-312] Post–Polio League for Information
Suite 204
5432 Connecticut Avenue NW
Washington, DC 20015
(202)653–5010

Porphyria
[7-313] American Porphyria Foundation
PO Box 11163
Montgomery, AL 36111
(205)265–2200

Pregnancy
American College of Obstetricians and Gynecologists
409 12th Street SW
Washington, DC 20024
(202)638–5577

Rare Diseases
[7-314] National Information Center for Orphan Drugs and Rare Diseases
PO Box 1133
Washington, DC 20013
(800)336–4797

[7-315] National Organization for Rare Disorders
PO Box 8923
New Fairfield, CT 06812
(203)746–6518

Respiratory Diseases
American College of Chest Physicians
911 Busse Highway
Park Ridge, IL 60068
(708)698–2200

American Lung Association
1740 Broadway
New York, NY 10019
(212)315–8700

Cystic Fibrosis Foundation
6931 Arlington Road
Bethesda, MD 20814
(301)951–4422

Retinitis Pigmentosa
[7-316] National Retinitis Pigmentosa Foundation
1401 Mt. Royal Avenue
Baltimore, MD 21217
(301)225–9400
(800)638–2300

Reye's Syndrome
[7-317] American Reye's Syndrome Association
Suite 203
701 Logan Street
Denver, CO 80209
(303)777–2592

[7-318] National Reye's Syndrome Foundation
426 North Lewis
Bryan, OH 43506
(800)233–7393

Rheumatism
American College of Rheumatology
Suite 480
17 Executive Park Drive NE
Atlanta, GA 30329
(404)633–3777

Sarcoidosis
[7-319] Sarcoidosis Family Aid and Research Foundation
760 Clinton Avenue
Newark, NJ 07108
(800)223–6429

Schizophrenia
American Academy of Clinical Psychiatrists
PO Box 3212
San Diego, CA 92103
(619)298–4782

American Psychiatric Association
1400 K Street NW
Washington, DC 20005
(202)682–6000

[7-320] National Alliance for the Mentally Ill
Suite 500
1901 North Fort Myer Drive
Arlington, VA 22209
(703)524–7600

Scleroderma
[7-321] United Scleroderma Foundation
PO Box 350
Watsonville, CA 95077
(408)728–2202
(800)722-HOPE

Scoliosis
[7-322] National Scoliosis Foundation
PO Box 547
93 Concord Avenue
Belmont, MA 02178
(617)489–0880

[7-323] The Scoliosis Association
PO Box 51353
Raleigh, NC 27609
(919)846–2639

Sexually Transmitted Diseases
[7-324] American Foundation for the Prevention of Venereal Disease
Suite 638
799 Broadway
New York, NY 10003
(212)759–2069

[7-325] American Public Health Association
1015 15th Street NW
Washington, DC 20005
(202)789–5600

[7-326] American Social Health Association
PO Box 13827
Research Triangle Park, NC 27709
(919)361–2742

Planned Parenthood Federation of America
810 Seventh Avenue
New York, NY 10019
(212)541–7800

SIECUS (Sex Information and Education Council of the U.S.)
Room 52
32 Washington Place
New York, NY 10003
(212)673–3850

Sickle Cell Disease
[7-327] Center for Sickle Cell Disease
Howard University
2121 Georgia Avenue NW
Washington, DC 20059
(202)636–7930

[7-328] National Association for Sickle Cell Disease
Suite 360
4221 Wilshire Boulevard
Los Angeles, CA 90010
(213)936–7205
(800)421–8453

Sinusitis
American Rhinological Society
Suite 105
2929 Baltimore Street
Kansas City, MO 64108
(816)561–4423

American Laryngological, Rhinological, and Otological Society
PO Box 155 Bethesda Church Road
East Greenville, PA 18041
(215)679–7180

Sjögren's Syndrome
[7-329] Sjögren's Syndrome Foundation
382 Main Street
Port Washington, NY 11050
(516)767–2866

Skin Cancer
American Academy of Dermatology
PO Box 3116
Evanston, IL 60201
(708)869–3954

American Cancer Society
1599 Clifton Road NE
Atlanta, GA 30329
(404)320–3333

[7-330] Skin Cancer Foundation
475 Park Avenue South
New York, NY 10016
(212)725–5176

Skin Disorders
American Academy of Dermatology
PO Box 3116
Evanston, IL 60201
(708)869–3954

[7-331] D.E.B.R.A. (Dystrophic Epidermolysis Bullosa Research Association) of
America
Suite 7-South
141 Fifth Avenue
New York, NY 10010
(212)995–2220

[7-332] National Foundation for Ectodermal Dysplasia
Suite 311
108 North First Street
Mascoutah, IL 62258
(618)566–2020

Society for Investigative Dermatology
Room 269, Bldg. 100
1001 Potrero Street
San Francisco, CA 94110
(415)647–3992

[7-333] Xeroderma Pigmentosum Registry
Department of Pathology
Medical Science Building, Room C 520
University of Medicine and Dentistry of New Jersey
New Jersey Medical School
185 South Orange Avenue
Newark, NJ 07103
(201)456–6255

Sleep Disorders
[7-334] American Sleep Disorders Association
604 Second Street SW
Rochester, MN 55902
(507)287-6006

Speech Disorders
[7-335] American Speech-Language-Hearing Association
10801 Rockville Pike
Rockville, MD 20852
(301)897-5700
(800)638-8255

[7-336] National Council on Stuttering
9242 Gross Point Road
Skokie, IL 60077
(708)677-8280

[7-337] Stuttering Resource Foundation
123 Oxford
New Rochelle, NY 10804
(800)232-4773

Spina Bifida
[7-338] Spina Bifida Association of America
Suite 540
1700 Rockville Pike
Rockville, MD 20852
(301)770-7222
(800)621-3141

Spinal Cord Injuries
American Academy of Neurology
Suite 335
2221 University Avenue SE
Minneapolis, MN 55414
(612)623-8115

[7-339] National Spinal Cord Injury Association
600 West Cummings Park
Woburn, MA 01801
(800)962-9629

[7-340] Spinal Cord Society
2410 Lakeview Drive
Fergus Falls, MN 56537
(218)739-5252

Sports Injuries

[7-341] American College of Sports Medicine
PO Box 1440
One Virginia Avenue
Indianapolis, IN 46206
(317)637–9200

American Orthopaedic Society for Sports Medicine
Suite 115
2250 East Devon
Des Plaines, IL 60618
(708)803–8700

[7-342] Women's Sports Foundation
Suite 728
342 Madison Avenue
New York, NY 10017
(800)227–3988

Sprue

Celiac Sprue Society
PO Box 31700
Omaha, NE 68131
(402)558–0600

Stroke

American Heart Association
7320 Greenville Avenue
Dallas, TX 75231
(214)373–6300

[7-343] National Stroke Association
300 East Hampden Avenue
Englewood, CO 80110
(303)762–9922

[7-344] The Stroke Foundation
898 Park Avenue
New York, NY 10021
(212)734–3461

Sudden Infant Death Syndrome (SIDS)

[7-345] American Sudden Infant Death Syndrome Institute
275 Carpenter Drive
Atlanta, GA 30328
(800)232-SIDS

[7-346] National Sudden Infant Death Syndrome Foundation
10500 Little Patuxent Parkway
Columbia, MD 21044
(301)964–8000
(800)221-SIDS

[7-347] Sudden Infant Death Syndrome Clearinghouse
8201 Greensboro
McLean, VA 22102
(703)821–8955

Tay-Sachs Disease
[7-348] National Tay-Sachs and Allied Diseases Association
385 Elliot Street
Newton, MA 02164
(617)964–5508

Temporomandibular Joint (TMJ) Syndrome
American Dental Association
211 East Chicago Avenue
Chicago, IL 60611
(312)440–2500

Thyroid Disorders
American Thyroid Association
Mayo Clinic
200 First Street SW
Rochester, MN 55905
(507)284–4738

Tinnitus
[7-349] American Tinnitus Association
PO Box 5
1618 SW First Street
Portland, OR 97207
(503)248–9985

Tourette's Syndrome
[7-350] Tourette's Syndrome Association
42–40 Bell Boulevard
Bayside, NY 11361
(800)237–0717

Trauma
American College of Emergency Physicians
PO Box 619911
Dallas, TX 75261
(214)550–0911

[7-351] American Trauma Society
Suite 188
1400 Mercantile Lane
Landover, MD 20785
(800)556–7890

Tuberous Sclerosis
[7-352] National Tuberous Sclerosis Association
Suite 660
4351 Garden City Drive
Landover, MD 20785
(800)225–6872

Urinary Incontinence
[7-353] HIP (Help for Incontinent People)
PO Box 544
Union, SC 29379
(803)585–8789

[7-354] Simon Foundation
PO Box 815
Wilmette, IL 60091
(800)23-SIMON

Vitiligo
[7-355] National Vitiligo Foundation
Texas American Bank Building
PO Box 6337
Tyler, TX 75711
(214)561–4700

Wegener's Granulomatosis
[7-356] Wegener's Granulomatosis Support Group
PO Box 1518
Platte City, MO 64079
(816)431–2096

ORGANIZATIONS ACCORDING TO INFORMATION
ABOUT SPECIFIC HEALTH PROCEDURES

Abdominal Surgery
American Society of Abdominal Surgeons
675 Main Street
Melrose, MA 02176
(617)665–6102

Acupuncture
[7-357] American Association for Acupuncture and Oriental Medicine
50 Maple Place
Manhasset, NY 11030
(516)627–0400

[7-358] National Commission for the Certification for Acupuncture
Suite 105
1424 16th Street NW
Washington, DC 20036
(202)232–1404

Amputation
[7-359] American Amputee Foundation
PO Box 55218, Hillcrest Station
Little Rock, AR 72225
(501)666–2523

[7-360] Amputee Services Association
6613 North Clark Street
Chicago, IL 60626
(312)274–2044

[7-361] National Odd Shoe Exchange
2242 West Keim Drive
Phoenix, AZ 85015
(602)246–8725

Artificial Insemination and In-Vitro Fertilization
American College of Obstetricians and Gynecologists
409 12th Street SW
Washington, DC 20024
(202)638–5577

American Fertility Society
Suite 210
2140 11th Avenue South
Birmingham, AL 35205
(205)933–8494

Biofeedback
[7-362] Association of Applied Physiology and Biofeedback
Suite 304
10200 West 44th Avenue
Wheat Ridge, CO 80303
(303)422–8436

Blood Transfusions
[7-363] American Association of Blood Banks
1117 North 19th Street
Arlington, VA 22209
(703)528–8200

[7-364] American Red Cross
17th and D Streets NW
Washington, DC 20006
(202)737–8300

Breast Feeding
American Academy of Pediatrics
141 Northwest Point Boulevard
Elk Grove Village, IL 60007
(708)228–5005
(800)433–9016

American College of Obstetricians and Gynecologists
409 12th Street SW
Washington, DC 20024
(202)638–5577

[7-365] La Leche League International
9616 Minneapolis Avenue
Franklin Park, IL 60131
(708)455–7730

Cataract Surgery
American Academy of Ophthalmology
655 Beach
San Francisco, CA 94120
(415)561–8500

[7-366] American Society of Cataract and Refractive Surgery
Suite 108
3700 Pender Drive
Fairfax, VA 22030
(703)591–2220

Cesarean Section
American College of Obstetricians and Gynecologists
409 12th Street SW
Washington, DC 20024
(202)638–5577

Colon Surgery
American Society of Colon and Rectal Surgery
Suite 1080
800 East Northwest Highway
Palatine, IL 60067
(708)359–9184

Contact Lenses
American Academy of Ophthalmology
655 Beach
San Francisco, CA 94120
(415)561–8500

[7-367] Contact Lens Association of Ophthalmologists
Suite 1
523 Decatur Street
New Orleans, LA 70130
(504)581–4000

CPR (Cardiopulmonary Resuscitation)
American Heart Association
7320 Greenville Avenue
Dallas, TX 75231
(214)373–6300

Cryosurgery
American College of Cryosurgery
1567 Maple Avenue
Evanston, IL 60201
(708)869–3954

Dental Care—Handicapped
[7-368] National Foundation of Dentistry for the Handicapped
Suite 1420
1600 Stout Street
Denver, CO 80202
(303)573–0264

Dialysis
American Kidney Fund
Suite 1010
6110 Executive Boulevard
Rockville, MD 20852
(800)638–8299

National Kidney Foundation
30 East 33rd Street
New York, NY 10016
(212)889–2210

Drug Testing
American College of Occupational Medicine
55 West Seegers Road
Arlington Heights, IL 60005
(708)228–6850

College of American Pathologists
325 Waukegan Road
Northfield, IL 60093
(708)446–8800

Epilepsy—Surgery
American Association of Neurological Surgeons
22 South Washington
Park Ridge, IL 60068
(708)692–9500

Epilepsy Foundation of America
Suite 406
4351 Garden City Drive
Landover, MD 20785
(301)459–3700

Gastrointestinal Endoscopy
American Society for Gastrointestinal Endoscopy
13 Elm Street
Manchester, MA 01944
(508)526–8330

Hand Surgery
American Association for Hand Surgery
Suite 210
2934 Fish Hatchery Road
Madison, WI 53713
(608)273–8940

American Society for Surgery of the Hand
3025 South Park Road
Aurora, CO 80014
(303)755–4588

Heart Surgery
American Association for Thoracic Surgery
13 Elm Street
Manchester, MA 01944
(508)526–8330

Society of Thoracic Surgeons
Suite 600
111 East Wacker Drive
Chicago, IL 60601
(312)644–6610

Hyperbaric Therapy
[7-369] Undersea and Hyperbaric Medical Society
9650 Rockville Pike
Bethesda, MD 20814
(301)571–1818

Hypnosis
[7-370] American Society of Clinical Hypnosis
Suite 336
2250 East Devon Avenue
Des Plaines, IL 60018
(708)297–3317

Immunization—Children
American Academy of Pediatrics
141 Northwest Point Boulevard
Elk Grove Village, IL 60007
(708)228–5005
(800)433–9016

Kidney Transplantation
American Association of Kidney Patients
Suite LL1
1 Davis Boulevard
Tampa, FL 33606
(813)251–0725

American Kidney Fund
Suite 1010
6110 Executive Boulevard
Rockville, MD 20852
(301)881–3052
(800)638–8299

National Kidney Foundation
30 East 33rd Street
New York, NY 10016
(212)889–2210

Larynx—Artificial
[7-371] American Laryngological Association
200 First Street SW
Rochester, MN 55905
(507)284–2369

Laser Surgery
American Academy of Ophthalmology
655 Beach Street
San Francisco, CA 94120
(415)561–8500

[7-372] American Society for Laser Medicine and Surgery
2404 Stewart Square
Wausau, WI 54401
(715)845–9283

Liposuction
[7-373] American Society of Lipo-Suction Surgery
1455 City Line Avenue
Philadelphia, PA 19151
(215)896–6677

American Society of Plastic and Reconstructive Surgeons
444 East Algonquin Road
Arlington Heights, IL 60005
(708)228–9900
(800)635–0635

Lithotripsy
National Kidney Foundation
30 East 33rd Street
New York, NY 10016
(212)889–2210

Mammography
American Cancer Society
1599 Clifton Road NE
Atlanta, GA 30329
(404)320–3333

American College of Radiology
1891 Preston White Drive
Reston, VA 22091
(703)648–8900

Neurological Surgery
American Association of Neurological Surgeons
22 South Washington
Park Ridge, IL 60068
(708)692–9500

Obesity—Surgery
American College of Gastroenterology
4222 King Street
Alexandria, VA 22302
(703)549–4440

American Gastroenterological Association
6900 Grove Road
Thorofare, NJ 08086
(609)848–9218

Gastroplasty Support Group
657 Irvington Avenue
Newark, NJ 07106
(201)374–1717

Orthopedic Therapy
American Academy of Orthopaedic Surgeons
222 South Prospect
Park Ridge, IL 60068
(708)823–7186

American Orthopaedic Association
222 South Prospect
Park Ridge, IL 60068
(708)698–1640

American Orthopaedic Society for Sports Medicine
70 West Hubbard
Chicago, IL 60610
(312)644–2623

Ostomy
[7-374] United Ostomy Association
Suite 120
36 Executive Park
Irvine, CA 92714
(714)476–0268

Pancreatic Transplants
American Diabetes Association
1660 Duke Street
Alexandria, VA 22314
(703)549–1500
(800)232–3472

Juvenile Diabetes Foundation
432 Park Avenue
New York, NY 10016
(212)889–7575
(800)223–1138

[7-375] American Pancreatic Association
Department of Surgery
University of Missouri Health Sciences Center
Columbia, MO 65212
(314)882–7942

Pediatric Surgery
American Pediatric Surgical Association
Children's Hospital National Medical Center
111 Michigan Avenue NW
Washington, DC 20010
(202)745–2153

Plastic Surgery
American Academy of Facial Plastic & Reconstructive Surgery
Suite 404
1101 Vermont Avenue NW
Washington, DC 20005
(202)842–4500
(800)332-FACE

American Association of Plastic Surgeons
811 Harvey, Johns Hopkins Hospitals
600 North Wolfe Street
Baltimore, MD 21205
(301)955–6897

American Society of Plastic and Reconstructive Surgeons
444 East Algonquin
Arlington Heights, IL 60005
(708)228–9900
(800)635–0635

Radiology—Therapeutic
[7-376] American Society for Therapeutic Radiology and Oncology
1891 Preston White Drive
Reston, VA 22091
(703)648–8903

Sinusitis—Surgery
American Academy of Otolaryngology—Head and Neck Surgery
1 Prince Street
Alexandria, VA 22314
(703)836–4444

Surgical Procedures—General
American College of Surgeons
55 East Erie Street
Chicago, IL 60611
(312)664–4050

International College of Surgeons
1516 North Lake Shore Drive
Chicago, IL 60610
(312)787–6274

Transcervical Balloon Tuboplasty
American College of Obstetricians and Gynecologists
409 12th Street SW
Washington, DC 20024
(202)638–5577

Ultrasound

[7-377] American Institute of Ultrasound in Medicine
Suite 504
4405 East-West Highway
Bethesda, MD 20814
(301)656–6117

Vascular Surgery

Society for Vascular Surgery
13 Elm Street
Manchester, MA 01944
(508)526–8330

Vasectomy

American Urological Association
1120 North Charles Street
Baltimore, MD 21201
(301)727–1100

X-Rays

American College of Radiology
1891 Preston White Drive
Reston, VA 22091
(703) 648–8900

Radiological Society of North America
2021 Spring Street
Oak Brook, IL 60521
(708)571–2670

ORGANIZATIONS ACCORDING TO OTHER HEALTH INFORMATION

Aging

[7-378] American Association for International Aging
Suite 443
1511 K Street NW
Washington, DC 20005
(202)638–6815

[7-379] American Geriatrics Society
770 Lexington
New York, NY 10021
(212)308–1414

[7-380] American Health Assistance Foundation
15825 Shady Grove Road
Rockville, MD 20850
(800)227–7998

[7-381] American Society on Aging
Suite 516
833 Market Street
San Francisco, CA 94103
(415)543–2617

[7-382] Asociación Nacional por Personas Mayores (National Association for Hispanic Elderly)
Suite 270
2727 West Sixth Street
Los Angeles, CA 90057
(213)487–1922

[7-383] CAPS (Children of Aging Parents)
2761 Trenton Road
Levittown, PA 19056
(215)945–6900

[7-384] Gerontological Society of America
Suite 350
1275 K Street NW
Washington, DC 20005
(202)842–1275

[7-385] National Center and Caucus on Black Aged (NCBA)
Suite 500
1424 K Street NW
Washington, DC 20005
(202)637–8400

[7-386] National Council of Senior Citizens
925 15th Street NW
Washington, DC 20005
(202)347–8800

[7-387] National Council on the Aging
West Wing 100
600 Maryland Avenue SW
Washington, DC 20024
(202)479–1200

[7-388] National Indian Council on Aging
PO Box 2088
Albuquerque, NM 87103
(505)766–2276

[7-389] National Pacific/Asian Resource Center on Aging
Suite 410
2033 Sixth Avenue
Seattle, WA 98121
(206)448–0313

[7-390] Older Women's League
Suite 300
730 11th Street NW
Washington, DC 20001
(202)783–6686

Alternative Therapies

[7-391] National Center for Homeopathy
Suite 42
1500 Massachusetts Avenue NW
Washington, DC 20005
(202)223–6182

[7-392] American Association of Naturopathic Physicians
PO Box 20386
Seattle, WA 98102
(206)323–7610

Captioning

National Captioning Institute
5203 Leesburg Pike
Falls Church, VA 22041
(703)998–2400

Child Abuse

[7-393] Clearinghouse on Child Abuse and Neglect
8201 Greensboro Drive
McLean, VA 22102
(703)821–2086

[7-394] National Committee for Prevention of Child Abuse
Suite 950
332 South Michigan Avenue
Chicago, IL 60604
(312)663–3520

Children's Health

American Academy of Pediatrics
141 Northwest Point Boulevard
Elk Grove Village, IL 60007
(708)228–5005
(800)433–9016

[7-395] American School Health Association
PO Box 708
Kent, OH 44240
(216)678–1601

[7-396] Association for the Care of Children's Health
3615 Wisconsin Avenue NW
Washington, DC 20016
(202)224–1801

[7-397] Children in Hospitals
31 Wilshire Park
Needham, MA 02192
(617)444–3877

[7-398] Children's Defense Fund
Suite 400
122 C Street NW
Washington, DC 20001
(202)628–8787

[7-399] Children's Hospice International
Suite 131
1101 King Street
Alexandria, VA 22314
(703)684–0330

[7-400] National Center for Education in Maternal and Child Health
38th and R Streets NW
Washington, DC 20057
(202)625–8400

[7-401] National Child Safety Council
PO Box 1368
Jackson, MI 49204
(800)222–1464

Consumer Health Issues
Bill of Rights for Patients
American Hospital Association
840 North Lake Shore Drive
Chicago, IL 60611
(312)280–6000

American Medical Association
515 North State Street
Chicago, IL 60610
(312)464–4818

Fraud
[7-402] National Council Against Health Fraud
PO Box 1276
Loma Linda, CA 92354
(714)824–4690

Health and Safety
[7-403] American Council on Science and Health
1995 Broadway
New York, NY 10023
(212)362–7044

[7-404] American Health Foundation
320 East 43rd Street
New York, NY 10017
(212)953–1900

[7-405] Center for Science in the Public Interest
1501 16th Street NW
Washington, DC 20036
(202)332–9110

[7-406] National Center for Health Education
30 East 29th Street
New York, NY 10016
(212)689–1886

[7-407] National Council on Patient Information and Education
Suite 810
666 11th Street NW
Washington, DC 20001
(202)347–6711

[7-408] Public Citizen Health Research Group
2000 P Street NW
Washington, DC 20036
(202)872–0320

Pesticides
[7-409] National Coalition Against the Misuse of Pesticides
530 7th Street SE
Washington, DC 20003
(202)543–5450

[7-410] Rachel Carson Council
8940 Jones Mill Road
Chevy Chase, MD 20815
(301)652–1877

Self-Help
[7-411] National Self-Help Clearinghouse
Room 620
25 West 43rd Street
New York, NY 10036
(212)642–2944

Drugs
[7-412] Drug Information Association
PO Box 3113
Maple Glen, PA 19002
(215)628–2288

National Information Center for Orphan Drugs and Rare Diseases
PO Box 1133
Washington, DC 20013
(800)336–4797

National Organization for Rare Disorders
PO Box 8923
New Fairfield, CT 06812
(203)746–6518

[7-413] U.S.P.C. (United States Pharmacopoeial Convention)
PO Box 5367, Twinbrook Station
Rockville, MD 20851
(800)227–8772

Dying
[7-414] American Association of Suicidology
2459 South Ash
Denver, CO 80222
(303)692–0985

[7-415] Compassionate Friends
PO Box 3696
Oakbrook, IL 60522
(708)990–0010

[7-416] Choice in Dying
250 West 57th Street
New York, NY 10107
(212)246–6973

[7-417] Grief Education Institute
2422 South Downing Street
Denver, CO 80210
(303)759–6048

[7-418] Hemlock Society
PO Box 11830
Eugene, OR 97440
(503)342–5748

Emergencies
American College of Emergency Physicians
PO Box 619911
Dallas, TX 75261
(214)550–0911

American Red Cross
17th and D Streets NW
Washington, DC 20006
(202)737–8300

[7-419] Medic Alert Foundation
2323 Colorado
Turlock, CA 95380
(209)668–3333

Wilderness Medical Society
PO Box 397
Point Reyes Station, CA 94956
(415)663–9107

Exercise and Fitness

[7-420] Aerobics and Fitness Association of America
Suite 310
15250 Ventura Boulevard
Sherman Oaks, CA 91403
(800)445–5950

American Heart Association
7320 Greenville Avenue
Dallas, TX 75231
(214)373–6300

[7-421] Aquatic Exercise Association
PO Box 497
Port Washington, WI 53074
(414)284–3416

[7-422] National Fitness Foundation
Suite 412
2250 East Imperial Highway
El Segundo, CA 90245
(213)640–0145

[7-423] President's Council on Physical Fitness and Sports
Suite 7103
450 5th Street NW
Washington, DC 20001
(202)272–3421

Health Insurance

[7-424] Health Insurance Association of America
1025 Connecticut Avenue NW
Washington, DC 20036
(202)223–7780

[7-425] National Association of Insurance Commissioners
Suite 1100
120 West 12th Street
Kansas City, MO 64105
(816)842–3600

[7-426] National Healthcare Anti–Fraud Association
Suite 800
1255 23rd Street NW
Washington, DC 20037
(202)659–5955

[7-427] National Insurance Consumer Organization
121 North Payne Street
Alexandria, VA 22314
(703)549–8050

Medical Records
American Medical Association
515 North State Street
Chicago, IL 60610
(312)464–4818

See previous listing for specific State Medical Society/Association.

Nutrition
[7-428] American Dietetic Association
Suite 800
216 West Jackson Boulevard
Chicago, IL 60606
(312)899–0040

Center for Science in the Public Interest
1501 16th Street NW
Washington, DC 20036
(202)332–9110

[7-429] Community Nutrition Institute
2001 S Street NW
Washington, DC 20009
(202)462–4700

[7-430] Public Voice for Food and Health Policy
Suite 522
1001 Connecticut Avenue NW
Washington, DC 20036
(202)659–5930

Rehabilitation
Programs
[7-431] American Coalition of Citizens with Disabilities
Suite 201
1201 15th Street NW
Washington, DC 20005
(202)785–4265

American Congress of Rehabilitation Medicine
Suite 1310
130 South Michigan Avenue
Chicago, IL 60603
(312)922–9368

American Physical Therapy Association
1111 North Fairfax Street
Alexandria, VA 22314
(703)684–2782

[7-432] Federation of the Handicapped
211 West 14th Street
New York, NY 10011
(212)206–4200

[7-433] National Rehabilitation Association
633 South Washington Street
Alexandria, VA 22314
(703)836–0850

[7-434] Rehabilitation International
25 East 21st Street
New York, NY 10010
(212)420–1500

Sports
American Alliance for Health, Physical Education, Recreation and Dance
Program for the Handicapped
1900 Association Drive
Reston, VA 22091
(703)476–3400

[7-435] Center for Dance Medicine
Room 200
41 East 42nd Street
New York, NY 10017
(212)661–8401

[7-436] National Wheelchair Athletic Association
Suite S
3617 Betty Drive
Colorado Springs, CO 80917
(303)597–8330

[7-437] National Wheelchair Basketball Association
University of Kentucky
110 Seaton Building
Lexington, KY 40506
(606)275–1623

[7-438] North American Riding for the Handicapped Association
Box 100
Ashburn, VA 22011
(703)478–1075

Travel
[7-439] Flying Wheels Travel
PO Box 382
143 West Bridge
Owatonna, MN 55060
(800)533–0363

[7-440] Mobility International
PO Box 3551
Eugene, OR 97403
(503)343–1284

[7-441] Society for the Advancement of Travel for the Handicapped
26 Court Street
Brooklyn, NY 11242
(718)858–5483

Reproduction
American College of Obstetricians and Gynecologists
409 12th Street SW
Washington, DC 20024
(202)638–5577

American Fertility Society
Suite 200
2140 11th Avenue South
Birmingham, AL 35205
(205)933–8494

[7-442] American Society for Psychoprophylaxis in Obstetrics (ASPO/Lamaze)
Suite 204
1840 Wilson Boulevard
Arlington, VA 22201
(703)524–7802

[7-443] Center for the Study of Multiple Birth
Suite 476
333 East Superior Street
Chicago, IL 60611
(312)266–9093

Fertility Research Foundation
Suite 103
1430 Second Avenue
New York, NY 10021
(212)744–5500

[7-444] International Childbirth Education Association
PO Box 20048
Minneapolis, MN 55420
(612)854–8660

[7-445] National Organization of Mothers of Twins Clubs
12404 Princess Jeanne NE
Albuquerque, NM 87112
(505)275–0955

Planned Parenthood Federation of America
810 Seventh Avenue
New York, NY 10019
(212)541–7800

[7-446] Surrogate Parent Foundation
Suite 750D
8383 Wilshire Boulevard
Beverly Hills, CA 90211
(213)824–4723

[7-447] Twinline
Suite 234
2131 University Avenue
Berkeley, CA 94704
(415)644–0861

Sick Building Syndrome
[7-448] National Safe Workplace Institute
Suite 1450
122 South Michigan Avenue
Chicago, IL 60603
(312)939–0690

Transplantation
Donations
[7-452] American Council on Transplantation
Suite 505
700 North Fairfax
Alexandria, VA 22314
(703)836–4301
(800)622–9010

Lion's Club International
Eye Donor Registration
300 22nd Street
Oakbrook, IL 60570
(708)986–1700

[7-449] Living Bank
PO Box 6725
Houston, TX 77265
(800)528–2971
(800)527–2971

[7-450] Medic Alert Organ Donor Program Foundation
PO Box 1009
Turlock, CA 95381
(209)668–3333

National Kidney Foundation
30 East 33rd Street
New York, NY 10016
(212)889–2210

National Society to Prevent Blindness
500 East Remington Road
Schaumberg, IL 60173
(708)843–2020

Experimental Status
American Medical Association
515 North State Street
Chicago, IL 60610
(312)464–4818

Tissue/Organ Transplantation
[7-451] American Association of Tissue Banks
Suite 220-A
1350 Beverly Road
McLean, VA 22101
(703)827–9582

American Council on Transplantation
Suite 505
700 North Fairfax
Alexandria, VA 22314
(703)836–4301
(800)622–9010

American Diabetes Association
1660 Duke Street
Alexandria, VA 22314
(703)549–1500
(800)232–3472

[7-453] American Society of Transplant Surgeons
716 Lee Street
Des Plaines, IL 60016
(708)824–5700

[7-454] Children's Transplant Association
PO Box 53699
Dallas, TX 75253
(214)287–8484

National Kidney Foundation
30 East 33rd Street
New York, NY 10016
(212)889–2210

Travel
[7-455] Healthcare Abroad
243 Church Street West
Vienna, VA 22180
(703)281–9500
(800)237–6615

International Association for Medical Assistance to Travelers
417 Center Street
Lewiston, NY 14092
(716) 754–4883

[7-456] Medical Passport Foundation
PO Box 820
De Land, FL 32720
(904) 734–0639

Travel Health Information
5827 West Washington Boulevard
Milwaukee, WI 53208
(414) 774–4600
(800) 433–5256

8

Where Should I Go to Find Information in the U.S. Department of Health and Human Services?

The Department of Health and Human Services is the federal department that is charged with responsibility for directing research activity and for gathering and disseminating information related to health. The passage of the 1966 Freedom of Information Act, along with the growing consumer movement in the United States, has led to an increase in requests from the public for information from the various agencies and offices within the department. To meet this demand for health information, many agencies have established information centers and clearinghouses to respond to these requests, as well as to respond to requests from health professionals. Information provided by these centers and clearinghouses varies by agency, with some providing a wide range of information and others providing only information related to the current research interests of the agency. The Department of Agriculture has also established an information center to respond to requests from the public for nutritional information.

This chapter provides examples of many commonly asked questions which can be answered by federal agencies. (For a more complete listing of services provided by these agencies, see Chapter 9.) Entries are listed alphabetically under the broad headings Information about Health Problems; Information about Health Procedures; and Other Health Related Information. Item entry numbers correspond to those used in Chapter 9.

WHERE SHOULD I GO TO FIND. . .   *TRY*

Information About Health Problems

a listing of organizations providing the most recent treatment and educational information about acquired immune deficiency syndrome (AIDS)? — National Aids Information Clearinghouse [9-8]

information about alcoholism prevention and treatment programs? — National Clearinghouse for Alcohol and Drug Information [9-12]

the latest research findings for the treatment of allergies? — National Institute of Allergy and Infectious Diseases [9-19]

information on the treatment for Alzheimer's disease? — National Institute of Neurological Disorders and Stroke [9-24] / National Institute of Mental health [9-23]

diagnosis and treatment information for asthma? — National Institute of Allergy and Infectious Diseases [9-19]

information about diet, exercise, and medications for the treatment of arthritis? — National Arthritis and Musculoskeletal and Skin Disease Information Clearinghouse [9-9]

the latest drug treatment methods for brain injuries and brain diseases? — National Institute of Neurological Disorders and Stroke [9-24]

the location of local community clinical cancer programs? — National Cancer Institute [9-10]

the latest diagnostic information for chronic fatigue syndrome? — National Institute of Allergy and Infectious Diseases [9-19]

information about the treatment for cirrhosis? — National Digestive Diseases Information Clearinghouse [9-14]

information about deafness prevention programs? — National Institute on Deafness and Other Communication Disorders Clearinghouse [9-21]

the latest research on dental problems and prevention of tooth decay? — National Institute of Dental Research [9-22]

WHERE SHOULD I GO TO FIND. . .	*TRY*
the latest research findings for the treatment of depression?	National Institute of Mental Health [9-23]
information on the complications of diabetes?	National Diabetes Information Clcaringhouse [9-13]
diagnostic and treatment information for chronic digestive disease?	National Digestive Diseases Information Clearinghouse [9-14]
educational materials for drug problems in the work place?	National Clearinghouse for Alcohol and Drug Information [9-12]
rehabilitation programs for drug abuse?	National Clearinghouse for Alcohol and Drug Information [9-12]
educational materials about the prevention of eating disorders?	Food and Nutrition Information Center [9-5]
information about drug therapy and surgical treatment for epilepsy?	National Institute of Neurological Disorders and Stroke [9-24]
the latest diagnostic methods and treatment for eye diseases?	National Eye Institute [9-15]
referral to rehabilitation agencies for the handicapped?	Clearinghouse on the Handicapped [9-2]
information on the latest treatment for head injuries?	National Institute of Neurological Disorders and Stroke [9-24]
educational materials on hearing disorders?	National Institute on Deafness and Other Communication Disorders Clearinghouse [9-21]
materials on the prevention of heart disease?	National Heart, Lung, and Blood Institute Information Center [9-17]
information on the prevention of hepatitis?	National Institute of Allergy and Infectious Diseases [9-19]
the latest information on drug treatment for herpes?	National Institute of Allergy and Infectious Diseases [9-19]
educational materials about diagnosis, treatment, and prevention of hypertension?	Center for Health Promotion and Education [9-1]

(*answer continues*)

WHERE SHOULD I GO TO FIND. . .   *TRY*

educational materials about diagnosis, treatment, and prevention of hypertension?	High Blood Pressure Information Center [9-7] National Heart, Lung, and Blood Institute Information Center [9-17]
information on the financial issues associated with kidney failure?	National Kidney and Urologic Diseases Information Clearinghouse [9-25]
information about the prevention of kidney stones?	National Kidney and Urologic Diseases Information Clearinghouse [9-25]
treatment and survival statistics for leukemia?	National Cancer Institute [9-10]
educational materials for the prevention of lung diseases?	National Heart, Lung, and Blood Institute Information Center [9-17] Center for Health Promotion and Education [9-1]
information on the diagnosis and treatment of lyme disease?	National Arthritis and Musculoskeletal and Skin Diseases Information Clearinghouse [9-9]
referral to a mental health facility for mental illness?	National Institute of Mental Health [9-23]
information on current treatment for muscular sclerosis?	National Institute of Neurological Disorders and Stroke [9-24]
educational materials for musculoskeletal disorders?	National Arthritis and Musculoskeletal and Skin Diseases Information Clearinghouse [9-9]
information on the diagnosis and treatment of muscular dystrophy?	National Institute of Neurological Disorders and Stroke [9-24]
information about the health risks of obesity?	Center for Health Promotion and Education [9-1] Food and Nutrition Information Center [9-5]
educational materials for the prevention of osteoporosis?	National Arthritis and Musculoskeletal and Skin Diseases Information Clearinghouse [9-9]

WHERE SHOULD I GO TO FIND. . .	*TRY*
information about the diagnosis and treatment of Parkinson's disease?	National Institute of Neurological Disorders and Stroke [9-24]
information about the treatment for enlargement of the prostate?	National Kidney and Urologic Diseases Information Clcaringhouse [9-25]
educational materials for the prevention of respiratory diseases?	National Heart, Lung, and Blood Institute Information Center [9-17]
referral to treatment programs for schizophrenia?	National Institute of Mental Health [9-23]
the latest research findings for the treatment of sickle cell disease?	National Sickle Cell Disease Program [9-27]
information about the psychosocial factors associated with skin diseases?	National Arthritis and Musculoskeletal and Skin Diseases Information Clearinghouse [9-9]
information about therapy for speech disorders?	National Institute on Deafness and Other Communication Disorders Clearinghouse [9-21]
the latest research findings in the treatment of spinal cord injuries?	National Institute of Neurological Disorders and Stroke [9-24]
educational materials on the treatment of sports injuries?	National Arthritis and Musculoskeletal and Skin Diseases Information Clearinghouse [9-9]
educational materials for stress reduction?	Center for Health Promotion and Education [9-1]
educational materials for the prevention of stroke?	National Institute of Neurological Disorders and Stroke [9-24]
educational materials concerning the prevention of ulcers?	National Digestive Diseases Information Clearinghouse [9-14]
information on the treatment for urinary incontinence?	National Kidney and Urologic Diseases Information Clearinghouse [9-25]
information on the latest treatment for venereal diseases?	National Institute of Allergy and Infectious Diseases [9-19]

WHERE SHOULD I GO TO FIND. . .   *TRY*

Information About Health Procedures

information about the safety of blood transfusions?

National Heart, Lung and Blood Institute Information Center [9-17]

information about bone marrow transplants for cancer therapy?

National Cancer Institute [9-10]

information about the use of endoscopy for the diagnosis of gastrointestinal diseases?

National Digestive Diseases Information Clearinghouse [9-14]

educational materials on laser surgery for retinal disorders?

National Eye Institute [9-15]

information about lithotripsy for gall stones?

National Digestive Diseases Information Clearinghouse [9-14]

information on lithotripsy for kidney stones?

National Kidney and Urologic Diseases Information Clearinghouse [9-25]

at what age and how often to have a mammography?

National Cancer Institute [9-10]

survival statistics for organ transplants?

National Institute of Allergy and Infectious Diseases [9-19]

information on the safety of radiologic tests?

Food and Drug Administration [9-4]

assistance in locating a surgeon for a second surgical opinion?

National Second Surgical Opinion Program [9-26]

information on pancreatic transplants?

National Diabetes Information Clearinghouse [9-13]

Other Health-Related Information

educational materials on health and aging?

National Institute on Aging [9-18]

information about the reliability of blood pressure devices?

High Blood Pressure Information Center [9-7]

WHERE SHOULD I GO TO FIND...	*TRY*
research on children's health and human development?	National Institute of Child Health and Human Development [9-20]
educational materials about cholesterol control?	National Cholesterol Education Program [9-11] National Heart, Lung, and Blood Institute Information Center [9-17]
information about fad diets?	Food and Nutrition Information Center [9-5]
the approval status of an experimental drug?	Food and Drug Administration [9-4]
information on the federal benefits for the handicapped?	Clearinghouse on the Handicapped [9-2]
toll-free numbers for organizations providing information about many health problems?	National Health Information Center [9-16]
the location of a HMO in my area that accepts MEDICARE recipients?	Health Care Financing Administration [9-6]
educational materials on health promotion?	National Health Information Center [9-16]
information about the safety of irradiated food?	Food and Nutrition Information Center [9-5]
the safety record for a medical device?	Food and Drug Administration [9-4]
the health hazards of certain occupations?	Clearinghouse for Occupational Safety and Health Information [9-3]
educational materials for quitting smoking?	Office of Smoking and Health [9-28] Center for Health Promotion and Education [9-1] National Heart, Lung, and Blood Institute Information Center [9-17]

9

Profiles of Clearinghouses and Information Centers of the U.S. Department of Health and Human Services

The clearinghouses and information centers listed in this chapter were established by the U.S. Department of Health and Human Services to promote the dissemination of information generated by its various agencies and institutes. The Food and Nutrition Information Center of the U.S. Department of Agriculture is also included.

These centers provide to both the general public and to health professionals information related to the agency's mission. In addition, the centers cooperate with other agencies and organizations in their efforts to collect and disseminate information that will increase knowledge about disease and promote disease prevention. Many agencies produce publications, such as fact sheets, posters, literature guides, and brochures, that are distributed through the information centers. Some agencies also provide, when appropriate, referral to health professionals, health institutions, or other agencies and organizations.

Entries for these government clearinghouses and information centers are listed alphabetically, providing the name, address, and telephone number of each agency, along with a brief description of the services and materials that are provided. Item entry numbers correspond to those used in Chapter 8.

[9-1] Center for Health Promotion and Education,
Centers for Disease Control
Building 1 South, Room SSB249
1600 Clifton Road NE
Atlanta, GA 30333
(404) 329–3492

Instituted by the Centers for Disease Control, the center collects and disseminates to health professionals and the general public educational materials related to the prevention of chronic disease and the promotion of health. Materials include information for AIDS school health education, as well as programs for addressing health risks associated with smoking, obesity, hypertension, and stress.

[9-2] Clearinghouse on the Handicapped
Sweitzer Building, Room 3132
330 Cancer Street SW
Washington, DC 20202
(202) 732–1244

This clearinghouse provides information on federal benefits, funding, and legislation related to the handicapped. Staff respond to questions from the handicapped by referral to organizations that provide information on their disabilities.

[9-3] Clearinghouse for Occupational Safety and Health Information
4676 Columbia Parkway
Cincinnati, OH 45226
(800) 356–4674

This clearinghouse responds to telephone inquiries from health professionals and the public on topics related to occupational health and safety. It provides brochures on the prevention of occupational diseases and answers specific questions related to chemicals, heat stress, and occupational injuries.

[9-4] Food and Drug Administration (FDA)
Office of Consumer Affairs, HFE-88
5600 Fishers Lane
Rockville, MD 20857
(301) 443–3170

The Office of Consumer Affairs serves as the clearinghouse for the FDA's consumer publications, in addition to responding to inquiries from the public. Printed materials and answers to specific questions are provided on a wide range of topics, including medical devices, cosmetics, pharmaceuticals, radiological safety, health fraud, and nutrition.

[9-5] Food and Nutrition Information Center
Room 304
National Agricultural Library
Beltsville, MD 20705
(301) 344–3719

This center provides information on nutrition, food science, and food technology for health professionals and for the public. Consumer materials include resource guides on nutrition, fad diets, vegetarianism, eating disorders, vitamin and mineral supplements, and food irradiation, as well as general nutritional information. Staff also respond to specific questions from the public.

[9-6] Health Care Financing Administration
200 Independence Avenue SW
Washington, DC 20201
(202) 245–6726

This agency responds to written or telephone requests from the general public for information about the MEDICARE program. It provides general brochures about MEDICARE, and referral to one of the ten regional MEDICARE offices in the United States. Answers to specific questions about MEDICARE benefits are also provided.

[9-7] High Blood Pressure Information Center
120/80 National Institutes of Health
9000 Rockville Pike
Bethesda, MD 20892
(301) 496–1809

This center provides information and publications to professionals and the public on the detection, diagnosis, and management of high blood pressure. Educational materials are available on topics such as the pathophysiology of high blood pressure, sodium, diet and exercise, and blood pressure measurement devices.

[9-8] National AIDS Information Clearinghouse
PO Box 6003
Rockville, MD 20850
(800) 458–5231

A service of the Centers for Disease Control, the National AIDS Information Clearinghouse (NAIC) collects and distributes current medical information on HIV and AIDS. NAIC staff answer inquiries by telephone, fax, or TTY/TTD in English, Spanish, or French, providing information about the 10,000 AIDS service and resource organizations, about educational materials, and about school health education. They will also send free educational materials upon request. Of special interest to health professionals is the AIDS Clinical Trials Information Service (ACTIS). Every clinical trial being conducted under the auspices of the National Institutes of Health and every private clinical trial approved by the Food and Drug Administration are covered by ACTIS. The toll-free number for ACTIS is (800)TRIALS-A.

[9-9] National Arthritis and Musculoskeletal and Skin Diseases Information Clearinghouse
PO Box AMS
Bethesda, MD 20892
(301) 468–3235

This clearinghouse serves as the resource center for the National Institute of Arthritis and Musculoskeletal and Skin Diseases. It collects and distributes information about these disorders in such areas as disease description, diagnosis, treatment, and prevention; patient education and rehabilitation; physical and occupational therapy; diet, exercise, and medication; psychosocial factors; and epidemiology and statistics. The staff provide referrals to other sources of information, as well as responding to requests for printed materials from the Clearinghouse.

[9-10] National Cancer Institute Cancer Information Service
Building 31, Room 10A-24
9000 Rockville Pike
Bethesda, MD 20892
(800) 4-CANCER

The Cancer Information Service is a program of the National Cancer Institute that provides information to professionals, cancer patients, and the public on topics such as cancer prevention, detection, diagnosis, and treatment. In addition to providing confidential answers to questions, staff also send free publications on a variety of topics related to specific types of cancer. Referrals are also made to community agencies and services available in the caller's area.

[9-11] National Cholesterol Education Program NCEP Information Center
National Heart, Lung, and Blood Institute, C-200
PO Box NCEP
Bethesda, MD 20892
(301) 230–1340

This center provides information to health professionals and to the general public by responding to written or telephone inquiries. Fact sheets and educational materials on cholesterol, the effects of cholesterol on health, and methods for lowering total blood cholesterol are distributed.

[9-12] National Clearinghouse for Alcohol and Drug Information
PO Box 2345
Rockville, MD 20852
(301) 468–2600

This clearinghouse provides a focus for the federal effort to gather and disseminate alcohol and drug information. The Clearinghouse responds to questions and distributes publications to both health professionals and the public on a broad range of topics that include alcohol and drug abuse; fetal alcohol syndrome; and alcohol and drug problems of the elderly and specific groups such as Native Americans, hispanics, and blacks.

[9-13] National Diabetes Information Clearinghouse
PO Box NDIC
Bethesda, MD 20892
(301) 468–2162

This clearinghouse responds to requests for information about diabetes and its complications. Educational materials are collected and distributed to health professionals, to people with diabetes and their families, and to the general public. The Clearinghouse provides information on a wide range of topics related to diabetes, including patient education materials, diabetes research and care, and statistical data from the National Diabetes Data Group about clinical and epidemiological characteristics of diabetes.

[9-14] National Digestive Diseases Information Clearinghouse
PO Box NDDIC
Bethesda, MD 20892
(301) 468–6344

This clearinghouse provides information about digestive diseases that include disorders of the esophagus, liver, stomach, gall bladder, and the intestines. Information is provided to health professionals, patients, and the public. Services include providing fact sheets about specific digestive diseases, providing referral service for health professionals and the public, providing information about research developments, and providing information on organizational and government activities related to digestive diseases.

[9-15] National Eye Institute Information Center
9000 Rockville Pike
Bethesda, MD 20892
(301) 496–5248

This center responds to mail or telephone inquiries from health professionals and the public on a wide range of topics related to eye diseases and eye disorders. Printed brochures and fact sheets about eye diseases and current research findings are distributed. Information is also distributed about current clinical studies, and on the procedure for referral by a physician to an ongoing clinical study.

[9-16] National Health Information Center
Office of Disease Prevention and Health Promotion
PO Box 1133
Washington, DC 20013
(800) 336–4797

This center serves as an information and referral center for persons with health questions by responding directly to inquiries or by referring questions to appropriate sources. It prepares and distributes publications and directories on health promotion and disease prevention, and maintains a resource file of other organizations that provide information to the public and health professionals on health topics.

[9-17] National Heart, Lung, and Blood Institute Information Center
Suite 530
4733 Bethesda Avenue
Bethesda, MD 20814
(301) 951–3260

This information center distributes publications to health professionals and to the public on a number of topics related to heart diseases, lung diseases, and blood resources by responding to mail and telephone requests. The major emphasis of the Institute's publications addresses public education and disease prevention in the areas of high blood pressure, cholesterol control, asthma, smoking cessation, and blood resources. Guidelines for treatment of specific diseases are also distributed.

Future publications will include information on obesity and a heart attack alert for health professionals.

[9-18] National Institute on Aging Information Center
Federal Building, Room 6C12
Bethesda, MD 20892
(301) 496–1752

This information center serves as the clearinghouse for the Institute by collecting and distributing information to health professionals and to the public on the broad topic of aging. In addition to distributing information about the current biomedical and behavioral research conducted at the Institute, a number of publications on aging are available, including safe use of medications, susceptibility to disease, memory loss, finding good medical care, and health quackery.

[9-19] National Institute of Allergy and Infectious Diseases
Public Information Office
9000 Rockville Pike
Bethesda, MD 20892
(301) 496–5717

This institute supports research on the causes, characteristics, prevention, and treatment of a number of diseases caused by bacteria, viruses, parasites, allergies, and by deficiencies or disorders of the body's immune mechanisms. Its information office responds to questions in areas of special emphasis of the Institute, which include asthma and allergic disease, venereal diseases, hepatitis, influenza and other viral respiratory infections, and organ transplantation.

[9-20] National Institute of Child Health and Human Development
Information Center
9000 Rockville Pike
Bethesda, MD 20892
(301) 496–5133

This information center distributes information related to the research findings of the Institute to other researchers, health professionals, and the general public. Staff answer questions and provide publications on topics such as child and maternal health, problems of human development (with special emphasis on mental retardation), the family structure, dynamics of human population, and the reproductive process.

[9-21] National Institute on Deafness and Other
Communication Disorders Clearinghouse
PO Box 37777
Washington, DC 20013
(800) 241–1044 (800) 241–1055 (TDD/TT)

The newest institute in the National Institutes of Health (NIH) complex has just established this clearinghouse. Staff reply to telephone and mail inquiries from professionals and the public by responding to questions and sending publications and educational materials on a wide range of topics related to disorders of hearing and other communication processes, including diseases affecting hearing, balance, voice, speech, language, taste, and smell.

[9-22] National Institute of Dental Research Information Center
Building 31, Room 2C-35
9000 Rockville Pike
Bethesda, MD 20892
(301) 496–4261

This information center responds to written and telephone inquiries from health professionals and the public. Educational materials and fact sheets will be sent on current research being conducted at the Institute, which covers a wide range of dental problems.

[9-23] National Institute of Mental Health Public Inquiries Branch
Parklawn Building, Room 15C-05
5600 Fishers Lane
Rockville, MD 20857
(301) 443–4513

This institute provides a focus for the federal effort to increase knowledge and develop effective strategies to promote mental health, and for the prevention and treatment of mental illness. The information center provides referral to mental health facilities and distributes publications on mental health and mental illness, including material on depression, schizophrenia, Alzheimer's disease, suicide, and rape.

[9-24] National Institute of Neurological Disorders and Stroke
9000 Rockville Pike
Bethesda, MD 20892
(301) 496–5751

This institute conducts research on human neurological disorders such as epilepsy, muscular dystrophy, multiple sclerosis, Parkinson's disease, and stroke. Research is also conducted on the treatment of head and spinal cord injuries. Information is disseminated to health professionals and to the public on topics receiving emphasis by the Institute.

[9-25] National Kidney and Urologic Diseases Information Clearinghouse
PO Box NKUDIC
Bethesda, MD 20892
(301) 468–6345

This clearinghouse serves as a resource and referral center to increase the knowledge and understanding of patients, health care professionals, and the public about kidney and urologic disease. It gathers and disseminates educational information produced by many sources related to prostate enlargement, kidney stones, urinary track infections, urinary incontinence, kidney failure, diabetes and kidney disease, transplantation, dialysis, and impotence.

[9-26] National Second Surgical Opinion Program
Health Care Financing Administration
200 Independence Avenue SW
Washington, DC 20201
(800) 638–6833

This program provides information and brochures for patients who must obtain a
second opinion before undergoing non-emergency surgery. A toll-free telephone
line is provided to help the public locate a surgeon on other specialist in their local-
ity for a second opinion.

[9-27] National Sickle Cell Disease Program
National Heart, Lung, and Blood Institute
Federal Building, Room 508
7550 Wisconsin Avenue
Bethesda, MD 20892
(301) 496–6931

This program provides publications and educational materials to the general public
on all aspects of sickle cell disease by responding to written or telephone inquiries.
Referral is also provided to one of the ten centers throughout the United States that
is conducting research and clinical studies on sickle cell disease for the Institute.

[9-28] Office on Smoking and Health Technical Information Center
Park Building, Room 1–16
5600 Fishers Lane
Rockville, MD 20857
(301) 443–1690

This information center publishes and distributes many publications on smoking to
health professionals and to the public. Consumer publications include smoking and
pregnancy, smoking and teenagers, smoking cessation, and smoking and health.
The Center also provides bibliographic and reference services to researchers.

10

Guide to State Sources of Health Information

Many health programs are governed by state laws and regulations rather than by federal laws. Programs regulating licensure of physicians and insurance companies, enforcement of local health laws, and the administration of the Medicaid cost containment programs are examples of these state regulatory functions. Individual state agencies or departments provide information about the regulation and enforcement of the various state health laws or answer questions related to public health regulations or services. On the following pages are the names of the state health regulatory agencies for insurance, MEDICAID, physician licensure, and public health. The names, addresses, and telephone numbers are included for the administrators of the agencies or departments responsible for these programs in each state. Listings for American Samoa, Guam, Puerto Rico, and the Virgin Islands follow listings for the states.

WHERE SHOULD I GO TO FIND . . .   *TRY*

| Insurance |

answers to questions, or to report a complaint, about a specific insurance company?

specific state insurance commissioners listed below.

Alabama

Mike Weaver, Commissioner
Insurance Department
Room 504
64 North Union Street
Montgomery, AL 36130
(205) 269–3550

(answer continues)

WHERE SHOULD I GO TO FIND. . .   *TRY*

answers to questions, or to report a
complaint, about a specific insurance
company?

Alaska

Paul Roller, Director
Division of Insurance
PO Box D
Juneau, AK 99811
(907)465–2515

Arizona

Susan Gallinger, Director
Department of Insurance
Suite 1100
3030 North Third Street
Phoenix, AZ 85012
(602)255–5400

Arkansas

Ron Taylor, Commissioner
Insurance Department
400 University Tower Building
12th Street and University Avenue
Little Rock, AR 72204
(501)371–1325

California

Roxani M. Gillespie, Commissioner
Department of Insurance
600 South Commonwealth Avenue
Los Angeles, CA 90005
(213)736–2551

Colorado

Joanne Hill, Commissioner
Division of Insurance
Suite 500
303 West Colfax Avenue
Denver, CO 80204
(303)866–6400

Connecticut

Peter F. Kelly, Commissioner
Department of Insurance
State Office Building
Hartford, CT 06106
(203)297–3802

WHERE SHOULD I GO TO FIND. . .   *TRY*

answers to questions, or to report a
complaint, about a specific insurance
company?

Delaware

David N. Levinson, Commissioner
Department of Insurance
Suite 100
841 Silver Lake Boulevard
Dover, DE 19901
(302)736–4251

District of Columbia

Marguerite Stokes, Administrator
Insurance Administration
Room 600
613 C Street NW
Washington, DC 20001
(202)727–8000

Florida

Tom Gallagher, Insurance Commissioner
State Capitol
Tallahassee, FL 32399
(904)488–3440

Georgia

Warren D. Evans, Insurance Commissioner
West Tower, 7th Floor
2 Martin Luther King, Jr. Drive
Atlanta, GA 30334
(404)656–2056

Hawaii

Robin Campaniano, Insurance
Commissioner
Division of Insurance
1010 Richards Street
Honolulu, HI 96813
(808)548–6522

Idaho

Anthony J. Fagiano, Acting Director
Department of Insurance
500 South 10th Street
Boise, ID 83720
(208)334–2250

(*answer continues*)

WHERE SHOULD I GO TO FIND. . .   *TRY*

Illinois

answers to questions, or to report a
complaint, about a specific insurance
company?

Stephen Selcke, Director
Department of Insurance
4th Floor
320 West Washington Street
Springfield, IL 62767
(217)782–4515

Indiana

John J. Dillon III, Commissioner
Department of Insurance
Suite 300
311 West Washington Street
Indianapolis, IN 46204
(317)232–2386

Iowa

William Hager, Commissioner
Insurance Division
Department of Commerce
Lucas State Office Building
Des Moines, IA 50319
(515)281–5705

Kansas

Fletcher Bell, Commissioner
Insurance Department
420 SW 9th Street
Topeka, KS 66612
(913)296–3071

Kentucky

Leroy Morgan, Commissioner
Department of Insurance
229 West Main Street
Frankfort, KY 40601
(502)564–6027

Louisiana

Douglas D. Green, Commissioner
Department of Insurance
PO Box 94214
Baton Rouge, LA 70804
(504)342–5322

WHERE SHOULD I GO TO FIND. . .   **TRY**

answers to questions, or to report a
complaint, about a specific insurance
company?

Maine

Joseph Edwards, Superintendent
Bureau of Insurance Regulations
Department
State House Station #34
Augusta, ME 04333
(207)289–3101

Maryland

John A. Donaho, Commissioner
Division of Insurance
501 St. Paul Place
Baltimore, MD 21202
(301)333–6300

Massachusetts

Thomas Gailey, Commissioner
Division of Insurance
100 Cambridge Street
Boston, MA 02202
(617)727–3357

Michigan

Shiraf Shah, Commissioner of Insurance
Licensing and Regulation Department
611 West Ottawa
Lansing, MI 48909
(517)373–9273

Minnesota

Michael Hatch, Commissioner
Department of Commerce
5th Floor, Metro Square Building
Seventh and Robert Street
St. Paul, MN 55101
(612)296–6848

Mississippi

George Dale, Commissioner
Department of Insurance
1804 Sillers Building
550 High Street
Jackson, MS 39201
(601)359–3569

(answer continues)

<u>*WHERE SHOULD I GO TO FIND. . .*</u>   <u>*TRY*</u>

answers to questions, or to report a
complaint, about a specific insurance
company?

Missouri

Lewis Malahn, Director
Division of Insurance
Box 690, Truman Building
Jefferson City, MO 65102
(314)751–2451

Montana

Andrea Bennett, Commissioner of
Insurance
PO Box 4009
Helena, MT 59604
(406)444–2040

Nebraska

William H. McCartney, Director
Department of Insurance
Suite 400
The Terminal Building
941 O Street
Lincoln, NE 68508
(402)471–2201

Nevada

David Gates, Commissioner
Insurance Division
201 South Fall Street
Carson City, NV 89701
(702)885–4270

New Hampshire

Louis E. Bergeron, Commissioner
Insurance Department
169 Manchester Street
Concord, NH 03301
(603)271–2261

New Jersey

Kenneth Merin, Commissioner
Department of Insurance
12th Floor
20 West State Street
Trenton, NJ 08625
(609)292–5360

WHERE SHOULD I GO TO FIND. . .   *TRY*

New Mexico

answers to questions, or to report a
complaint, about a specific insurance
company?

Fabian Chavez, Superintendent
State Insurance Board
Room 428, Pera Building
Santa Fe, NM 87503
(505)827–4297

New York

James Corcoran, Superintendent
Insurance Department
Agency Building #1
Empire State Plaza
Albany, NY 12224
(518)474–4550

North Carolina

James E. Long, Commissioner
Department of Insurance
430 North Salisbury Street
Raleigh, NC 27603
(919)733–7343

North Dakota

Earl R. Pomeroy, Commissioner
Insurance Department
5th Floor, State Capitol
600 East Boulevard
Bismarck, ND 58505
(701)224–2440

Ohio

George Fabe, Director
Department of Insurance
2100 Stella Court
Columbus, OH 43266
(614)481–5728

Oklahoma

Gerald Grimes, Commissioner
Insurance Department
408 Will Rogers Boulevard
Oklahoma City, OK 73105
(405)521–2828

(*answer continues*)

WHERE SHOULD I GO TO FIND...	*TRY*

answers to questions, or to report a complaint, about a specific insurance company?

Oregon

Ted Kulongoski, Director
Department of Insurance and Finance
21 Labor and Industries Building
Salem, OR 97310
(503)378–4120

Pennsylvania

Peter Smith, Commissioner
Insurance Department
13th Floor, Strawberry Square
Harrisburg, PA 17120
(717)787–5173

Rhode Island

Robert Jones, Director
Department of Business Regulation
100 North Main Street
Providence, RI 02903
(401)277–2246

South Carolina

John G. Richards, Commissioner
Department of Insurance
1612 Marion Street
Columbia, SC 29201
(803)737–6117

South Dakota

Jeff Stingley, Secretary
Division of Insurance
State Capitol
910 Sioux
Pierre, SD 57501
(605)773–3563

Tennessee

Elaine McReynolds, Commissioner
Department of Commerce and Insurance
Suite 1400
1808 West End Road
Nashville, TN 37219
(615)741–2241

Texas

A. W. Pogue, Commissioner
Board of Insurance
1100 San Jacinto Boulevard
Austin, TX 78701
(512)463–6464

WHERE SHOULD I GO TO FIND. . .

answers to questions, or to report a
complaint, about a specific insurance
company?

TRY

Utah

Harold Yancy, Commissioner
Department of Insurance
160 East 300 South
Salt Lake City, UT 84111
(801)530–6400

Vermont

Gretchen Babcock, Commissioner
Department of Banking and Insurance
120 State Street
Montpelier, VT 05602
(802)828–3301

Virginia

Elizabeth B. Lacey, Chairman
State Corporation Commission
13th Floor
1220 Bank Street
Richmond, VA 23219
(804)786–3603

Washington

Richard C. Marquardt, Commissioner
Office of Insurance Commissioner
Insurance Building
Olympia, WA 98504
(206)753–7301

West Virginia

Hanley Clark, Commissioner
Division of Insurance
2100 Washington Street East
Charleston, WV 25305
(304)348–3394

Wisconsin

Robert D. Haase, Commissioner
Office of Insurance
PO Box 7873
123 West Washington Avenue
Madison, WI 53707
(608)266–3585

Wyoming

Gordon Taylor, Commissioner
Insurance Department
Herschler Building
Cheyenne, WY 82002
(307)777–7401

(*answer continues*)

<u>*WHERE SHOULD I GO TO FIND. . .*</u>   *TRY*

American Samoa

answers to questions, or to report a
complaint, about a specific insurance
company?

Fanene S. Scanlan, Insurance
Commissioner
Office of the Governor
Pago Pago, AS 96799
(684) 633–2225

Guam

Joaquin G. Blaz, Director
Department of Revenue and Taxation
855 West Marine Drive
Agana, GU 96910
(617) 477–5143

Puerto Rico

Miguel A. Villafana, Commissioner
Insurance Commission
PO Box 8330
Santurce, PR 00910
(809) 722–8686

Virgin Islands

Derek M. Hodge, Lieutenant Governor
18 Kangens Glade
St. Thomas, VI 00802
(809) 774–2991

| Medicaid |

answers to questions about the
administration of Medicaid programs, or
reports from Medicaid cost containment
councils regarding costs of certain medical
procedures in my area?

the specific administrator for your state
listed below.

Alabama

Carol Herrman, Commissioner
Medicaid Agency
2500 Fairlane Drive
Montgomery, AL 36130
(205) 277–2710

WHERE SHOULD I GO TO FIND. . .

TRY

answers to questions about the
administration of Medicaid programs, or
reports from Medicaid cost containment
councils regarding costs of certain medical
procedures in my area?

Alaska

Kim Busch, Director
Division of Medicaid Assistance
Health and Social Services Department
PO Box H–07
Juneau, AK 99811
(907)465–3355

Arizona

Leonard Kirschner, Director
Arizona Health Care Cost Containment
System
801 East Jefferson
Phoenix, AZ 85034
(602)234–3655

Arkansas

Kenny Whitlock, Deputy Director
Economic and Medical Services Division
Department of Human Services
PO Box 1437, Slot 316
Little Rock, AR 72203
(501)682–8375

California

Sally Lu, Chief
Medi-Cal Operations Division
Department of Human Services
Room 1540
714 P Street
Sacramento, CA 95814
(916)324–2681

Colorado

Garry Toerber, Director
Division of Medical Assistance
Department of Social Services
Room 617
1575 Sherman Street
Denver, CO 80203
(303)866–5901

(*answer continues*)

WHERE SHOULD I GO TO FIND. . .   *TRY*

Connecticut

answers to questions about the
administration of Medicaid programs, or
reports from Medicaid cost containment
councils regarding costs of certain medical
procedures in my area?

Sally Bowles, Director
Medical Care Administration
Department of Income Maintenance
110 Bartholomew Avenue
Hartford, CT 06106
(203)566–2934

Delaware

Phyllis T. Hazel, Administrator
Division of Economic Services
Health and Social Services Department
PO Box 906
New Castle, DE 19720
(302)421–6139

District of Columbia

Lee Partridge, Chief
Office of Health Care Financing
Department of Human Services
1331 H Street NW
Washington, DC 20005
(202)727–0735

Florida

Thomas W. Arnold, Deputy Assistant
Secretary for Medicaid
Health and Rehabilitative Services
1317 Winewood Boulevard
Tallahassee, FL 32399
(904)488–3560

Georgia

Aaron J. Johnson, Jr., Commissioner
Department of Medical Assistance
2 Martin Luther King, Jr. Drive NE
Atlanta, GA 30334
(404)656–4479

Hawaii

Earl Motooka, Health Care Administrator
Health Care Administration Division
Department of Human Services
Room 817
820 Mililani
Honolulu, HI 96813
(808)548–6584

WHERE SHOULD I GO TO FIND...   *TRY*

answers to questions about the
administration of Medicaid programs, or
reports from Medicaid cost containment
councils regarding costs of certain medical
procedures in my area?

Idaho

Allen Korhonen, Administrator
Division of Welfare
Department of Health and Welfare
450 West State Street
Boise, ID 83720
(208)334–5747

Illinois

Phil Bradley, Director
Department of Public Aid
100 South Grand Avenue
Springfield, IL 62762
(217)782–6716

Indiana

Gary Kizer-Sheeley, Director
Medicaid Division
Department of Public Welfare
702 State Office Building
Indianapolis, IN 46204
(317)232–4324

Iowa

Donald L. Herman, Chief
Medical Services Bureau
Department of Human Services
Hoover State Office Building
Des Moines, IA 50319
(515)281–8621

Kansas

Kathryn Klassen, Director of Medical Services
Division of Medical Programs
Department of Social and Rehabilitative
Services
6th Floor
State Office Building
Topeka, KS 66612
(913)296–3981

Kentucky

Ray Butler, Commissioner
Department for Medicaid Services
Cabinet for Human Resources
275 East Main Street
Frankfort, KY 40621
(502)564–4321

(answer continues)

<u>*WHERE SHOULD I GO TO FIND...*</u>   <u>*TRY*</u>

Louisiana

answers to questions about the
administration of Medicaid programs, or
reports from Medicaid cost containment
councils regarding costs of certain medical
procedures in my area?

Howard Prejean, Assistant Secretary
Eligibility Determination Office
Health and Human Resources Department
PO Box 9465
Baton Rouge, LA 70804
(504)342–3950

Maine

Douglas Hall, Acting Director
Bureau of Income Maintenance
Department of Human Services
State House Station #11
Augusta, ME 04333
(207)289–2415

Maryland

Douglas H. Morgan, Assistant Secretary
Medical Care Programs
Health and Mental Hygiene Department
201 West Preston Street
Baltimore, MD 21201
(301)225–6536

Massachusetts

Bruce Bullen, Associate Commissioner
Medical Payments
Department of Public Welfare
180 Tremont Street
Boston, MA 02111
(617)574–0100

Michigan

Kevin Seitz, Director
Medical Services Administration
Department of Social Services
PO Box 30037
Lansing, MI 48909
(517)334–7262

Minnesota

Robert C. Baird, Director
Health Care Programs Division
Department of Human Services
444 Lafayette Road
St. Paul, MN 55101
(612)296–2766

WHERE SHOULD I GO TO FIND. . .

TRY

answers to questions about the administration of Medicaid programs, or reports from Medicaid cost containment councils regarding costs of certain medical procedures in my area?

Mississippi

Clinton Smith, Director
Division of Medicaid
Office of the Governor
239 North Lamar Street
Jackson, MS 39202
(601)359–6050

Missouri

Donna Checkett, Director
Division of Medical Services
Department of Social Services
615 Howerton Court
Jefferson City, MO 65109
(314)751–3425

Montana

John Donwen, Administrator
Economic Assistance Division
Social and Rehabilitative Services
Department
111 Sanders Street
Helena, MT 59601
(406)444–4540

Nebraska

Robert Seiffert, Administrator
Medical Services
Department of Social Services
PO Box 95026
Lincoln, NE 68509
(402)471–3121

Nevada

April Hess, Deputy Administrator
Medicaid Division
Department of Human Resources
2527 North Carson Street
Carson City, NV 89710
(702)885–4698

New Hampshire

Robert Pliskin, Director
Division of Human Services
Department of Health and Welfare
6 Hazen Drive
Concord, NH 03301
(603)271–4321

(*answer continues*)

<u>*WHERE SHOULD I GO TO FIND. . .*</u>   <u>*TRY*</u>

answers to questions about the
administration of Medicaid programs, or
reports from Medicaid cost containment
councils regarding costs of certain medical
procedures in my area?

New Jersey

Saul M. Kilstein, Director
Division of Medical Assistance and Health
Services
Department of Human Services
Trenton, NJ 08625
(609)588–2600

New Mexico

Bruce Weydemeyer, Chief
Medical Assistance Division
Department of Human Services
Pera Building
Santa Fe, NM 87503
(505)827–4315

New York

Cesar Perales, Commissioner
Department of Social Services
40 North Pearl Street
Albany, NY 12243
(518)474–9475

North Carolina

Barbaras D. Matula, Director
Division of Medical Assistance
Department of Human Resources
1985 Umstead Drive
Raleigh, NC 27603
(919)733–2060

North Dakota

Richard Myatt, Director
Medical Services Division
Department of Human Services
Judicial Wing, State Capitol
600 East Boulevard
Bismarck, ND 58505
(701)224–2321

Ohio

John E. Boyle, Chief
Division of Medical Assistance
Department of Human Services
30 East Broad Street
Columbus, OH 43266
(614)466–2365

WHERE SHOULD I GO TO FIND. . .

answers to questions about the administration of Medicaid programs, or reports from Medicaid cost containment councils regarding costs of certain medical procedures in my area?

TRY

Oklahoma

Phillip Watson, Director
Department of Human Services
PO Box 25352
Oklahoma City, OK 73125
(405)521–3646

Oregon

Jean Thorne, Manager
Adult Family Services Division
Department of Human Resources
203 Public Service Building
Salem, OR 97310
(503)378–2263

Pennsylvania

Eileen M. Schoen, Deputy Secretary for
Medical Assistance
Department of Public Health
515 Health and Welfare Building
Harrisburg, PA 17120
(717)787–1870

Rhode Island

Anthony Barile, Associate Director Medical
Services
Department of Social and Rehabilitative
Services
600 New London Avenue
Cranston, RI 02920
(401)464–3575

South Carolina

Andy Laurent, Executive Director
Health and Human Services Finance
Commission
PO Box 8206
Columbia, SC 29202
(803)253–6100

South Dakota

Ervin Schumacher, Director
Office of Medical Services
Department of Social Services
Kneip Building
Pierre, SD 57501
(605)773–3495

(answer continues)

WHERE SHOULD I GO TO FIND. . .   TRY

answers to questions about the
administration of Medicaid programs, or
reports from Medicaid cost containment
councils regarding costs of certain medical
procedures in my area?

Tennessee

Manny Martinez, Director
Medicaid Administration
Department of Health and Environment
Terra Building
Nashville, TN 37219
(615)741–0213

Texas

Ron Lindsey, Commissioner
Department of Human Services
PO Box 2960
Austin, TX 78769
(512)450–3030

Utah

Rod Betit, Director
Division of Health Care Financing
Department of Health
288 North 1460 West
Salt Lake City, UT 84116
(801)538–6151

Vermont

Elmo Sassorossi, Director
Medical Services Division
Department of Social Welfare
Waterbury Office Complex
Waterbury, VT 05676
(802)241–2880

Virginia

Bruce U. Kozlowski, Director
Department of Medical Assistance Services
600 East Broad Street
Richmond, VA 23219
(804)786–7933

Washington

Ron Kero, Director
Division of Medical Assistance
Social and Health Services Department
Twon Square Building B
Olympia, WA 98504
(206)753–1777

WHERE SHOULD I GO TO FIND. . .   ## TRY

West Virginia

answers to questions about the administration of Medicaid programs, or reports from Medicaid cost containment councils regarding costs of certain medical procedures in my area?

Helen M. Condry
Division of Medical Services
Department of Human Services
1900 Washington East
Charleston, WV 25305
(304) 348–8990

Wisconsin

John Torphy, Administrator
Division of Health
Health and Social Services Department
PO Box 309
Madison, WI 53701
(608) 266–1511

Wyoming

Kenneth C. Kamis, Director
Medical Assistance
Health and Medical Services Division
Hathaway Building
Cheyenne, WY 82002
(307) 777–7531

American Samoa

Iotama Saleapaga
Department of Health
Pago Pago, AS 96799
(684) 633–2732

Guam

Leticia Espaldon, Director
Department of Public Health and Social
Services
PO Box 2816
Agana, GU 96910
(671) 734–2931

U.S. Virgin Islands

Rita Dudley, Assistant Commissioner
Department of Health
St. Thomas Hospital
St. Thomas, VI 00802
(809) 774–0117

WHERE SHOULD I GO TO FIND...   *TRY*

Physician Licensure

answers to questions about physician licensure, or to report a complaint about a physician in my area?

the specific administrator for your state listed below.

Alabama

Larry D. Dixon, Executive Director
Alabama State Board of Medical Examiners
PO Box 946
Montgomery, AL 36102
(205)261–4116

Alaska

Pam Ventgen, Executive Secretary
Alaska State Medical Board
Suite 722
3601 C Street
Anchorage, AK 99503
(907)561–2878

Arizona

Douglas N. Cerf, Executive Director
Arizona Board of Medical Examiners
Suite 300
2001 West Camelback Road
Phoenix, AZ 85015
(602)255–3751

Arkansas

Joe Verser, M.D.
Arkansas State Medical Board
PO Box 102
Harrisburg, AR 72432
(501)578–2448

California

Kenneth Wagstaff, Executive Director
Medical Board of California
Verification Department
1430 Howe Avenue
Sacramento, CA 95825
(916)920–6393

WHERE SHOULD I GO TO FIND. . .   *TRY*

Colorado

answers to questions about physician
licensure, or to report a complaint about a
physician in my area?

Thomas J. Beckett, Program Administrator
Board of Medical Examiners
Room 132
1525 Sherman Street
Denver, CO 80203
(303)866–2468

Connecticut

Joseph Gillen, Section Chief
Connecticut Division of Medical Quality
Assurance
150 Washington Street
Hartford, CT 06106
(203)566–7398

Delaware

Rosemarie S. Vanderhoogt, Administrative
Officer
Delaware Board of Medical Practice
PO Box 1401
Dover, DE 19903
(302)736–4522

District of Columbia

John P. Hopkins, Executive Director
District of Columbia Board of Medicine
Room 202
605 G Street SW
Washington, DC 20001
(202)727–9794

Florida

Dorothy Faircloth, Executive Director
Florida Board of Medical Examiners
Suite 110
1940 North Monroe Street
Tallahassee, FL 32399

Georgia

Andrew Watry, Executive Director
Composite State Board of Medical
Examiners
Room 300
166 Pryor Street SW
Atlanta, GA 30303
(404)656–3913

(*answer continues*)

WHERE SHOULD I GO TO FIND. . .   *TRY*

answers to questions about physician
licensure, or to report a complaint about a
physician in my area?

Hawaii

John Tamashiro
Board of Medical Examiners
PO Box 3469
Honolulu, HI 96801
(808)548–4392

Idaho

Donald L. Deleski, Executive Director
State Board of Medicine
Suite 103
500 South 10th Street
Boise, ID 83720
(208)334–2822

Illinois

Nikki Zollar, Director
Department of Professional Regulation
320 West Washington Street
Springfield, IL 62786
(217)785–0820

Indiana

Patrick J. Turner, Board Administrator
Indiana Health Professions Services Bureau
Suite 1020, Box 82067
One American Square
Indianapolis, IN 46282
(317)232–2960

Iowa

William S. Vanderpool, Executive Director
Board of Medical Examiners
State Capitol Complex
Executive Hills West
1209 East Court Avenue
Des Moines, IA 50319
(515)281–5171

Kansas

Susan Lambrecht, Licensing Supervisor
Board of Healing Arts
Landon State Office Building
Suite 553
900 SW Jackson
Topeka, KS 66612
(913)296–7413

WHERE SHOULD I GO TO FIND. . .

TRY

answers to questions about physician licensure, or to report a complaint about a physician in my area?

Kentucky

C. William Schmidt, Executive Director
State Board of Medical Licensure
Suite 222
400 Sherburn Lane
Louisville, KY 40207
(502)896–1516

Louisiana

Paula M. Mensen, Administrative Services Assistant
Louisiana State Board of Medical Examiners
Suite 100
830 Union Street
New Orleans, LA 70112
(504)524–6763

Maine

David R. Hedrick, Executive Director
Maine Board of Registration in Medicine
State House Station #137
Augusta, ME 04333
(207)289–3601

Maryland

J. Michael Compton, Executive Director
Maryland Board of Physician Quality Assurance
4201 Patterson Avenue
Baltimore, MD 21215
(301)764–4777

Massachusetts

Barbara Neuman, Executive Director
Massachusetts Board of Registration and Discipline in Medicine
10 West Street
Boston, MA 02111
(617)727–3086

Michigan

Marcia Malouin, Licensing Supervisor
Michigan Board of Medicine
Bureau of Health Services
611 West Ottawa Street
Lansing, MI 48909
(517)373–0680

(answer continues)

WHERE SHOULD I GO TO FIND. . .   *TRY*

answers to questions about physician
licensure, or to report a complaint about a
physician in my area?

Minnesota

H. Leonard Boche, Executive Director
Board of Medical Examiners
2700 University Avenue, West
St. Paul, MN 55114
(612)642–0538

Mississippi

Frank Jay Morgan, Jr., M.D., Executive
Officer
Mississippi State Board of Medical
Licensure
2688-D Insurance Center Drive
Jackson, MS 39216
(601)354–6645

Missouri

Gary R. Clark, Executive Secretary
Missouri State Board of Registration of the
Healing Arts
PO Box 4
Jefferson City, MO 65102
(314)751–0171

Montana

Carol Berger Norling, Administrative
Assistant
Montana State Board of Medical Examiners
1424 9th Avenue
Helena, MT 59620
(406)444–4284

Nebraska

Katherine A. Brown, Associate Director
Nebraska State Board of Medical Examiners
PO Box 95007
301 Centennial Mall South
Lincoln, NE 68509
(402)471–2115

Nevada

David K. Boston, Executive Director
Nevada State Board of Medical Examiners
Suite 301
1105 Terminal Way
Reno, NV 89510
(702)329–2559

WHERE SHOULD I GO TO FIND. . .   *TRY*

New Hampshire

answers to questions about physician   William T. Wallace, M.D., Executive
licensure, or to report a complaint about a   Secretary
physician in my area?   Board of Registration in Medicine
                                                   Health and Welfare Building
                                                   6 Hazen Drive
                                                   Concord, NH 03301
                                                   (603)271–4503

                                                   New Jersey

                                                   Charles A. Janousek, Executive Secretary
                                                   New Jersey Board of Medical Examiners
                                                   Room 602
                                                   28 West State Street
                                                   Trenton, NJ 08608
                                                   (609)292–4843

                                                   New Mexico

                                                   Bill Schmidt, Executive Secretary
                                                   New Mexico State Board of Medical
                                                   Examiners
                                                   Lamy Building, Room 129
                                                   491 Old Santa Fe Trail
                                                   Santa Fe, NM 87504
                                                   (505)827–7317

                                                   New York

                                                   Thomas Monahan, Associate Executive
                                                   Secretary
                                                   State Board for Medicine
                                                   State Education Department
                                                   Cultural Education Center
                                                   Empire State Plaza
                                                   Albany, NY 11230
                                                   (518)474–3841

                                                   North Carolina

                                                   Bryant D. Paris, Jr., Executive Secretary
                                                   North Carolina Board of Medical Examiners
                                                   1313 Navajo Drive
                                                   Raleigh, NC 27609
                                                   (919)876–3885

                                                   (*answer continues*)

<u>*WHERE SHOULD I GO TO FIND. . .*</u>   <u>*TRY*</u>

North Dakota

answers to questions about physician
licensure, or to report a complaint about a
physician in my area?

Rolf P. Sletten, Executive Secretary
Treasurer
Board of Medical Examiners
Suite C–10
418 East Broadway Avenue
Bismarck, ND 58501
(701)223–9485

Ohio

Raymond Q. Bumgarner
Ohio State Medical Board
77 South High Street
Columbus, OH 43266
(614)466–3934

Oklahoma

Carole A. Smith, Administrator
Oklahoma State Board of Medical
Examiners
PO Box 18256
Oklahoma City, OK 73118
(405)848–6841

Oregon

John J. Ulwelling, Executive Secretary
Board of Medical Examiners
Crown Plaza
Suite 620
1500 SW First Avenue
Portland, OR 97201
(503)229–5770

Pennsylvania

Loretta M. Frank, Administrative Assistant
Pennsylvania State Board of Medicine
Bureau of Professional and Occupational
Affairs
PO Box 2649
Harrisburg, PA 17105
(717)787–2381

WHERE SHOULD I GO TO FIND. . .   *TRY*

Rhode Island

answers to questions about physician
licensure, or to report a complaint about a
physician in my area?

Milton Hamolsky, M.D., Chief
Administrative Officer
Rhode Island Board of Licensure and
Discipline
Department of Health
Room 205
75 Davis Street
Providence, RI 02908
(401)277–3855

South Carolina

Stephen S. Seeling, J.D., Executive Director
South Carolina State Board of Medical
Examiners
PO Box 12245
Columbia, SC 29211
(803)734–8901

South Dakota

Robert D. Johnson, Executive Secretary
South Dakota State Board of Medical and
Osteopathic Examiners
1323 South Minnesota Avenue
Sioux Falls, SD 57105
(605)336–1965

Tennessee

Louise Blair, Regulatory Board
Administrator
Tennessee Board of Medical Examiners
283 Plus Park Boulevard
Nashville, TN 37219
(615)367–6231

Texas

G. Valter Brindley, Jr., M.D., Executive
Director
Texas State Board of Medical Examiners
PO Box 13562 Capitol Station
Austin, TX 78711
(512)452–1078

(*answer continues*)

WHERE SHOULD I GO TO FIND. . .   *TRY*

Utah

answers to questions about physician   David E. Robinson, Director
licensure, or to report a complaint about a   Utah Division of Occupational and
physician in my area?   Professional Licensing
                                              160 East 300 South
                                              Salt Lake City, UT 84110
                                              (801)530–6628

Vermont

Vera A. Jones
Vermont State Board of Medical Practice
Redstone Building
26 Terrace Street
Montpelier, VT 05602
(802)828–2674

Virginia

Hilary H. Connor, M.D., Executive Director
Virginia State Board of Medicine
1601 Rolling Hills Drive
Richmond, VA 23229
(804)662–9960

Washington

Sherman Cox, D.D.S., Executive Secretary
Washington Board of Medical Examiners
1300 South Quince
Olympia, WA 98504
(206)753–3129

West Virginia

Ronald D. Walton, Executive Director
West Virginia Board of Medicine
Suite 104
101 Dee Drive
Charleston, WV 25311
(304)348–2921

Wisconsin

Deanna Zychowski, Executive Secretary
Wisconsin Medical Examining Board
PO Box 8935
Madison, WI 53708
(608)266–2811

WHERE SHOULD I GO TO FIND. . .

TRY

answers to questions about physician licensure, or to report a complaint about a physician in my area?

Wyoming

Beverly Hacher, Executive Secretary
Wyoming State Board of Medical Examiners
Room 343 Barrett Building
2301 Central Avenue
Cheyenne, WY 82002
(307)777–6463

Guam

Tina T. Blas, R.N., Administrator
Guam Board of Medical Examiners
Department of Public Health and Social
Services
PO Box 2816
Agana, Guam 96910
(671)734–2951

Puerto Rico

Pablo Valentin Torres, J.D., Executive Director
Puerto Rico Board of Medical Examiners
Call Box 13969
Santurce, PR 00908
(809)723–1617

Virgin Islands

Jane Aubain, Administrative Assistant
Virgin Islands Board of Medical Examiners
48 Sugar Estate
St. Thomas, VI 00802
(809)776–8311

Public Health

a state's school immunization requirements, how to obtain a chest x-ray, and other information about the state's public health laws?

specific state health departments listed below.

Alabama

Cloud Earl Fox, Director
State Health Officer
Department of Public Health
Room 381
434 Monroe Street
Montgomery, AL 36130
(205)242–5052

(answer continues)

WHERE SHOULD I GO TO FIND. . .   *TRY*

Alaska

a state's school immunization
requirements, how to obtain a chest x-ray,
and other information about the state's
public health laws?

Myra Munson, Commissioner
Department of Health and Social Services
PO Box H–01
Juneau, AK 99811
(907)465–3030

Arizona

Ted Williams, Director
Department of Health Services
Room 407
1740 West Adams Street
Phoenix, AZ 85007
(602)542–1024

Arkansas

Tom S. Butler, Acting Director
Department of Health
4815 West Markham Street
Little Rock, AR 72205
(501)661–2111

California

Kenneth Kizer, Director
Department of Health Services
Room 1253
714 P Street
Sacramento, CA 95814
(916)445–1248

Colorado

Joel Kohn, Acting Director
Department of Health
4210 East 11th Avenue
Denver, CO 80220
(303)320–8333

Connecticut

Frederick G. Adams, Commissioner
Department of Health Services
150 Washington Street
Hartford, CT 06106
(203)566–2038

WHERE SHOULD I GO TO FIND. . .

TRY

a state's school immunization requirements, how to obtain a chest x-ray, and other information about the state's public health laws?

Delaware

Lyman J. Olsen, Director
Division of Public Health
Health and Social Services Department
PO Box 637
Dover, DE 19901
(302)736–4701

District of Columbia

Reed V. Tuckson, Commissioner
Commission of Public Health
Department of Human Services
12th Floor
1660 L Street NW
Washington, DC 20036
(202)673–7700

Florida

Charles Mahan, Deputy Secretary for Health
Health and Rehabilitative Services
1317 Winewood Boulevard
Tallahassee, FL 32399
(904)487–2705

Georgia

James W. Alley, Director
Public Health Division
Department of Human Resources
878 Peachtree Street NE
Atlanta, GA 30309
(404)894–7505

Hawaii

John Lewin, Director
Department of Health
1250 Punchbowl Street
Honolulu, HI 96813
(808)548–6505

Idaho

Richard P. Donovan, Director
Department of Health and Welfare
Statehouse
Boise, ID 83720
(208)334–5700

(answer continues)

WHERE SHOULD I GO TO FIND. . .	***TRY***

Illinois

a state's school immunization
requirements, how to obtain a chest x-ray,
and other information about the state's
public health laws?

John Lumpkin, M.D., Director
Department of Public Health
535 West Jefferson Street
5th Floor
Springfield, IL 62761
(217)782–4977

Indiana

Woodrow Myers Jr., Commissioner
State Board of Health
1330 W. Michigan Street
Indianapolis, IN 46206
(317)633–8400

Iowa

Mary L. Ellis, Commissioner
Department of Health
Lucas State Office Building
Des Moines, IA 50319
(515)281–5605

Kansas

Charles Konigsberg, Jr., Director
Division of Health
Department of Health and Environment
Room 1052
Landon State Office Building
Topeka, KS 66620
(913)296–1343

Kentucky

Carlos Hernandez, Commissioner
Department for Health Services
Cabinet for Human Services
275 East Main Street
Frankfort, KY 40601
(502)564–3970

Louisiana

Joel L. Nitzkin, M.D., Assistant Secretary
Office of Public Health
Department of Health and Hospitals
325 Loyola Avenue
New Orleans, LA 70112
(504)568–5052

WHERE SHOULD I GO TO FIND. . .   *TRY*

Maine

a state's school immunization
requirements, how to obtain a chest x-ray,
and other information about the state's
public health laws?

H. Rollin Ives, Commissioner
Department of Human Services
State House Station #11
Augusta, ME 04333
(207) 289–2736

Maryland

Adele Wilzack, Secretary
Department of Health and Mental Hygiene
201 West Preston Street
Annapolis, MD 21201
(301) 225–6500

Massachusetts

Deborah Prothrow-Stith, Commissioner
Department of Public Health
Executive Office of Human Services
150 Tremont Street
Boston, MA 02111
(617) 727–2700

Michigan

Raj Weiner, Director
Department of Public Health
3500 North Logan
PO Box 30035
Lansing, MI 48909
(517) 335–8024

Minnesota

Mary Madonna Ashton, Commissioner
Department of Health
717 Delaware Street SE
Minneapolis, MN 55440
(612) 623–5460

Mississippi

Alton Cobb
State Health Officer
Department of Health
2423 North State Street
Jackson, MS 39216
(601) 354–6646

(answer continues)

WHERE SHOULD I GO TO FIND. . .   *TRY*

a state's school immunization
requirements, how to obtain a chest x-ray,
and other information about the state's
public health laws?

Missouri

Bob Harmon, Director
Department of Health
PO Box 570
Jefferson City, MO 65102
(314)751–6001

Montana

J. Dale Taliaferro, Administrator
Health Services Division
Health and Environmental Sciences
Capitol Station
Helena, MT 59620
(406)444–2037

Nebraska

Gregg Wright, Director
Department of Health
301 Centennial Mall South
PO Box 95007
Lincoln, NE 68509
(402)471–2133

Nevada

Mylo C. Florence, Administrator
Health Division
Department of Human Resources
505 East King Street
Carson City, NV 89710
(702)885–4740

New Hampshire

William T. Wallace, Director
Division of Public Health Services
Department of Health and Human Services
6 Hazen Drive
Concord, NH 03301
(603)271–4501

New Jersey

Molly Joel Coye, Commissioner
Department of Health
John Fitch Plaza
Trenton, NJ 08625
(609)292–7834

WHERE SHOULD I GO TO FIND. . .

TRY

a state's school immunization requirements, how to obtain a chest x-ray, and other information about the state's public health laws?

New Mexico

Carla L. Muth, Deputy Secretary
Department of Health and Environment
Room N4100
1190 St. Francis Drive
Santa Fe, NM 87503
(505)984–2000

New York

David Axelrod, Commissioner
Department of Health
Empire State Plaza
Corning Tower Building
Albany, NY 12237
(518)474–2011

North Carolina

Ron Levine, Director
Division of Health Services
Department of Human Resources
225 North McDowell Street
Raleigh, NC 27603
(919)733–3446

North Dakota

Robert M. Wentz, State Health Officer
Department of Health
State Capitol
600 East Boulevard
Bismarck, ND 58505
(701)224–2372

Ohio

Ronald L. Fletcher, Director
Department of Health
246 North High Street
Columbus, OH 43266
(614)466–2253

Oklahoma

Joan Leavitt, Commissioner
Department of Health
1000 NE 10th Street
PO Box 53551
Oklahoma City, OK 73152
(405)271–4200

(*answer continues*)

WHERE SHOULD I GO TO FIND. . .	*TRY*

a state's school immunization
requirements, how to obtain a chest x-ray,
and other information about the state's
public health laws?

Oregon

Kristine Gebbie, Administrator
Health Division
Department of Human Resources
1400 SW 5th Avenue
Portland, OR 97201
(503)229–5032

Pennsylvania

N. Mark Richards, Secretary
Department of Health
802 Health and Welfare Building
Harrisburg, PA 17120
(717)787–6436

Rhode Island

H. Denman Scott, Director
Department of Health
75 Davis Street
Providence, RI 02908
(401)277–2231

South Carolina

Michael D. Jarrett, Commissioner
Health and Environmental Control
2600 Bull Street
Columbia, SC 29201
(803)734–4880

South Dakota

Charles Anderson, Secretary
Department of Health
Foss Building
Pierre, SD 57501
(605)773–3361

Tennessee

J. W. Luna, Commissioner
Department of Health and Environment
344 Cordell Hull Building
Nashville, TN 37219
(615)741–3111

Texas

Robert Bernstein, Commissioner
Department of Health
1100 West 49th Street
Austin, TX 78756
(512)458–7375

WHERE SHOULD I GO TO FIND. . .   *TRY*

a state's school immunization
requirements, how to obtain a chest x-ray,
and other information about the state's
public health laws?

Utah

Suzanne Dandoy, Executive Director
Department of Health
PO Box 2500
288 North 1460 West
Salt Lake City, UT 84116
(801)538–6111

Vermont

Roberta Coffin, Commissioner
Department of Health
60 Main Street
Burlington, VT 05401
(802)863–7280

Virginia

C. M. G. Buttery, Commissioner
Department of Health
400 James Madison Building
109 Governor Street
Richmond, VA 23219
(804)786–3561

Washington

Kristine Gebbie, Secretary
Department of Health
1112 Quince Street SE
M/S: ET–21
Olympia, WA 98504
(206)753–5871

West Virginia

Tounja Willis-Miller, Secretary
Health and Human Resources Department
State Capitol Complex
Room B–617, Bldg. 6
Charleston, WV 25305
(304)348–2400

Wisconsin

John Torphy, Administrator
Division of Health
Health and Social Services Department
PO Box 309
Madison, WI 53701
(608)266–1511

(*answer continues*)

<u>*WHERE SHOULD I GO TO FIND. . .*</u>   <u>*TRY*</u>

a state's school immunization
requirements, how to obtain a chest x-ray,
and other information about the state's
public health laws?

Wyoming

R. Larry Meuli, Administrator
Health and Medical Services Division
Health and Social Services Department
Hathaway Building
Cheyenne, WY 82002
(307)777–7121

American Samoa

Iotamo Saleapaga, Director
Department of Health
Pago Pago, AS 96799
(684)633–2732

Guam

Leticia Espaldon, Director
Department of Public Health and Social
Services
PO Box 2816
Agana, GU 96910
(671)734–2931

Puerto Rico

Enrique Mendez Grau, Secretary
Department of Health
PO Box 9342
Santurce, PR 00908
(809)767–6060

U. S. Virgin Islands

Alfred O. Heath, Commissioner
Department of Health
St. Thomas Hospital
St. Thomas, VI 00802
(809)774–0117

I

Directory of Print Publishers

Adolescent Medicine, Inc.
No. 306
1001 3rd Street, SW
Washington, DC 20024
(202)332–7700

American Academy of Allergy and
    Immunology
611 East Wells Street
Milwaukee, WI 53202
(414)272–6071
(800)822–2762

American Allergy Association
PO Box 7273
Menlo Park, CA 94026
(415)322–1663

American Association of Retired Persons
1909 K Street, NW
Washington, DC 20049
(202)662–4842

American Board of Medical Specialties
Suite 805
One Rotary Center
Evanston, IL 60201
(708)491–9091

American Camping Association
Bradford Woods
5000 State Road, 67 North
Martinsville, IN 46151
(317)342–8456

American Chiropractic Association
1701 Clarendon Boulevard
Arlington, VA 22209
(703)276–8800

American Council on Transplantation
Suite 505
700 North Fairfax Street
Alexandria, VA 22314
(703)836–4301
(800)223–4483

American Dental Association
211 East Chicago Avenue
Chicago, IL 60611
(312)440–2639

American Diabetes Association
National Service Center
1660 Duke Street
Alexandria, VA 22314
(703)549–1500
(800)232–2172

American Health Assistance Foundation
Suite 140
15825 Shady Grove Road
Rockville, MD 20850
(301)948–3244
(800)227–7998

American Health Consultants, Inc.
67 Peachtree Park Drive NE
Atlanta, GA 30309
(404)351–4523

American Medical Association
515 North State Street
Chicago, IL 60610
(312)464–0183
(312)464–5000

American National Standards Institute
1430 Broadway
New York, NY 10018
(212)354–3300

American Osteopathic Association
142 East Ontario Street
Chicago, IL 60611
(312)380–5800

American Psychiatric Association
Division of Publications and Marketing
1400 K Street NW
Washington, DC 20005
(202) 682–6000

Andrews Publications, Inc.
PO Box 200
Edgemont, PA 19028
(215)353–2565
(800)345–1101

Anxiety Disorders Association of America
Suite 513
6000 Executive Blvd.
Rockville, MD 20852
(900)737–3400
(301)231–9350

Arco Publishing Co.
Order Department
200 Old Tappan Road
Old Tappan, NJ 07675
(201)767–5937

Arthritis Health Professions Association
1314 Spring Street NW
Atlanta, GA 30309
(404)872–7100

Aspen Publishers, Inc.
1600 Research Boulevard
Rockville, MD 20850
(301)251–5554
(800)638–8437

Association for Research of Childhood
  Cancer, Inc.
PO Box 251
Buffalo, NY 14225
(716)684–8864

Association of Birth Defect Children
Suite 270
5400 Diplomat Circle
Orlando, FL 32810
(407)629–1466

Barrett Book Co.
1123 High Ridge Road
Stamford, CT 06905
(203)322–8270

The Body Press
Suite 650
11150 Olympic Boulevard
Los Angeles, CA 90064
(213)477–4118
(800)421–0892

R. R. Bowker Co.
121 Chanlon Road
New Providence, NJ 07974
(800)521–8110

Buraff Publications, Inc.
Suite 1000
1350 Connecticut Avenue NW
Washington, DC 20036
(202)862–0946

Bureau of National Affairs, Inc.
1231 25th Street NW
Washington, DC 20037
(202)452–4200
(800)372–1033

Butterworth-Heinemann Publishers
80 Montvale Avenue
Stoneham, MA 02180
(800)366–2665

Cambridge Information Group Directories,
  Inc.
7200 Wisconsin Avenue
Bethesda, MD 20814
(301)961–6750
(800)843–7751

Carroll Publishing Co.
1058 Thomas Jefferson Street NW
Washington, DC 20007
(202)333–8620

Cancer Guidance Institute
1323 Forbes Avenue
Pittsburgh, PA 15219
(412)261–2211

CD Publications
No. 100
8555 16th Street
Silver Spring, MD 20910
(301)588–6380

Chelsea House Publishers
95 Madison Avenue
New York, NY 10016
(212)683–4400
(800)848–2665

Chilton Book Co.
201 King of Prussia Road
Radnor, PA 19089
(215)964–4000
(800)695–1214

CIBA-GEIGY, Inc.
Medical Education and Communications
30 B Vreeland Road
Florham Park, NJ 07932
(201)822–4995
(800)631–1162

Consumers Union of U.S., Inc.
9180 LeSaint Drive
Fairfield, OH 45014
(513)860–1178

Council of State Governments
Iron Works Pike
PO Box 11910
Lexington, KY 40578
(606)252–2291

Crown Publishers, Inc.
201 East 50th Street
New York, NY 10022
(212)572–2068

Marcel Dekker, Inc.
270 Madison Avenue
New York, NY 10016
(212)696–9000
(800)228–1160

Doubleday & Company
Order Department
PO Box 5071
Des Plaines, IL 60017
(800)223–6834, Ext. 479

Dun's Marketing Services
3 Sylvan Drive
Parsippany, NJ 07054
(201)605–6000
(800)526–0651

Facts On File, Inc.
460 Park Avenue South
New York, NY 10016
(212)683–2244
(800)322–8755

Families in Action National Drug
  Information Center
Suite 300
3845 North Druid Hills Road
Decatur, GA 30033
(404)325–5799

Fisher Books
PO Box 38040
Tucson, AZ 85740
(602)292–9080
(800)255–1514

Fulfillment Etc., Inc.
9300 Oak Street NE
St. Petersburg, FL 33702
(201)768–0201

Gale Research Co., Inc.
835 Penobscot Building
Detroit, MI 48226
(313)961–2242
(800)877–4253

Harper & Row, Publishers
See HarperCollins Publishers

HarperCollins Publishers
Order Department
1000 Keystone Industrial Park
Scranton, PA 18512
(717)343–4761
(800)242–7737
(800)982–4377 (in PA)

Hearst Books
105 Madison Avenue
New York, NY 10016
(212)889–3050

Henry Holt and Co.
115 West 18th Street
New York, NY 10011
(212)886–9200
(800)488–5233

Houghton Mifflin Co.
Order Department
Wayside Road
Burlington, MA 01803
(617)272–1500
(800)225–3362

Hunter House, Inc.
c/o Publisher's Services
Box 2510
Novato, CA 94948
(415)883–3530

IBS Press
744 Pier Avenue
Santa Monica, CA 90405
(213)450–6485

Impulse Publishing
PO Box 3321
Danbury, CT 06831
(203)790–8430

Institute for Labor and Mental Health
3137 Telegraph Avenue
Oakland, CA 94609
(415)653–6166

LaSenda Publishers
1590 Via Chaparral
Fallbrook, CA 92028
(619)723–1407

Lawman Press
PO Box 1468
Mount Shasta, CA 96067

Lea & Febiger
200 Chester Field Parkway
Malvern, PA 19355
(215)251–2230
(800)638–0672

J. P. Lippincott Co.
227 East Washington Square
Philadelphia, PA 19106
(215)238–4200
(800)441–4526
(800)982–4377 (in PA)

McGraw-Hill Publishing Co.
Order Department
Princeton Road
Hightstown, NJ 08520
(609)426–5254

Macmillan Publishing Co.
Order Department
Front & Brown Streets
Riverside, NJ 08075
(609)461–6500
(800)257–5755

Marquis Who's Who
Macmillan Directory Division
3002 Glenview Road
Wilmette, IL 60091
(708)441–2387
(800)621–9669

Medical Economics Data
5 Paragon Drive
Montvale, NJ 07645
(201)358–7200
(800)526–4870

Merck & Co., Inc.
PO Box 2000
Rahway, NJ 07065
(908)855–4558

Meredith Corporation
1716 Locust Street
Des Moines, IA 50336
(515)284–3000
(800)678–8091

Mountain Home Publishing
PO Box 829
Ingram, TX 78025
(512)367–4492
(800)527–3044

National Academy Press
2101 Constitution Avenue NW
Washington, DC 20418
(202)334–3313
(800)624–6242

National Foundation for Ileitis and Colitis,
   Inc.
444 Park Avenue South
New York, NY 10016
(212)685–3440
(800)343–3637

National Headache Foundation
5252 North Western Avenue
Chicago, IL 60625
(312) 878–7715
(800)843–2256
(800)523–8858 (in IL)

National Library of Medicine
8600 Rockville Pike
Bethesda, MD 20894
(301)496–6308
(800)638–8480

National Register Publishing Co.
3004 Glenview Road
Wilmette, IL 60091
(708)256–6067
(800)323–6772

National Spinal Cord Injury Association
600 West Cummings Park
Woburn, MA 01801
(617)935–2722
(800)962–9629

New American Library
375 Hudson Street
New York, NY 10014
(212)366–2000

W. W. Norton & Co.
500 Fifth Avenue
New York, NY 10110
(212)354–5500
(800)233–4830

Oryx Press
Suite 700
4041 North Central
Phoenix, AZ 85012
(602)265–2651
(800)279–6799.

Oxbridge Communications, Inc.
Suite 636
150 Fifth Avenue
New York, NY 10011
(212)741–0231

Palmer College of Chiropractic
1000 Brady Street
Davenport, IA 52803
(319)326–9600

Parkinson's Disease Foundation
650 West 168th Street
New York, NY 10032
(212)923–4700
(800)457–6676

Pedipress, Inc.
125 Red Gate Lane
Amherst, MA 01002
(413)549–7798
(800)344–5864

Phillips Publishing Co.
7811 Montrose Road
Potomac, MD 20854
(301)340–2100
(800)722–9000

Phobia Society of America
See Anxiety Disorders Association of
   America

PM, Inc.
PO Box 2468
Van Nuys, CA 91404
(818) 873–4399

Practice Management Information
   Corporation
Suite 300
4727 Wilshire Boulevard
Los Angeles, CA 90010
(708)920–0700
(800)633–7467

Prentice Hall Press
Order Department
200 Old Tappan Road
Old Tappan, NJ 07675
(201)767–5937
(800)223–2348

Price Stern Sloan, Inc.
Suite 650
11150 Olympic Boulevard
Los Angeles, CA 90064
(213)477–4118
(800)421–0892

Prometheus Books
700 East Amherst Street
Buffalo, NY 14215
(716)837–2475
(800)421–0351

PSG Publishing Co.
PO Box 6
545 Great Road
Littleton, MA 01460
(508)486–8971

Public Citizen's Health Research Group
Suite 700
2000 P Street NW
Washington, DC 20036
(202)872–0320

Putnam Publishing Group
200 Madison Avenue
New York, NY 10016
(212)951–8400
(800)631–8571

Quinlan Publishing Co.
23 Drydock Avenue
Boston, MA 02210
(617)542–0071
(800)229–2084

Quintessence Publishing Co.
551 N. Kimberly Drive
Carol Stream, IL 60188
(708)682–3223
(800)621–0387

Random House, Inc.
Order Department
400 Hahn Road
Westminster, MD 21157
(301)848–1900
(800)733–3000

Rittenhouse Book Distributors
511 Feheley Drive
King of Prussia, PA 19406
(215)277–1414
(800)345–6425

Rodale Press
33 East Minor Street
Emmaus, PA 18098
(215)967–5171
(800)527–8200

Royal Society of Medicine
7 East 60th Street
New York, NY 10022
(212)371–1150

W. B. Saunders Co.
Order Department
6277 Sea Harbor Drive
Orlando, FL 32821
(800)545–2522

Scott, Foresman & Co.
1900 East Lake Avenue
Glenview, IL 60025
(708)729–3000
(800)782–2665

Charles Scribner's Sons
Order Department
Front & Brown Streets
Riverside, NJ 08075
(609)461–6500
(800)257–5755

Simon & Schuster, Inc.
Order Department
200 Old Tappan Road
Old Tappan, NJ 07675
(201)767–5937
(800)223–2336

Skin Cancer Foundation
Suite 2402
245 Fifth Avenue
New York, NY 10016
(212)725–5176

M. Lee Smith, Publishers & Printers
Box 2678, Arcade Station
Nashville, TN 37219
(615)242–7395

Springhouse Corporation
See Springhouse Publishing Co.

Springhouse Publishing Co.
1111 Bethlehem Pike
Springhouse, PA 19477
(215)646–8700
(800)346–7844

Summit Books
Order Department
200 Old Tappan Road
Old Tappan, NJ 07675
(201)767–5937
(800)223–2336

Superintendent of Documents
U.S. Government Printing Office
Washington, DC 20402–9322
(202)783–3238

Jeremy P. Tarcher, Inc.
Suite 200
5858 Wilshire Boulevard
Los Angeles, CA 90036
(213)935–9980
(800)325–5525 (distributor)

Charles C Thomas, Publisher
2600 South First Street
Springfield, IL 62794
(217)789–8980

University Press of Hawaii
See University of Hawaii Press

University of Hawaii Press
2840 Kolowalu Street
Honolulu, HI 96822
(808)956–8697
Fax (808)988–6052

Van Nostrand Reinhold Co.
Order Department
7625 Empire Drive
Florence, KY 41042
(606)525–6600

Warner Books, Inc.
666 Fifth Avenue
New York, NY 10103
(212)484–3115
(800)733–3000

Williams & Wilkins
PO Box 1496
Baltimore, MD 21203
(800)638–0672

H. W. Wilson Co.
950 University Avenue
Bronx, NY 10452
(212)588–8400
(800)367–6770
(800)462–6060 (in New York)

II

Directory of Computer Database Publishers and Vendors

American Association of Retired Persons
National Gerontology Resource Center
1909 K Street NW
Washington, DC 20049
(202)728–4895
AGELINE

American Psychological Association
1400 North Uhle Street
Arlington, VA 22201
(800)336–4980
PSYCINFO

American Society of Hospital Pharmacists
4630 Montgomery Avenue
Bethesda, MD 20814
(301)657–3000
CONSUMER DRUG INFORMATION

BRS Information Technologies
8000 Westpark Drive
McLean, VA 22102
(703)442–0900
(800)289–4277
COMPREHENSIVE CORE MEDICAL
  LIBRARY

CRI Inc.
Suite 600
1400 I Street NW
Washington, DC 20005
(202)842–7600
ALCOHOL AND ALCOHOL PROBLEMS
  SCIENCE DATABASE

Combined Health Information Database
National Institutes of Health
Box NDIC (CHID)
Bethesda, MD 20892
(301)468–2162
COMBINED HEALTH INFORMATION
  DATABASE

Cumulative Index to Nursing and Allied
  Health Literature
Information Systems
1509 Wilson Terrace
PO Box 871
Glendale, CA 91209
(818)409–8005
NURSING AND ALLIED HEALTH

DIALOG Information Services, Inc.
3460 Hillview Avenue
Palo Alto, CA 94304
(800)334–2564

ECRI
5200 Butler Pike
Plymouth Meeting, PA 19462
(215)825–6000
HEALTH DEVICES ALERTS
HEALTH DEVICES SOURCEBOOK

Elsevier Science Publishers
North American Database Department
655 Avenue of the Americas
New York, NY 10010
(212)633–3971
EMBASE

Gale Research Inc.
835 Penobscot Building
Detroit, MI 48226
(800)377–4253
ENCYCLOPEDIA OF ASSOCIATIONS

IFI/Plenum Data Company
302 Swann Avenue
Alexandria, VA 22301
(800)368–3093
MENTAL HEALTH ABSTRACTS

Information Access Company
362 Lakeside Drive
Foster City, CA 94404
(800)227–8431
HEALTH PERIODICALS DATABASE
HEALTH REFERENCE CENTER
MAGAZINE INDEX

Maxwell Electronic Publishing
124 Mount Auburn Street
Cambridge, MA 02138
(800)342–1338
AIDS KNOWLEDGE BASE

National Cancer Institute
R. A. Block International Cancer
 Information Center
9030 Old Georgetown Road
Bethesda, MD 20892
(301)496–7403
PDQ: PATIENT INFORMATION FILE
PDQ; PROTOCOL FILE

National Cancer Institute
 in cooperation with
  National Library of Medicine
8600 Rockville Pike
Bethesda, MD 20894
(301)496–6193
(800)638–8480
CANCERLIT

National Library of Medicine
MEDLARS Management Section
8600 Rockville Pike
Bethesda, MD 20894
(301)496–6193
(800)638–8480
AIDSLINE
BIOETHICSLINE
CANCERLIT
DIRLINE
HEALTH PLANNING AND
 ADMINISTRATION
MEDLINE
TOXLINE

National Rehabilitation Information Center
Macro Systems Inc.
Suite 935
8455 Colesville Road
Silver Springs, MD 20910
(800)346–2742
REHABDATA

Scientific Medicine, Inc.
415 Madison Avenue
New York, NY 10017
(212)754–0805
SCIENTIFIC AMERICAN MEDICINE

Sport Information Resource Center
1600 James Naismith Drive
Gloucester, Ontario K 1B 5N4
(613)748–5658
SPORT

U.S. Department of Health and Human
   Services
Office of Smoking and Health
Park Building, Room 1–16
5600 Fishers Lane
Rockville, MD 20857
(301)443–1690
SMOKING AND HEALTH

U.S. National Institute for Occupational
   Safety and Health
Technical Information Center
4676 Columbia Parkway
Cincinnati, OH 45226
(800)356–4674
OCCUPATIONAL SAFETY AND
   HEALTH

III

Directory of Non-Governmental Health Organizations

AHEPA Cooley's Anemia Foundation
1707 L Street NW
Washington, DC 20036
(202)628–4974
(800)759–1515

Academy of Psychosomatic Medicine
5824 Magnolia
Chicago, IL 60660
(312)784–2025

Acoustic Neuroma Association
PO Box 398
Carlisle, PA 17013
(717)249–4783

Aerobics and Fitness Association of America
Suite 310
15250 Ventura Boulevard
Sherman Oaks, CA 91403
(800)445–5950

AL-ANON Family Group Headquarters
7th Floor
1372 Broadway
New, York, NY 10018
(212)302–7240

Alaska State Medical Association
4107 Laurel Street
Anchorage, AK 99508
(907)562–2662

Alcohol Education for Youth
1500 Western Avenue
Albany, NY 12203
(514)456–3800

Alcoholics Anonymous World Services
468 Park Avenue South
New York, NY 10016
(212)686–1100

Alzheimer's Disease Education and
    Referral Center
Suite 304
8737 Colesville Road
Silver Spring, MD 20910
(301)495–3311

Alzheimer's Disease and Related Disorders
    Association
70 East Lake Street
Chicago, IL 60601
(800)621–0379

American Academy of Allergy and
  Immunology
611 East Wells Street
Milwaukee, WI 53202
(414)272–6071
(800)822–2762

American Academy for Cerebral Palsy and
  Developmental Medicine
PO Box 11086
1910 Byrd Avenue
Richmond VA 23230
(804)282–0036

American Academy of Child and
  Adolescent Psychiatry
3615 Wisconsin Avenue NW
Washington, DC 20016
(202)996–7300

American Academy of Clinical Psychiatrists
PO Box 3212
San Diego, CA 92103
(619)298–4782

American Academy of Dermatology
PO Box 3116
Evanston, IL 60201
(708)869–3954

American Academy of Disability Evaluating
  Physicians
PO Box 4313
Arlington Heights, IL 60006
(708)228–6095

American Academy of Facial Plastic and
  Reconstructive Surgery
Suite 404
1101 Vermont Avenue NW
Washington, DC 20005
(202)842–4500
(800)332-FACE

American Academy of Neurology
Suite 335
2221 University Avenue SE
Minneapolis, MN 55414
(612)623–8115

American Academy of Ophthalmology
655 Beach Street
San Francisco, CA 94120
(415)561–8500

American Academy of Orthopaedic
  Surgeons
222 South Prospect
Park Ridge, IL 60068
(708)823–7186

American Academy of Otolaryngic Allergy
Suite 745
8455 Colesville Road
Silver Spring, MD 20910
(301)588–1800

American Academy of Otolaryngology—
  Head and Neck Surgery
1 Prince Street
Alexandria, VA 22314
(703)836–4444

American Academy of Pain Medicine
5700 Old Orchard Road
Skokie, IL 60077
(708)966–9510

American Academy of Pediatrics
141 Northwest Point Boulevard
Elk Grove Village, IL 60007
(708)228–5005
(800)433–9016

American Academy of Physical Medicine
  and Rehabilitation
Suite 1300
122 South Michigan Avenue
Chicago, IL 60603
(312)922–9366

American Academy of Psychoanalysis
Suite 206
30 East 40th Street
New York, NY 10016
(212)679–4105

American Alliance for Health, Physical
  Education, Recreation and Dance
  Program for the Handicapped
1900 Association Drive
Reston, VA 22091
(703)476–3400

American Amputee Foundation
PO Box 55218, Hillcrest Station
Little Rock, AR 72225
(501)666–2523

American Association for the Accreditation
  of Ambulatory Plastic Surgery Facilities
1202 Allanson Road
Mundelein, IL 60060
(708)949–6058

American Association for Acupuncture and
  Oriental Medicine
50 Maple Place
Manhasset, NY 11030
(516)627–0400

American Association of Blood Banks
1117 North 19th Street
Arlington, VA 22209
(703)528–8200

American Association of Colleges of
  Nursing
Suite 530
One Dupont Circle NW
Washington, DC 20036
(202)463–6930

American Association for Hand Surgery
Suite 210
2934 Fish Hatchery Road
Madison, WI 53713
(608)273–8940

American Association of Homes for the
  Aging
Suite 400
1129 20th Street NW
Washington, DC 20036
(202)296–5960

American Association for International
  Aging
Suite 443
1511 K Street NW
Washington, DC 20005
(202)638–6815

American Association of Kidney Patients
Suite LL1
1 Davis Blvd.
Tampa, FL 33606
(813)251–0725

American Association of Naturopathic
  Physicians
PO Box 20386
Seattle, WA 98102
(206)323–7610

American Association of Neurological
  Surgeons
22 South Washington
Park Ridge, IL 60068
(708)692–9500

American Association of Plastic Surgeons
811 Harvey, Johns Hopkins Hospitals
600 North Wolfe Street
Baltimore, MD 21205
(301)955–6897

American Association for the Study of
  Headache
PO Box 5136
San Clemente, CA 92672
(714)498–1846

American Association for the Study of Liver
  Disease
6900 Grove Road
Thorofare, NJ 08086
(609)848–1000

American Association of Suicidology
2459 South Ash
Denver, CO 80222
(303)692–0985

American Association for Thoracic Surgery
13 Elm Street
Manchester, MA 01944
(508)526–8330

American Association of Tissue Banks
Suite 220-A
1350 Beverly Road
McLean, VA 22101
(703)827–9582

American Back Society
Suite 401
2647 East 14th Street
Oakland, CA 94601
(415)536–9929

American Board of Allergy and
   Immunology
University City Science Center
3624 Market Street
Philadelphia, PA 19104
(215)349–9466

American Board of Anesthesiology
100 Constitution Plaza
Hartford, CT 06103
(203)522–9857

American Board of Colon and Rectal
   Surgery
Suite 410
875 Telegraph Road
Taylor, MI 48180
(313)295–1740

American Board of Dermatology
Henry Ford Hospital
Detroit, MI 48202
(313)871–8739

American Board of Emergency Medicine
Suite D
200 Woodland Pass
East Lansing, MI 48823
(517)332–4800

American Board of Family Practice
2228 Young Drive
Lexington, KY 40505
(606)269–5626

American Board of Internal Medicine
University City Science Center
3624 Market Street
Philadelphia, PA 19104
(215)243–1500
(800)441-ABIM

American Board of Medical Specialities
Suite 805
One Rotary Center
Evanston, IL 60201
(708)491–9091

American Board of Neurological Surgery
Smith Tower, Suite 2139
6550 Fannin Street
Houston, TX 77030
(713)790–6015

American Board of Nuclear Medicine
Room 12–200
900 Veteran Avenue
Los Angeles, CA 90024
(213)825–6787

American Board of Obstetrics and
   Gynecology
Suite 305
4225 Roosevelt Way NE
Seattle, WA 98105
(206)547–4884

American Board of Ophthalmology
Suite 241
111 Presidential Boulevard
Bala Cynwyd, PA 19004
(215)664–1175

American Board of Orthopedic Surgery
Suite 1150
737 North Michigan Avenue
Chicago, IL 60611
(312)664–9444

American Board of Otolaryngology
Suite 936
5615 Kirby Drive
Houston, TX 77005
(713)528–6200

American Board of Pathology
PO Box 25915
5401 West Kennedy Boulevard
Tampa, FL 33622
(813)286–2444

American Board of Pediatrics
111 Silver Cedar Court
Chapel Hill, NC 27514
(919)929–0461

American Board of Physical Medicine and
 Rehabilitation
Suite 674
Norwest Center
21 First Street SW
Rochester, MN 55902
(507)282–1776

American Board of Plastic Surgery
Suite 400, 7 Penn Center
1635 Market Street
Philadelphia, PA 19103
(215)587–9322

American Board of Preventive Medicine
Department of Community Medicine
Wright State University School of Medicine
PO Box 927
Dayton, OH 45401
(513)278–6915

American Board of Psychiatry and
 Neurology
Suite 335
500 Lake Cook Road
Deerfield, IL 60015
(708)945–7900

American Board of Radiology
Suite 440
300 Park Street
Birmingham, MI 48009
(313)645–0600

American Board of Surgery
Suite 860
1617 John F. Kennedy Boulevard
Philadelphia, PA 19103
(215)568–4000

American Board of Thoracic Surgery
Suite 803
1 Rotary Center
Evanston, IL 60201
(708)475–1520

American Board of Urology
Suite 150
31700 Telegraph Road
Birmingham, MI 48010
(313)646–9720

American Brittle Bone Society
1256 Merrill Drive
West Chester, PA 19382
(215)692–6248

American Burn Association
Suite B10
1130 East McDowell Road
Phoenix, AZ 85006
(602)239–2391

American Cancer Society
1599 Clifton Road NE
Atlanta, GA 30329
(404)320–3333

American Chiropractic Association
1701 Clarendon Boulevard
Arlington, VA 22201
(703)276–8800

American Cleft Palate-Craniofacial
  Association
1218 Grandview Avenue
Pittsburgh, PA 15211
(412)481–1376

American Cleft Palate Foundation
1218 Grandview Avenue
Pittsburgh, PA 15211
(800)242–5338

American Coalition of Citizens with
  Disabilities
Suite 201
1201 15th Street NW
Washington, DC 20005
(202)785–4265

American College of Allergy and
  Immunology
Suite 1080
800 East Northwest Highway
Palatine, IL 60067
(708)359–2800

American College of Cardiology
9111 Old Georgetown Road
Bethesda, MD 20814
(301)897–5400

American College of Chest Physicians
911 Busse Highway
Park Ridge, IL 60068
(708)698–2200

American College of Cryosurgery
1567 Maple Avenue
Evanston, IL 60201
(708)869–3954

American College of Emergency Physicians
PO Box 619911
Dallas, TX 75261
(214)550–0911

American College of Gastroenterology
4222 King Street
Alexandria, VA 22302
(703)549–4440

American College of Nurse-Midwives
Suite 1000
1522 K Street NW
Washington, DC 20005
(202)289–0171

American College of Obstetricians and
  Gynecologists
409 12th Street SW
Washington, DC 20024
(202)638–5577

American College of Occupational
  Medicine
55 West Seegers Road
Arlington Heights, IL 60005
(708)228–6850

American College of Radiology
1891 Preston White Drive
Reston, VA 22091
(703)648–8900

American College of Rheumatology
Suite 480
17 Executive Park Drive NE
Atlanta, GA 30329
(404)633–3777

American College of Sports Medicine
PO Box 1440
One Virginia Avenue
Indianapolis, IN 46206
(317)637–9200

American College of Surgeons
55 East Erie Street
Chicago, IL 60611
(312)664–4050

American Congress of Rehabilitation
  Medicine
Suite 1310
130 South Michigan Avenue
Chicago, IL 60603
(312)922–9368

American Council of the Blind
Suite 1100
1010 Vermont Avenue NW
Washington, DC 20005
(202)393–3666
(800)424–8666

American Council of Blind Parents
14400 Cedar
University Heights, OH 44121
(216)381–1822

American Council for Drug Education
5820 Hubbard Drive
Rockville, MD 20852
(301)984–5700

American Council of Life Insurance
Department 190
1001 Pennsylvania Avenue NW
Washington, DC 20004
(202)624–2000

American Council on Science and Health
1995 Broadway
New York, NY 10023
(212)362–7044

American Council on Transplantation
Suite 505
700 North Fairfax
Alexandria, VA 22314
(703)836–4301
(800)622–9010

American Deafness and Rehabilitation
  Association
PO Box 251554
Little Rock, AR 72225
(501)375–6643

American Dental Association
211 East Chicago Avenue
Chicago, IL 60611
(312)440–2500

American Diabetes Association
1660 Duke Street
Alexandria, VA 22314
(703)549–1500
(800)232–3472

American Dietetic Association
Suite 800
2165 West Jackson Boulevard
Chicago, IL 60606
(312)899–0040

American Epilepsy Society
Suite 304
179 Allyn Street
Hartford, CT 06130
(203)246–6566

American Fertility Society
Suite 200
2140 11th Avenue South
Birmingham, AL 35205
(205)933–8494

American Foundation for the Prevention of
  Venereal Disease
Suite 638
799 Broadway
New York, NY 10003
(212)759–2069

American Gastroenterological Association
6900 Grove Road
Thorofare, NJ 08086
(609)848–1000

American Geriatrics Society
770 Lexington
New York, NY 10021
(212)308–1414

American Hair Loss Council
4500 South Broadway
Tyler, TX 75703
(214)581–8717

American Health Assistance Foundation
15825 Shady Grove Road
Rockville, MD 20850
(800)227–7998

American Health Foundation
320 East 43rd Street
New York, NY 10017
(212)953–1900

American Heart Association
7320 Greenville Avenue
Dallas, TX 75231
(214)373–6300

American Hepatitis Association
30 East 40th Street
New York, NY 10011
(212)599–5070

American Holistic Medical Association
2002 Eastlake Avenue East
Seattle, WA 98102
(206)322–6842

American Hospital Association
840 North Lake Shore Drive
Chicago, IL 60611
(312)280–6000

American Institute of Ultrasound in
  Medicine
Suite 504
4405 East-West Highway
Bethesda, MD 20814
(301)656–6117

American Kidney Fund
Suite 1010
6110 Executive Boulevard
Rockville, MD 20852
(301)881–3052
(800)638–8299

American Laryngological Association
200 First Street SW
Rochester, MN 55906
(507)284–2369

American Laryngological, Rhinological,
  and Otological Society
PO Box 155
Bethesda Church Road
East Greenville, PA 18041
(215)679–7180

American Leprosy Foundation
Suite 210
11600 Nebel Street
Rockville, MD 20852
(301)984–1336

American Leprosy Missions
One Broadway
Elmwood Park, NJ 07407
(201)794–8650
(800)543–3131

American Liver Foundation
1425 Pompton Avenue
Cedar Grove, NJ 07009
(201)256–2550
(800)223–0179

American Lung Association
1740 Broadway
New York, NY 10019
(212)315–8700

American Medical Association
515 North State Street
Chicago, IL 60610
(312)464–4818

American Medical Records Association
Suite 1400
919 North Michigan Avenue
Chicago, IL 60611
(312)787–2672

American Medical Writers Association
Suite 410
5282 River Road
Bethesda, MD 20816
(301)493–0003

American Narcolepsy Association
PO Box 1187
San Carlos, CA 94070
(415)591–7979

American Nurses Association
2420 Pershing Road
Kansas City, MO 64108
(816)474–5720

American Optometric Association
243 North Lindbergh Boulevard
St. Louis. MO 63141
(314)991–4100

American Orthopaedic Association
222 South Prospect
Park Ridge, IL 60068
(708)698–1640

American Orthopaedic Society for Sports
  Medicine
70 West Hubbard
Chicago, IL 60610
(312)644–2623

American Osteopathic Association
142 East Ontario
Chicago, IL 60611
(312)280–5800

American Otological Society
Loyola University of Chicago Medical
  Center
Building 105, Room 1870
2160 South First Avenue
Maywood, IL 60153
(708)216–9183

American Pain Society
PO Box 186
Skokie, IL 60076
(708)475–7300

American Pancreatic Association
Department of Surgery
University of Missouri Health Sciences
  Center
Columbia, MO 65212
(314)882–7942

American Parkinson Disease Association
116 John Street
New York, NY 10038
(800)223–2732

American Pediatric Surgical Association
Children's Hospital National Medical
  Center
111 Michigan Avenue NW
Washington, DC 20010
(202)745–2153

American Pharmaceutical Association
2215 Constitution Avenue NW
Washington, DC 20037
(202)628–4410

American Physical Therapy Association
111 North Fairfax Street
Alexandria, VA 22314
(703)684–2784

American Podiatric Medical Association
9312 Old Georgetown Road
Bethesda, MD 20814
(301)571–9200

American Porphyria Foundation
PO Box 11163
Montgomery, AL 36111
(205)265–2200

American Psychiatric Association
1400 K Street NW
Washington, DC 20005
(202)682–6000

American Psychoanalytic Association
309 49th Street
New York, NY 10017
(212)752–0450

American Psychological Association
1200 17th Street NW
Washington, DC 20036
(202)955–7600

American Public Health Association
1015 15th Street NW
Washington, DC 20005
(202)789–5600

American Red Cross
17th and D Streets NW
Washington, DC 20006
(202)737–8300

American Reye's Syndrome Association
Suite 203
701 Logan Street
Denver, CO 80209
(303)777–2592

American Rhinological Society
Suite 105
2929 Baltimore Street
Kansas City, MO 64108
(816)561–4423

American School Health Association
PO Box 708
Kent, OH 44240
(216)678–1601

American Sleep Disorders Association
604 Second Street SW
Rochester, MN 55902
(507)287–6006

American Social Health Association
PO Box 13827
Research Triangle Park, NC 27709
(919)361–2742

American Society of Abdominal Surgeons
675 Main Street
Melrose, MA 02176
(617)665–6102

American Society on Aging
Suite 516
833 Market Street
San Francisco, CA 94103
(415)543–2617

American Society of Allied Health
   Professions
Suite 700
1101 Connecticut Avenue NW
Washington, DC 20036
(202)857–1150

American Society of Cataract and
   Refractive Surgery
Suite 108
3700 Pender Drive
Fairfax, VA 22030
(703)591–2220

American Society of Clinical Hypnosis
Suite 336
2250 East Devon Avenue
Des Plaines, IL 60018
(708)297–3317

American Society of Colon and Rectal
   Surgery
Suite 1080
800 East Northwest Highway
Palatine, IL 60067
(708)359–9184

American Society for Dermatologic Surgery
PO Box 3116
Evanston, IL 60204
(708)869–3954
(800)441-ASDS

American Society for Gastrointestinal
   Endoscopy
13 Elm Street
Manchester, MA 01944
(508)526–8330

American Society of Hematology
6900 Grove Road
Thorofare, NJ 08086
(609)845–0003

American Society for Laser Medicine and
  Surgery
2404 Stewart Square
Wausau, WI 54401
(715)845–9283

American Society of Lipo-Suction Surgery
1455 City Line Avenue
Philadelphia, PA 19151
(215)896–6677

American Society of Maxillofacial Surgeons
444 East Algonquin Road
Arlington Heights, IL 60005
(708)228–9900

American Society of Plastic and
  Reconstructive Surgeons
444 East Algonquin Road
Arlington Heights, IL 60005
(708)228–9900
(800)635–0635

American Society for Psychoprophylaxis in
  Obstetrics
(ASPO/Lamaze)
Suite 204
1840 Wilson Boulevard
Arlington, VA 22201
(703)524–7802

American Society for Surgery of the Hand
3025 South Parker Road
Aurora, CO 80014
(303)755–4588

American Society for Therapeutic
  Radiology and Oncology
1891 Preston White Drive
Reston, VA 22091
(703)648–8903

American Society of Transplant Surgeons
716 Lee Street
Des Plaines, IL 60016
(708)824–5700

American Speech-Language-Hearing
  Association
10801 Rockville Pike
Rockville, MD 20852
(301)897–5700
(800)638–8255

American Sudden Infant Death Syndrome
  Institute
275 Carpenter Drive
Atlanta, GA 30328
(800)232-SIDS

American Thyroid Association
Mayo Clinic
200 First Street SW
Rochester, MN 55905
(507)284–4738

American Tinnitus Association
PO Box 5
1618 SW First Street
Portland, OR 97207
(503)248–9985

American Trauma Society
Suite 188
1400 Mercantile Lane
Landover, MD 20785
(800)556–7890

American Urological Association
1120 North Charles Street
Baltimore, MD 21201
(301)727–1100

Amputee Services Association
6613 North Clark Street
Chicago, IL 60626
(312)274–2044

Amyotrophic Lateral Sclerosis Association
Suite 321
21021 Ventura Boulevard
Woodland Hills, CA 91364
(818)990–2151

Anorexia Nervosa and Related Eating
  Disorders
PO Box 5102
Eugene, OR 97405
(503)344–1144

Anxiety Disorders Association of America
Suite 513
6000 Executive Boulevard
Rockville, MD 20852
(301)231–9350
(900)737–3400

Aquatic Exercise Association
PO Box 497
Port Washington, WI 53074
(414)284–3416

Arizona Medical Association
810 West Bethany Home Road
Phoenix, AZ 85013
(602)246–8901

Arkansas Medical Society
Suite 300
10 Corporate Hill
PO Box 5776
Little Rock, AR 72215
(501)224–8967

Arthritis Foundation
1314 Spring Street NW
Atlanta, GA 30309
(404) 872–7100

Asbestos Information Association of North
  America
Suite 509
1745 Jefferson Davis Highway
Arlington, VA 22202
(703)979–1150

Asbestos Victims of America
2715 Porter Street
Soquel, CA 95073
(408)476–3646

Asociación de Médicos Mexicanos
  (Mexican Medical Association)
Santiago Papasquiaro
140 Sur Zana Industrial
Gomez Palacio, DGO, Mexico

Asociación Nacional por Personas Mayores
  (National Association for Hispanic
  Elderly)
Suite 270
2727 West Sixth Street
Los Angeles, Ca 90057
(213)487–1922

Association of American Medical Colleges
Suite 200
One DuPont Circle NW
Washington, DC 20036
(202)828–0400

Association of Applied Physiology and
  Biofeedback
Suite 304
10200 West 44th Avenue
Wheat Ridge, CO 80303
(303)422–8436

Association of Birth Defect Children
Suite 270
5400 Diplomat Circle
Orlando, FL 32810
(407)629–1466

Association for the Care of Children's
  Health
3615 Wisconsin Avenue NW
Washington, DC 20016
(202)224–1801

Association for Macular Diseases
210 East 64th Street
New York, NY 10021
(212)605–3719

Association of Medical Illustrators
2692 Huguenot Springs Road
Midlothian, VA 23113
(804)794–2908

Asthma and Allergy Foundation of America
Suite 305
1717 Massachusetts Avenue NW
Washington, DC 20036
(202)265–0265

BASH (Bulimia Anorexia Self-Help)
Deaconess Hospital
6150 Oakland Avenue
St. Louis, MO 63139
(314)768–3838
(800)762–3334

British Medical Association
BMA House, Tavistock Square
London, WC1H 9JP, England
(01)387–4499

California Medical Association
221 Main Street
PO Box 7690
San Francisco, CA 94120
(415)541–0900

Canadian Medical Association
1867 Alta Vista Drive
PO Box 8650
Ottawa, Ontario K16 0G8
(613)731–9331

Candelighters Childhood Cancer
   Foundation
Suite 1001
1901 Pennsylvania Avenue NW
Washington, DC 20006
(202)659–5136

Candida Research and Information
   Foundation
Box 2719
Castro Valley, CA 94546
(415)582–2179

CAPS (Children of Aging Parents)
2761 Trenton Road
Levittown, PA 19056
(215)945–6900

Care Medico
660 First Avenue
New York, NY 10016
(212)686–3110

Celiac Sprue Society
PO Box 31700
Omaha, NE 68131
(402)558–0600

Center for Dance Medicine
Room 200
41 East 42nd Street
New York, NY 10017
(212)661–8401

Center for Science in the Public Interest
1501 16th Street NW
Washington, DC 20036
(202)332–9110

Center for Sickle Cell Disease
Howard University
2121 Georgia Avenue NW
Washington, DC 20059
(202)636–7930

Center for the Study of Multiple Birth
Suite 476
333 East Superior Street
Chicago, IL 60611
(312)266–9093

Children in Hospitals
31 Wilshire Park
Needham, MA 02192
(617)444–3877

Children's Defense Fund
Suite 400
122 C Street NW
Washington, DC 20001
(202)628–8787

Children's Hospice International
Suite 131
1101 King Street
Alexandria, VA 22314
(703)684–0330

Children's Transplant Association
PO Box 53699
Dallas, TX 75253
(214)287–8484

Choice in Dying
200 Varick Street
New York, NY 10014
(212)366–5540

Chronic Fatigue Immune Dysfunction
  Syndrome Association
PO Box 220398
Charlotte, NC 28222
(704)362–2343

Chronic Fatigue Immune Dysfunction
  Syndrome Society
PO Box 230108
Portland, OR 97223
(503)684–5261

Citizens for the Treatment of High Blood
  Pressure
Suite 904
888 17th Street NW
Washington, DC 20006
(202)466–4553

Clearinghouse on Child Abuse and Neglect
8201 Greensboro Drive
McLean, VA 22102
(703)821–2086

College of American Pathologists
325 Waukegan Road
Northfield, IL 60093
(708)446–8800

Colorado Medical Society
PO Box 17550
Denver, Co 80217
(303)779–5455

Community Nutrition Institute
2001 S Street NW
Washington, DC 20009
(202)462–4700

Compassionate Friends
PO Box 3696
Oakbrook, IL 60522
(708)990–0010

Connecticut State Medical Society
160 St. Ronan Street
New Haven, CT 06511
(203)865–0587

Contact Lens Association of
  Ophthalmologists
Suite 1
523 Decatur Street
New Orleans, LA 70130
(504)581–4000

Cornelia De Lange Syndrome Foundation
60 Dyer Avenue
Collinsville, CT 06022
(800)223–8355

Council of Better Business Bureaus
4200 Wilson Boulevard
Arlington, VA 22203
(703)276–0100

Council on Teaching Hospitals
One DuPont Circle NW
Washington, DC 20036
(202)828–0490

Cri du Chat Syndrome Society
11609 Oakmont
Overland Park, KS 66210
(913)469–8900

Cystic Fibrosis Foundation
6931 Arlington Road
Bethesda, MD 20814
(301)951–4422

D.E.B.R.A. (Dystrophic Epidermolysis
  Bullosa Research Association) of America
Suite 7-South
141 Fifth Avenue
New York, NY 10010
(212)995–2220

Deafness Research Foundation
9 East 38th Street
New York, NY 10016
(212)684–6559 (TDD/TT)
(800)535–3323

Drug Information Association
PO Box 3113
Maple Glen, PA 19002
(215)628–2288

EAR Foundation
2000 Church Street
Nashville, TN 37236
(615)329–7809
(800)545-HEAR

Endocrine Society
9650 Rockville Pike
Bethesda, MD 20814
(301)571–1802

Endometriosis Association
8585 North 76th Place
Milwaukee, WI 53223
(414)355–2200
(800)992-ENDO

Epilepsy Foundation of America
Suite 406
4351 Garden City Drive
Landover, MD 20785
(301)459–3700

Eye Bank Association of America
Suite 308
1725 Eye Street NW
Washington, DC 20006
(202)775–4999

Familial Polyposis Registry
Department of Colorectal Surgery
Cleveland Clinic Foundation
9500 Euclid Avenue
Cleveland, OH 44195
(216)444–6470

Federation of the Handicapped
211 West 14th Street
New York, NY 10011
(212)206–4200

Fertility Research Foundation
Suite 103
1430 Second Avenue
New York, NY 10021
(212)744–5500

Florida Medical Association
760 Riverside Avenue
PO Box 2411
Jacksonville, FL 32203
(904)356–1571

Flying Wheels Travel
PO Box 382
143 West Bridge
Owatonna, MN 55060
(800)533–0363

Fragile X Foundation
PO Box 300233
Denver, CO 80220
(800)835–2246

Friedreich's Ataxia Group in America
PO Box 11116
Oakland, CA 94611
(415)655–0833

Gastroplasty Support Group
657 Irvington Avenue
Newark, NJ 07106
(201)374–1717

Gerontological Society of America
Suite 350
1275 K Street NW
Washington, DC 20005
(202)842-1275

Grief Education Institute
2422 South Downing Street
Denver, CO 80210
(303)759-6048

Guam Medical Society
PO Box 8718
Tamuning, GU 96911
(671)646-5824

Guide Dog Foundation for the Blind
   Training Center
371 East Jericho Turnpike
Smithtown, NY 11787
(516)265-2121

Hawaii Medical Association
1360 South Beretania Street
Honolulu, HI 96814
(808)536-7702

Health Insurance Association of America
1025 Connecticut Avenue NW
Washington, DC 20036
(202)223-7780

Healthcare Abroad
243 Church Street West
Vienna, VA 22180
(703)281-9500
(800)237-6615

Helen Keller National Center for
   Deaf-Blind Youths and Adults
111 Middle Neck Road
Sands Point, NY 11050
(516)944-8900

Hemlock Society
PO Box 11830
Eugene, OR 97440
(503)342-5748

Hemochromatosis Research Foundation
PO Box 8569
Albany, NY 12208
(518)489-0972

HIP (Help for Incontinent People)
PO Box 544
Union, SC 29379
(803)585-8789

Human Growth Foundation
4720 Montgomery Lane
Bethesda, MD 20814
(301)656-7540

Huntington's Disease Society of America
140 West 22nd Street
New York, NY 10011
(212)242-1968
(800)345-4372

Idaho Medical Association
PO Box 2668
Boise, ID 83701
(208)344-7888

Illinois State Medical Society
Suite 700
20 North Michigan Avenue
Chicago, IL 60602
(312)782-1654

Indiana State Medical Association
3935 North Meridian Street
Indianapolis, IN 46208
(317)925-7545

International Association for Medical
   Assistance to Travelers
417 Center Street
Lewiston, NY 14092
(716)754-4883

International Association for the Study of
   Pain
Suite 306
909 NE 43rd Street
Seattle, WA 98105
(206)547-6409

International Childbirth Education
  Association
PO Box 20048
Minneapolis, MN 55420
(612)854–8660

International College of Surgeons
1516 North Lake Shore Drive
Chicago, IL 60610
(312)787–6274

International Hearing Dog Association
5901 East 89th Avenue
Henderson, CO 80640
(303)287–3277

International Ménière's Disease Research
  Institute
Suite 400
300 East Hampden Avenue
Englewood, CO 80110
(800)637–6646

Iowa Medical Society
1001 Grand Avenue
West Des Moines, IA 50265
(515)223–1401

Iron Overload Diseases Association
Suite 911
224 Datura Street
West Palm Beach, FL 33401
(407)659–5616

Joint Commission on Accreditation of
  Health Care
Organizations (JCAHO)
One Renaissance Boulevard
Oakbrook Terrace, IL 60181
(708)916–5600

Juvenile Diabetes Foundation
432 Park Avenue
New York, NY 10016
(212)889–7575
(800)223–1138

Kansas Medical Society
1300 Topeka Avenue
Topeka, KS 66612
(913)235–2383

Kentucky Medical Association
3532 Ephraim McDowell Drive
Louisville, KY 40205
(502)459–9790

La Leche League International
9616 Minneapolis Avenue
Franklin Park, IL 60131
(708)455–7730

Leukemia Society of America
733 Third Avenue
New York, NY 10017
(212)573–8484

Lion's Clubs International
300 22nd Street
Oakbrook, IL 60570
(708)986–1700

Living Bank
PO Box 6725
Houston, TX 77265
(800)528–2971
(800)527–2971

Louisiana State Medical Society
1700 Josephine Street
New Orleans, LA 70113
(504)561–1033

Lupus Foundation of America
Suite 203
1717 Massachusetts Avenue NW
Washington, DC 20036
(202)328–4550
(800)558–0121

Lyme Borreliosis Foundation
PO Box 462
Tolland, CT 06084
(203)871–2900

Maine Medical Association
PO Box 190
Manchester, ME 04351
(207)622–3374

March of Dimes Birth Defects Foundation
1275 Mamaroneck Avenue
White Plains, NY 10605
(914)428–7100
(800)533–9255

Massachusetts Medical Society
1440 Main Street
Waltham, MA 02154
(617)893–4610

Medic Alert Foundation
2323 Colorado
Turlock, CA 95380
(209)668–3333

Medic Alert Organ Donor Program
  Foundation
PO Box 1009
Turlock, CA 95381
(209)668–3333

Medical Association of Georgia
938 Peachtree Street NE
Atlanta, GA 30309
(404)876–7535

Medical Association of the State of Alabama
19 South Jackson Street
PO Box 1900
Montgomery, AL 36102
(202)263–6441

Medical & Chirurgical Faculty of the State
  of Maryland
1211 Cathedral Street
Baltimore, MD 21201
(301)539–0872

Medical Passport Foundation
PO Box 820
De Land, FL 32720
(904)734–0639

Medical Society of Delaware
1925 Lovering Avenue
Wilmington, DE 19806
(302)658–7596

Medical Society of the District of Columbia
Suite 400
1701 L Street NW
Washington, DC 20036
(202)466–1800

Medical Society of New Jersey
2 Princess Road
Lawrenceville, NJ 08648
(609)896–1766

Medical Society of the State of New York
420 Lakeville Road
Lake Success, NY 11042
(516)488–6100

Medical Society of Virginia
4205 Dover Road
Richmond, VA 23221
(804)353–2721

Michigan Medical Society
120 West Saginaw
East Lansing, MI 48823
(517)337–1351

Minnesota Medical Association
Suite 400
2221 University Avenue SE
Minneapolis, MN 55414
(612)378–1875

Mississippi State Medical Association
735 Riverside Drive
Jackson, MS 39202
(601)354–5433

Missouri State Medical Association
113 Madison Street
PO Box 1028
Jefferson City, MO 65102
(314)636–5151

Mobility International
PO Box 3551
Eugene, OR 97403
(503)343–1284

Montana Medical Association
2021 11th Avenue
Helena, MT 59601
(406)443–4000

Muscular Dystrophy Association
810 Seventh Avenue
New York, NY 10019
(212)586–0808

Myasthenia Gravis Foundation
Suite 1352
53 West Jackson
Chicago, IL 60604
(800)541–5454

Narcolepsy and Cataplexy Foundation of
America
Suite 2D
1410 New York Avenue
New York, NY 10021
(212)628–6315

Narcotics Anonymous
PO Box 9999
Van Nuys, CA 91409
(818)780–3951

Narcotics Educational Foundation of
America
5055 Sunset Boulevard
Los Angeles, CA 90027
(213)663–5171

National Alliance of Blind Students
Suite 1100
1010 Vermont Avenue NW
Washington, DC 20005
(800)424–8666

National Alliance of Breast Cancer
Organizations
1180 Avenue of the Americas
New York, NY 10036
(212)719–0154

National Alliance for the Mentally Ill
Suite 500
1901 North Fort Myer Drive
Arlington, VA 22209
(703)524–7600

National Alopecia Areata Foundation
Suite 216
714 C Street
San Rafael, CA 94901
(415)456–4644

National Association to Aid Fat Americans
PO Box 188620
Sacramento, CA 95818
(916)443–0303

National Association of Anorexia Nervosa
and Associated Disorders
Box 271
Highland Park, IL 60035
(708)831–3438

National Association of Disability Examiners
3299 K Street NW
Washington, DC 20007
(202)965–1544

National Association of Insurance
Commissioners
Suite 1100
120 West 12th Street
Kansas City, MO 64105
(816)842–3600

National Association for Sickle Cell Disease
Suite 360
4221 Wilshire Boulevard
Los Angeles, CA 90010
(213)936–7205
(800)421–8453

National Asthma Center
National Jewish Center for Immunology
  and Respiratory Medicine
1400 Jackson Street
Denver, CO 80206
(800) 222-Lung

National Brain Research Association
1439 Rhode Island Avenue NW
Washington, DC 20005
(202) 483-6272

National Brain Tumor Foundation
Suite 510
323 Geary Street
San Francisco, CA 94102
(415) 296-0404

National Captioning Institute
5203 Leesburg Pike
Falls Church, VA 22014
(703) 998-2400

National Center and Caucus on Black Aged
  (NCBA)
Suite 500
1424 K Street NW
Washington, DC 20005
(202) 637-8400

National Center for Education in Maternal
  and Child Health
38th and R Streets NW
Washington, DC 20057
(202) 625-8400

National Center for Health Education
30 East 29th Street
New York, NY 10016
(212) 689-1886

National Center for Homecare Education
  and Research
350 Fifth Avenue
New York, NY 10011
(212) 560-3300

National Center for Homeopathy
Suite 42
1500 Massachusetts Avenue NW
Washington, DC 20005
(202) 223-6182

National Child Safety Council
PO Box 1368
Jackson, MI 49204
(800) 222-1464

National Chronic Pain Outreach
  Association
8222 Wycliffe Court
Manassas, VA 22110
(703) 368-7353

National Coalition Against the Misuse of
  Pesticides
530 7th Street SE
Washington, DC 20003
(202) 543-5450

National Commission for the Certification
  for Acupuncture
Suite 105
1424 16th Street NW
Washington, DC 20036
(202) 232-1404

National Committee for Prevention of
  Child Abuse
Suite 950
332 South Michigan Avenue
Chicago, IL 60604
(312) 663-3520

National Council Against Health Fraud
PO Box 1276
Loma Linda, CA 92354
(714) 824-4690

National Council on the Aging
West Wing 100
600 Maryland Avenue SW
Washington, DC 20024
(202) 479-1200

National Council on Alcoholism
12 West 21st Street
New York, NY 10010
(212)206–6770
(800)NCA-CALL

National Council for International Health
Suite 600
1701 K Street, NW
Washington, DC 20006
(202)833–5900

National Council on Patient Information
  and Education
Suite 810
666 11th Street NW
Washington, DC 20001
(202)347–6711

National Council of Senior Citizens
925 15th Street NW
Washington, DC 20005
(202)347–8800

National Council on Stuttering
9242 Gross Point Road
Skokie, IL 60077
(708)677–8280

National Depressive and Manic Depressive
  Association
Suite 2812
222 South Riverside Plaza
Chicago, IL 60606
(312)993–0066

National Down's Syndrome Society
141 Fifth Avenue
New York, NY 10010
(212)460–9330
(800)221–4602

National Easter Seal Society
70 East Lake Street
Chicago, IL 60601
(312)726–6200

National Eye Research Foundation
Suite 207A
910 Skokie Boulevard
Northbrook, IL 60062
(708)564–4652

National Federation of Parents for
  Drug-Free Youth
Suite 200
8730 Georgia Avenue
Silver Spring, MD 20910
(301)585–5437

National Fitness Foundation
Suite 412
2250 East Imperial Highway
El Segundo, CA 90245
(213)640–0145

National Foundation of Dentistry for the
  Handicapped
Suite 1420
1600 Stout Street
Denver, CO 80202
(303)573–0264

National Foundation for Ectodermal
  Dysplasia
Suite 311
108 North First Street
Mascoutah, IL 62258
(618)566–2020

National Foundation for Ileitis and Colitis
444 Park Avenue South
New York, NY 10016
(212)685–3440

National Foundation for Infectious Diseases
Suite 750
4733 Bethesda Avenue
Bethesda, MD 20814
(301)656–0003

National Gaucher Foundation
1424 K Street NW
Washington, DC 20005
(202)393–2777

National Head Injury Foundation
333 Turnpike Road
Southborough, MA 01772
(508)485–9950

National Headache Foundation
5252 North Western Avenue
Chicago, IL 60625
(312)878–7715
(800)843–2256

National Health Council
Suite 1118
350 Fifth Avenue
New York, NY 10018
(212)268–8900

National Healthcare Anti-Fraud Association
Suite 800
1255 23rd Street NW
Washington, DC 20037
(202)659–5955

National Hearing Aid Society
20361 Middlebelt
Livonia, MI 48152
(800)521–5247

National Hemophilia Foundation
110 Green Street
New York, NY 10012
(212)219–8180

National Hypoglycemia Association
PO Box 120
Ridgewood, NJ 07451
(201)670–1189

National Indian Council on Aging
PO Box 2088
Albuquerque, NM 87103
(505)766–2276

National Information Center for Orphan
  Drugs and Rare Diseases
PO Box 1133
Washington, DC 20013
(800)336–4797

National Insurance Consumer Organization
121 North Payne Street
Alexandria, VA 22314
(703)549–8050

National Kidney Foundation
30 East 33rd Street
New York, NY 10016
(212)889–2210

National League of Nursing
10 Columbus Circle
New York, NY 10019
(212)582–1022

National Leukemia Association
Suite 536
585 Stewart Avenue
Garden City, NY 11530
(516)222–1944

National Lipid Diseases Foundation
1201 Corbin Street
Elizabeth, NJ 07201
(201)527–8000

National Lupus Erythematosus Foundation
5430 Van Nuys Boulevard
Van Nuys, CA 91401
(818)885–8787

National Marfan Foundation
382 Main Street
Port Washington, NY 11050
(516)883–8712

National Multiple Sclerosis Society
205 East 42nd Street
New York, NY 10017
(212)986–3240
(800)624–8236

National Neurofibromatosis Foundation
Suite 7-S
141 Fifth Avenue
New York, NY 10010
(800)323–7938

National Odd Shoe Exchange
2242 West Keim Drive
Phoenix, AZ 85015
(602)246–8725

National Organization of Mothers of Twins
  Clubs
12404 Princess Jeanne NE
Albuquerque, NM 87112
(505)275–0955

National Organization for Rare Disorders
PO Box 8923
New Fairfield, CT 06812
(203)746–6518

National Osteoporosis Foundation
Suite 822
1625 I Street NW
Washington, DC 20006
(202)223–2226

National Pacific/Asian Resource Center on
  Aging
Suite 410
2033 Sixth Avenue
Seattle, WA 98121
(206)448–0313

National Parent-Teachers Association
700 North Rush Street
Chicago, IL 60610
(312)787–0977

National Parkinson Association
1501 NW 9th Avenue
Miami, FL 33136
(305)547–6666
(800)327–4545

National Rehabilitation Association
633 South Washington Street
Alexandria, VA 22314
(703)836–0850

National Retinitis Pigmentosa Foundation
1401 Mt. Royal Avenue
Baltimore, MD 21217
(301)225–9400
(800)638–2300

National Reye's Syndrome Foundation
426 North Lewis
Bryan, OH 43506
(800)233–7393

National Safe Workplace Institute
Suite 1450
122 South Michigan Avenue
Chicago, IL 60603
(312)939–0690

National Scoliosis Foundation
PO Box 547
93 Concord Avenue
Belmont, MA 02178
(617)489–0880

National Self-Help Clearinghouse
Room 620
25 West 43rd Street
New York, NY 10036
(212)642–2944

National Society for Children and Adults
  with Autism
Suite 1017
1234 Massachusetts Avenue NW
Washington, DC 20005
(202)783–0125

National Society to Prevent Blindness
500 East Remington Road
Schaumberg, IL 60173
(708)843–2020

National Spinal Cord Injury Association
600 West Cummings Park
Woburn, MA 01801
(617)935–2722
(800)962–9629

National Stroke Association
300 East Hampden Avenue
Englewood, Co 80110
(303)762–9922

National Sudden Infant Death Syndrome
Foundation
10500 Little Patuxent Parkway
Columbia, MD 21044
(301)964–8000
(800)221-SIDS

National Tay-Sachs and Allied Diseases
Association
385 Elliot Street
Newton, MA 02164
(617)964–5508

National Tuberous Sclerosis Association
Suite 660
4351 Garden City Drive
Landover, MD 20785
(800)225–6872

National Vitiligo Foundation
Texas American Bank Building
PO Box 6337
Tyler, TX 75711
(214)561–4700

National Wheelchair Athletic Association
Suite S
3617 Betty Drive
Colorado Springs, CO 80917
(303)597–8330

National Wheelchair Basketball Association
University of Kentucky
110 Seaton Building
Lexington, NY 40506
(606)275–1623

Nebraska Medical Association
1512 FirstTier Bank Building
Lincoln, NE 68508
(402)474–4472

Nevada State Medical Association
Suite 101
3660 Baker Lane
Reno, NV 89509
(702)825–6788

New Hampshire Medical Society
4 Park Street
Concord, NH 03301
(603)224–1909

New Mexico Medical Society
Suite 400
7770 Jefferson Street NE
Albuquerque, NM 87109
(505)828–0237

North American Riding for the
Handicapped Association
Box 100
Ashburn, VA 22011
(703)478–1075

North Carolina Medical Society
222 North Person Street
PO Box 27167
Raleigh, NC 27611
(919)833–3836

North Dakota Medical Association
PO Box 1198
Bismarck, ND 58502
(701)223–9475

The OCD Foundation
PO Box 9573
New Haven, CT 06535
(203) 772–0565

Ohio State Medical Association
1500 Lake Shore Drive
Columbus, OH 43204
(614)486–2401

Oklahoma State Medical Association
601 NW Expressway
Oklahoma City, OK 73118
(405)843–9571

Older Women's League
Suite 300
730 11th Street NW
Washington, DC 20001
(202)783–6686

Oregon Medical Association
5210 SW Corbett Street
Portland, OR 97201
(503)226–1555

Orton Dyslexia Society
724 York Road
Baltimore, MD 21204
(301)296–0232
(800)ABCD-123

Osteogenesis Imperfecta Foundation
PO Box 14807
Clearwater, FL 34629
(813)855–7077

Paget's Disease Foundation
165 Cadman Plaza East
Brooklyn, NY 11201
(718)596–1043

Parkinson Support Group of America
11376 Cherry Hill Road
Beltsville, MD 20705
(301)937–1545

PASS Group (Panic Attack Sufferers'
  Support Group)
PO Box 1614
Williamsville, NY 14221
(716)689–4399

Pennsylvania Medical Society
777 East Park Drive
PO Box 8820
Harrisburg, PA 17105
(717)558–7750

Planned Parenthood Federation of America
810 Seventh Avenue
New York, NY 10019
(212)541–7800

Polio Survivors Association
12720 La Reina Avenue
Downey, CA 90242
(213)923–0034

Post-Polio League for Information
Suite 204
5432 Connecticut Avenue NW
Washington, DC 20015
(202)653–5010

Potsmokers Anonymous
316 East Third Street
New York, NY 10009
(212)254–1777

Premenstrual Syndrome Action
PO Box 16292
Irvine, CA 92716
(714)854–4407

President's Council on Physical Fitness and
  Sports
Suite 7103
450 5th Street NW
Washington, DC 20001
(202)272–3421

Public Citizen Health Research Group
2000 P Street NW
Washington, DC 20036
(202)872–0320

Public Voice for Food and Health Policy
Suite 522
1001 Connecticut Avenue NW
Washington, DC 20036
(202)659–5930

Puerto Rico Medical Association
Box 9387
Santurce, PR 00908
(809)721–6969

Rachel Carson Council
8940 Jones Mill Road
Chevy Chase, MD 20815
(301)652–1877

Radiological Society of North America
2021 Spring Street
Oakbrook, IL 60521
(708)571-2670

Rehabilitation International
25 East 21st Street
New York, NY 10010
(212)420-1500

Resolve
PO Box 474
Belmont, MA 02178
(617)484-2424

Rhode Island Medical Society
106 Francis Street
Providence, RI 02903
(401)331-3207

Royal College of Physicians
11 St. Andrew's Place
London NW1 4LE, England
(01)935-1174

Royal College of Surgeons
35-43 Lincoln's Inn Fields
London WC2A 3PN, England
(01)405-3474

Sarcoidosis Family Aid and Research
   Foundation
760 Clinton Avenue
Newark, NJ 07108
(800)223-6429

The Scoliosis Association
PO Box 51353
Raleigh, NC 27609
(919)846-2639

SHHH (Self Help for Hard of Hearing
   People)
7800 Wisconsin Avenue
Bethesda, MD 20814
(301)657-2248

SIECUS (Sex Information and Education
   Council of the U.S.)
Room 52
32 Washington Place
New York, NY 10003
(212)673-3850

Simon Foundation
PO Box 815
Wilmette, IL 60091
(800)23-SIMON

Sjögren's Syndrome Foundation
382 Main Street
Port Washington, NY 11050
(516)767-2866

Skin Cancer Foundation
475 Park Avenue South
New York, NY 10016
(212)725-5176

Society for the Advancement of Travel for
   the Handicapped
26 Court Street
Brooklyn, NY 11242
(718)858 5183

Society for Investigative Dermatology
Room 269, Building 100
1001 Potrero Street
San Francisco, CA 94110
(415)647-3992

Society of Thoracic Surgeons
Suite 600
111 East Wacker Drive
Chicago, IL 60601
(312)644-6610

Society for Vascular Surgery
13 Elm Street
Manchester, MA 01944
(508)526-8330

South Carolina Medical Association
PO Box 11188
Columbia, SC 29211
(803)798-6207

South Dakota State Medical Association
1323 South Minnesota Avenue
Sioux Falls, SD 57105
(605)336–1965

Spina Bifida Association of America
Suite 540
1700 Rockville Pike
Rockville, MD 20852
(301)770–7222
(800)621–3141

Spinal Cord Society
2410 Lakeview Drive
Fergus Falls, MN 56537
(218)739–5252

State Medical Society of Wisconsin
PO Box 1109
Madison, WI 53701
(608)257–6781

The Stroke Foundation
898 Park Avenue
New York, NY 10021
(212)734–3461

Stuttering Resource Foundation
123 Oxford
New Rochelle, NY 10804
(800)232–4773

Sudden Infant Death Syndrome
  Clearinghouse
8201 Greensboro
McLean, VA 22102
(703)821–8955

Surrogate Parent Foundation
Suite 750D
8383 Wilshire Boulevard
Beverly Hills, CA 90211
(213)824–4723

Tennessee Medical Association
112 Louise Avenue
Nashville, TN 37203
(615)327–1451

Texas Medical Association
1801 North Lamar Boulevard
Austin, TX 78701
(512)477–6704

Tourette's Syndrome Association
42–40 Bell Boulevard
Bayside, NY 11361
(800)237–0717

Travel Health Information Service
5827 West Washington Boulevard
Milwaukee, WI 53208
(414)774–4600
(800)433–5256

Twinline
Suite 234
2131 University Avenue
Berkeley, CA 94704
(415)644–0861

U.S.P.C. (United States Pharmacopeial
  Convention)
PO Box 5367, Twinbrook Station
Rockville, MD 20851
(800)227–8772

Undersea and Hyperbaric Medical Society
9650 Rockville Pike
Bethesda, MD 20814
(301)571–1818

United Cerebral Palsy Association
7 Penn Plaza
New York, NY 10001
(212)268–6655
(800)USA-5UCP

United Ostomy Association
Suite 120
36 Executive Park
Irvine, CA 92714
(714)476–0268

United Scleroderma Foundation
PO Box 350
Watsonville, CA 95077
(408)728–2202
(800)722-HOPE

Utah Medical Association
540 East 500 Street South
Salt Lake City, UT 84102
(801)355–7477

Vermont State Medical Society
Box H
136 Main Street
Montpelier, VT 05601
(802)223–7898

Virgin Islands Medical Society
PO Box 5986
St. Croix, VI 00823
(809)778–5305

Washington State Medical Association
Suite 900
2033 Sixth Avenue
Seattle, WA 98121
(206)441–9762

Wegener's Granulomatosis Support Group
PO Box 1518
Platte City, MO 64079
(816)431–2096

West Virginia State Medical Association
PO Box 4106
Charleston, WV 25364
(304)925–0342

Wilderness Medical Society
PO Box 397
Point Reyes Station, CA 94956
(415)663–9107

Women's Sports Foundation
Suite 720
342 Madison Avenue
New, York, NY 10017
(800)227–3988

Wyoming Medical Society
PO Drawer 4009
Cheyenne, WY 82003
(307)635–2424

Xeroderma Pigmentosum Registry
Department of Pathology
Medical Science Building, Room C 520
University of Medicine and Dentistry of
    New Jersey
New Jersey Medical School
185 South Orange Avenue
Newark, NJ 07103
(201)456–6255

Y-Me Breast Cancer Support Program
18220 Harwood Avenue
Homewood, IL 60430
(708)799–8228
(800)221–2141

Index

Numbers following the entries refer to page numbers, not to item numbers in the chapters. For additional references to some diseases and disorders listed separately in this index, see also "Diseases and disorders (children and adolescent) explained" or "Diseases and disorders (adult) explained."

A

AARP Bulletin, 145
Abbreviations and Acronyms, 31–33
Abdomen, chiropractic recommendations for exercising muscles in the, 94
Abdominal surgery explained, 102–103, 192
ABMS Compendium of Certified Medical Specialists, 121
Abstracting services, 87
Academy of Psychosomatic Medicine, 221
Accessibility Standards, 38
Acne
    drugs for treating, 21
    drugs that cause, 21
    explained, 21, 154, 180
Acoustic neuroma, 42, 180
Acoustic Neuroma Association, 225
Acronyms, Initialisms, and Abbreviations Dictionary, 119
Acupuncture
    as therapy for selected health conditions, 15
    explained, 15, 192
    source of names of practitioners, 84
Adolescent Medicine—Newsletter, 146
Advantages to the Early Removal of Impacted Wisdom Teeth, 110
Adverse drug interactions
    a guide to, 57, 157
    probability of, 57
Aerobics and Fitness Association of America, 269
AGELINE, 165
Aging, 196
    educational materials on health of the, 282
    health problems of the, organizations specializing in providing help for, 196
Aging Action Alert, 146
Aging Process, The, 13
Agoraphobia, 42, 180
AHEPA Cooley's Anemia Foundation, 232
AHPA Newsletter, 146
Aiding the sick or injured child, 22
AIDS
    dental care guidelines, 37, 154
    drug-nutrient interactions associated with treatment, 58

drug therapies for, 156
evaluating hospice facilities for AIDS patients, 158
explained, 23, 46, 154, 180–181
in children, social and psychological concerns, 23
information sources, 79
literature on, 88
newsletter *re* laws, regulations, and political developments, 73
newsletters, 28, 53, 73
nutritional program for managing the chronic malnutrition that accompanies, 46
organizations providing services regarding, 8, 278
patients
    availability of federal and state disability benefits for, 78
Durable Power of Attorney for Health Care, 72
guidelines for home care providers, 75
home care for, 27, 51
prevention, 155
psychological factors, 160
related skin conditions, 45
related terms defined, 32
symptoms and their management, 23, 46
testing, policy issues, 159
Aids Information Sourcebook, 121
AIDS KNOWLEDGE BASE, 166
AIDS Letter, The, 146
AIDS Policy and Law, 146
AIDS: A Self-Care Manual, 110
AIDS and Women: A Sourcebook, 107
AIDSLINE, 166
Airline menus, calorie content, 64
AL-ANON Family Group Headquarters, 225
Alaska State Medical Association, 208
ALCOHOL AND ALCOHOL PROBLEMS SCIENCE DATABASE, 166
Alcohol and drug rehabilitation centers, evaluative profiles, 75
Alcohol Education for Youth, 226
Alcohol-free medications, 55
Alcohol prevention programs and treatment centers, directory and/or descriptive information, 74, 278
Alcohol treatment centers, guidelines for selecting, 74
Alcoholic beverages

Alcoholic beverages (*continued*)
  alcohol content, 66
  calorie content, 65
Alcoholics Anonymous World Services, 226
Alcoholism
  drug therapy for, 156
  effects on the body, 44
  nutritional program for treating, 68
  organizations for the prevention and treatment of, 181
  psychological factors, 160
  symptoms, 44
  therapeutic procedures, 44, 155
Allergen characteristics of different U.S. regions, 24, 48
Allergen-free diets, food-product manufacturers, 67
Allergen-free food products, manufacturers of, 12
Allergens and Foods, 63
Allergens in foreign countries, 51
Allergic diseases, drugs used to treat, 55
Allergies
  answers to questions about, 24, 48
  diagnostic methods, 181
  distinguished from respiratory illnesses, 48
  in children explained, 23
  latest research findings for treatment of, 278
  newsletters, 28, 53
Allergy clinics, directory, 81
Allergy emergencies, 24, 48
Allergy Encyclopedia, The, 130
Allergy-free meals, recipes, 71
Allergy-related terms defined, 33
Allergy in the World: A Guide for Physicians and Travelers, 130
Allied health professions, educational requirements, 179
Alternative health care
  journal articles about, 152
  organizations for identifying practitioners, addresses and telephone numbers, 6
  professionals, sources for names of, 84
Alternative Therapies, 196
Alternatives, 146
Alternatives in Healing, 130–131
Alzheimer patient
  guide for achieving a balanced daily diet, 68
  how to maintain sufficient food intake, 68
Alzheimer's Disease and Related Disorders Association, 226
Alzheimer's disease
  answers to questions about, 50
  caring for the patient, 50, 158
  current research on, 181, 278
  Education and Referral Center, 226
  materials on diagnosis and treatment, 157, 278
  newsletter, 53
  patients, answers to legal questions about, 72
  rating scale for assessing progression, 42
  symptoms, 50
  treatment centers, directory, 81
Alzheimer's Research Review, 146
American Academy for Cerebral Palsy and Developmental Medicine, 231
American Academy of Allergy and Immunology, 217
American Academy of Child and Adolescent Psychiatry, 220
American Academy of Clinical Psychiatrists, 220
American Academy of Dermatology, 218
American Academy of Disability Evaluating Physicians, 218
American Academy of Facial Plastic & Reconstructive Surgery, 223

American Academy of Neurology, 219
American Academy of Ophthalmology, 220
American Academy of Orthopaedic Surgeons, 223
American Academy of Otolaryngic Allergy, 217
American Academy of Otolaryngology—Head and Neck Surgery, 223
American Academy of Pain Medicine, 245
American Academy of Pediatrics, 220
American Academy of Physical Medicine and Rehabilitation, 221
American Academy of Psychoanalyisis, 221
American Alliance for Health, Physical Education, Recreation and Dance, 225
American Amputee Foundation, 255
American Association for the Accreditation of Ambulatory Plastic Surgery Facilities, 204
American Association for Acupuncture and Oriental Medicine, 254
American Association for Hand Surgery, 222
American Association for International Aging, 263
American Association of Blood Banks, 255
American Association of Colleges of Nursing, 207
American Association of Homes for the Aging, 205
American Association of Kidney Patients, 240
American Association of Naturopathic Physicians, 265
American Association of Neurological Surgeons, 223
American Association of Plastic Surgeons, 223
American Association for the Study of Headache, 238
American Association for the Study of Liver Disease, 239
American Association of Suicidology, 268
American Association for Thoracic Surgery, 224
American Association of Tissue Banks, 274
American Back Society, 228
American Board of Allergy and Immunology, 214
American Board of Anesthesiology, 214
American Board of Colon and Rectal Surgery, 214
American Board of Dermatology, 214
American Board of Emergency Medicine, 215
American Board of Family Practice, 215
American Board of Internal Medicine, 215
American Board of Medical Specialties, 214
American Board of Neurological Surgery, 215
American Board of Nuclear Medicine, 215
American Board of Obstetrics and Gynecology, 215
American Board of Ophthalmology, 215
American Board of Orthopedic Surgery, 215
American Board of Otolaryngology, 216
American Board of Pathology, 216
American Board of Pediatrics, 216
American Board of Physical Medicine and Rehabilitation, 216
American Board of Plastic Surgery, 216
American Board of Preventive Medicine, 216
American Board of Psychiatry and Neurology, 216
American Board of Radiology, 216
American Board of Surgery, 217
American Board of Thoracic Surgery, 217
American Board of Urology, 217
American Brittle Bone Society, 245
American Burn Association, 231
American Cancer Society, 231
American Cancer Society Cancer Book: Prevention, Detection, Diagnosis, Treatment, Rehabilitation, Cure, The, 110–111
American Cancer Society Cookbook, The, 131
American Chiropractic Association, 205
American Chiropractic Association, Membership Directory, 121
American Cleft Palate-Craniofacial Association, 232

American Cleft Palate Foundation, 232
American Coalition of Citizens with Disabilities, 270
American College of Allergy and Immunology, 217
American College of Cardiology, 217
American College of Chest Physicians, 217
American College of Cryosurgery, 222
American College of Emergency Physicians, 218
American College of Gastroenterology, 218
American college of Nurse-Midwives, 206
American College of Obstetricians and Gynecologists, 206
American College of Occupational Medicine, 219
American College of Radiology, 221
American College of Rheumatology, 221
American College of Sports Medicine, 252
American College of Surgeons, 222
American Congress of Rehabilitation Medicine, 221
American Council for Drug Education, 235
American Council of Blind Parents, 229
American Council of the Blind, 229
American Council of Life Insurance, 225
American Council on Science and Health, 266
American Council on Transplantation, 273
American Deafness and Rehabilitation Association, 233
American Dental Association, 206
American Dental Directory, 121–122
American Diabetes Association, 234
American Dietetic Association, 270
American Epilepsy Society, 236
American Fertility Society, 237
American Foundation for the Prevention of Venereal Disease, 248
American Gastroenterological Association, 219
American Geriatrics Society, 263
American Hair Loss Council, 238
American Health Assistance Foundation, 263
American Health Foundation, 267
American Heart Association, 230
American Hepatitis Association, 239
American Holistic Medical Association, 219
American Hospital Association, 204
American Institute of Ultrasound in Medicine, 263
American Kidney Fund, 240
American Laryngological Association, 259
American Laryngological, Rhinological, and Otological Society, 220
American Leprosy Foundation, 241
American Leprosy Missions, 241
American Liver Foundation, 239
American Lung Association, 233
American Medical Association, 205
American Medical Association Encyclopedia of Medicine, The, 131
American Medical Directory: Directory of Physicians in the United States, Puerto Rico, Virgin Islands, Certain Pacific Islands and U.S. Physicians Temporarily Located in Foreign Countries, 122
American Medical Records Association, 206
American Medical Writers Association, 206
American Narcolepsy Association, 243
American National Standard for Buildings and Facilities—Providing Accessibility and Usability for Physically Handicapped People, 150
American Nurses Association, 207
American Optometric Association, 207
American Orthopaedic Association, 220
American Orthopedic Society for Sports Medicine, 220
American Osteopathic Association, 207
American Otological Society, 220
American Pain Society, 245

American Pancreatic Association, 261
American Parkinson Disease Association, 246
American Pediatric Surgical Association, 223
American Pharmaceutical Association, 207
American Physical Therapy Association, 207
American Podiatric Medical Association, 208
American Porphyria Foundation, 246
American Psychiatric Association, 220
American Psychoanalytic Association, 221
American Psychological Association, 208
American Public Health Association, 249
American Red Cross, 255
American Reye's Syndrome Association, 247
American Rhinological Society, 222
American School Health Association, 265
American Sign Language for medical and dental terms, 33
American Sleep Disorders Association, 251
American Social Health Association, 249
American Society of Abdominal Surgeons, 222
American Society on Aging, 264
American Society of Allied Health Professions, 205
American Society of Cataract and Refractive Surgery, 256
American Society of Clinical Hypnosis, 259
American Society of Colon and Rectal Surgery, 222
American Society for Dermatologic Surgery, 224
American Society for Gastrointestinal Endoscopy, 219
American Society of Hematology, 219
American Society for Laser Medicine and Surgery, 259
American Society of Lipo-Suction Surgery, 260
American Society of Maxillofacial Surgeons, 223
American Society of Plastic and Reconstructive Surgeons, 224
American Society for Psychoprophylaxis in Obstetrics, 272
American Society for Surgery of the Hand, 223
American Society for Therapeutic Radiology and Oncology, 262
American Society of Transplant Surgeons, 274
American Speech-Language-Hearing Association, 251
American Sudden Infant Death Syndrome Institute, 252
American Thyroid Association, 218
American Tinnitus Association, 253
American Trauma Society, 253
American Urological Association, 224
Amputation, support groups, 192
Amputee Services Association, 255
Amyotrophic lateral sclerosis (ALS), 42, 181
Amyotrophic Lateral Sclerosis Association, 227
Anatomical features, explanations and illustrations, 16–17, 153
Anatomical Illustrations and Explanations, 16–17
Anatomy and physiology, normal, 153
Anatomy of the Human Body, 131
Anorexia Nervosa and Associated Disorders, 227
Anorexia Nervosa and Related Eating Disorders, 227
Anorexia nervosa/bulimia, support groups, 181
Anxiety Disorders Association of America, 225
APGAR system explained, 19
Aquatic Exercise Association, 269
Arizona Medical Association, 208
Arkansas Medical Society, 208
AROCC Newsletter, 146–147
Arthritis
　explained, 47, 154
　newsletter, 53
　questions to ask about, 52
　treatment for, 278
　water therapy for, 181

Arthritis Foundation, 227
Artificial insemination, success rates, 192
Artificial larynx, recent research on, 194
Asbestos Information Association of North America, 228
Asbestos Victims of America, 228
Asbestosis, support group, 182
Asociación de Médicos Mexicanos, 214
Asociación Nacional por Personas Mayores, 264
Assessment and Reporting, 61
Assessments (medical equipment and supplies), 82
Association of American Medical Colleges, 205
Association of Applied Physiology and Biofeedback, 255
Association of Birth Defect Children, 229
Association of Birth Defect Children—Newsletter, 147
Association for the Care of Children's Health, 265
Association for Macular Diseases, 242
Association of Medical Illustrators, 206
Associations and Organizations, 5–8
Associations for diseases and disorders, addresses and telephone numbers, 5–6, 152, 224–254
Associations, membership lists of professional health, 6
Asthma and Allergy Advocate, 147
Asthma
  current therapy information for, 182, 278
  explained, 24, 154
  inhalation devices for children with, 24
  literature regarding children with, 88
  medications used to treat, 24
  minimizing dust in a child's room, 24
  preparing for a second medical opinion for a child with, 27
  questions to ask about, 28, 52
  asthma-related terms defined, 32
  selecting a physician for a child with, 27
Asthma and Allergy Foundation of America, 226
Asthma clinics, directory, 81
Athletes, diseases and medical disorders affecting, 93
Athletes and drugs, parents/coaches guidelines, 56
Atlas of Human Anatomy, 131
Audiology, rehabilitation programs, 81
Autism, 42, 182
Ayurvedic medicine, source of names of practitioners, 84

B

Baby bottles, care of, 31
Baby foods, calorie content, 64
Back
  chiropractic recommendations for exercising muscles in the, 94
  exercises for maintaining the, 94
  proper care of, 50
Back pain
  prevention of, 49
  treatment exercises, 50
Back problems
  current therapy information for, 182
  newsletter, 53
Back Pain Monitor, 147
Back tooth replacement, 37
Barrier-free standards for persons with disabilities, 38
BASH (Bulimia Anorexia Self-Help), 227
Basic food group daily servings for young children, 30
Bedtime problems, guidelines, 30
Behavior disorders
  guidelines for finding and applying to treatment centers, 82

treatment centers, directory, 82
Behavioral problems of children, determining when professional help is needed, 26
Behavioral problems of youth, 21
Bell's Palsy, 42, 182
Best Hospitals in America, The, 122
BIOETHICSLINE, 166
Biofeedback
  latest research findings on, 192
  source of names of practitioners, 84
Biomedical journals, 87
Birth control, latest research on, 200
Birth defects
  current research, 182
  newsletter, 28
Bladder disorders
  diagnostic tests used and explained, 20, 41
  drugs used to treat, 25, 49
  explained, 25, 49, 154
Bland diet for ambulatory patients, 71
Blindness, support groups, 182
Blood autotransfusions, 153
Blood and blood vessel disorders explained, 45, 154
Blood glucose levels, regulation of, 43
Blood glucose monitoring kits, 43
Blood groups explained, 17
Blood pressure devices, reliability of, 282
Blood pressure, high, diet and exercise therapy for, 182
Blood pressure monitoring, 41
Blood sugar measurement procedure, 43
Blood sugar variations during menstrual cycle, 43
Blood sugars, numerical computations for normalizing, 43
Blood supply safety, 153
Blood transfusions, safety of, 193, 282
Blue Book of Optometrists, The, 122
Blue Cross and Blue Shield Plans, 11
Board certification, meaning of, in, 176
  allergy and immunology, 176
  anesthesiology, 176
  colon and rectal surgery, 176
  dermatology, 176
  emergency medicine, 176
  family practice, 176
  internal medicine, 176
  neurological surgery, 176
  neurology, 177
  nuclear medicine, 177
  obstetrics and gynecology, 177
  ophthalmology, 177
  orthopedic surgery, 177
  otolaryngology, 177
  pathology, 177
  pediatrics, 177
  physical medicine and rehabilitation, 177
  plastic surgery, 177
  preventive medicine, 177
  psychiatry, 177
  radiology, 177
  surgery, 177
  thoracic surgery, 177
  urology, 177
Body and Sports, The, 92–93
Body components and their functions during sports, 92
Bone marrow transplantation, 201, 282
Bone mass, exercises that will help increase, 95
Books in Print, 107
Brain injuries/diseases, latest drug treatment methods, 278
Brain-injury centers, listing, 97

Brain (neurological) surgery explained, 102–103, 260
Brand-name drugs, generic names of, 58–59
Brand names of generic drugs, 59
Breast-feeding, benefits, 193
Breast-feeding guidelines, 70, 193
Breast-feeding and use of therapeutic drugs, 60–61
Bridges and dentures explained, 34
British Medical Association, 214
Bureaus of vital records and statistics, by state, 11
Burns, latest treatment techniques, 183

C

Caffeine content of foods, 65
Calcium, high, sample menus with, 71
California Medical Association, 208
Call the doctor, when to, 22
Calorie Factor: The Dieter's Companion, The, 131–132
Calorie requirements daily for young children, 30
Calories
    how to calculate the number needed, 69
    how to reduce intake, 70
Camps, summer, for children with disabilities, directory, 79
Canadian Medical Association, 213
Cancer, bone marrow transplants, 201, 282
Cancer, breast, support groups for, 79, 183
Cancer Challenge, The, 147
Cancer
    chemicals causing, 164
    in children, newsletter, 28
    in children, treatment of, 25, 154, 155, 161
    Comprehensive Cancer Centers, directory, 80
    different types explained, 45, 154, 155
    location of local clinical programs, 278
    newest surgical techniques for treatment, 164
    newsletter, 28, 29, 53
    nutritional guidelines and recipes that may reduce
        the risk of, 68
    patients, nutritional guidelines and recipes for, 68
    pediatric treatment centers, 80
    questions to ask about, 28, 52
    research studies on treatment of, 155
    skin, prevention, 45, 190
    survival rates by cancer type, 46, 183, 187
    therapy, admission to drug treatment protocol for,
        156
    treatment protocol for children, location of and
        entry criteria, 162
CANCERLIT, 166
Candlelighters Childhood Cancer Foundation, 231
Candida Research and Information Foundation, 231
Candidiasis, diet therapy for, 183
CAPS (Children of Aging Parents), 264
Capsules, identification of, 55
Captioning for the hearing impaired, 197
Car seats for young children, how to use, 31, 197
Carbohydrate content per serving, 65
Carbohydrate meals, recipes for low, 71
Cardiac Alert, 147
Cardiovascular fitness, relative effectiveness of exercising methods for achieving, 94
Cardiovascular fitness program, designing a, 94
Care Centers (*re* the elderly), 13
Care Medico, 207
Caregivers, 147
Caring for the Alzheimer Patient: A Practical Guide, 111
Caring for the disabled, newsletter, 39
Caring for a sick child at home, 27

CAT or CT explained, 40–41
Cataracts
    surgical procedure explained, 103, 193
    symptoms and removal procedures explained, 47
Celiac sprue, 42, 183, 191
Celiac Sprue Society, 231
Center for Dance Medicine, 271
Center for Health Promotion and Education, 285–286
Center for Science in the Public Interest, 267
Center for Sickle Cell Disease, 249
Center for the Study of Multiple Birth, 272
Cerebral palsy, 42, 183
Certifying and Licensing Boards and Agencies, 8–10
Cesarean section, guidelines, 193
Change Your Smile, 132
Chemicals causing cancer, 164
Chemotherapy, side effects, 25, 46
Child abuse
    causes and symptoms, 30
    reporting procedures, 197
Child care, types available, 73
Child care arrangements, types of, 18
Child care centers, how to evaluate, 18
Child Care Services, 18
Child development schedule, 25, 161
Child health, newsletters, 28
Child psychology, articles on, 161
Childbirth
    calculating due-date, 99
    educational materials on, 200
    guidelines for selecting a hospital, 76
    procedure to follow during emergency, 101
    process explained, 101
Childbirth emergency, what to do, 62
Children in Hospitals, 266
Children in Sports, 93
Children With Asthma: A Manual for Parents, 111
Children's Defense Fund, 266
Children's health and human development, research
    on, 283
Children's Hospice International, 266
Children's Transplant Association, 274
Chiropractic as therapy for selected health conditions,
    15
Chiropractic health care explained, 14
Chiropractic Therapy, 14–15
Chiropractor, guidelines for selecting, 14
Chiropractors
    education and training, 14, 179
    national directory, 83
Chiropractors: Listings, 83
Choice in Dying, 268
Cholesterol content of foods, 65
Cholesterol
    explained, 65
    guidelines for lowering, 70, 283
    high and low, explained, 44
Chronic digestive disease, diagnosis and treatment, 279
Chronic Fatigue Immune Dysfunction Syndrome Association, 231
Chronic Fatigue Immune Dysfunction Syndrome Society, 232
Chronic fatigue syndrome, 183, 278
Cirrhosis, treatment for, 278
Citizens for the Treatment of High Blood Pressure, 230
Civil rights, organizations that provide information on
    the legal and civil rights of persons with disabilities, 7
Civil rights for the disabled, 72
Clearinghouse on Child Abuse and Neglect, 265

Clearinghouse on the Handicapped, 286

Clearinghouse for Occupational Safety and Health Information, 286

Cleft palate, 42, 183

Code of Federal Regulations, 143

Codes of professional ethics, examples, 159

Cold medicines, basic ingredients, 55

Colicky baby, care for, 22

Colitis, 42, 183

College of American Pathologists, 237

Colon surgery explained, 102–103, 193

Colorado Medical Society, 208

Columbia University College of Physicians and Surgeons Complete Guide to Early Child Care, 132

Columbia University College of Physicians and Surgeons Complete Guide to Pregnancy, 132

Columbia University College of Physicians and Surgeons Complete Home Medical Guide, 132

COMBINED HEALTH INFORMATION DATABASE, 167

Community Nutrition Institute, 270

Comparing Therapeutic Alternatives, 15

Compassionate Friends, 268

Complaints against an insurance company, where to report, 293–302

Complete Book of Cosmetic Surgery: A Candid Guide for Men, Women, and Teens, The, 133

Complete Book of Medical Tests, The, 133

Complete Book of Natural Medicines, The, 133

Complete Guide to Early Child Care. See *Columbia University College of Physicians and Surgeons Complete Guide to Early Child Care*

Complete Guide to Medical Tests, 133–134

Complete Guide to Pregnancy. See *Columbia University College of Physicians and Surgeons Complete Guide to Pregnancy*

Complete Guide to Prescription and Non-Prescription Drugs, 134

Complete Guide to Sports Injuries, 134

Complete Guide to Symptoms, Illness and Surgery, 134

Complete Home Medical Guide. See *Columbia University College of Physicians and Surgeons Complete Home Medical Guide*

Complete Parent's Guide to Telephone Medicine, The, 134–135

Comprehensive Cancer Centers, directory, 80

COMPREHENSIVE CORE MEDICAL LIBRARY, 167

Computer databases, medical, bibliography of, 87, 165–171

Computerized aides for persons with disabilities, 38

Confusion About Chiropractors, The, 111

Connecticut State Medical Society, 209

CONSUMER DRUG INFORMATION, 167

Consumer Guide to Modern Cataract Surgery, 111

Consumer Health Information Source Book, The, 108

Consumer Health and Nutrition Index, 106

Consumer Sourcebook, 122–123

Contact Lens Association of Ophthalmologists, 257

Contact lenses, latest research on, 193

Continuing care explained, 74

Continuing care plans, cost-comparison worksheet for determining affordability, 74

Continuing Care Retirement Communities, 74

Continuing care retirement communities
  checklists for selecting, 74
  directory with descriptive profiles, 74
  listing by geographic area, 74

Conventional medicine as therapy for selected health conditions, 15

Cooley's Anemia, 42, 183

Cornelia De Lange syndrome, 183

Cornelia De Lange Syndrome Foundation, 232

Coronary artery disease, questions to ask about, 52

Cosmetic dentistry explained, 36

Cosmetic surgeon, guidelines for selecting, 86

Cosmetic Surgery, 102

Cosmetic surgery
  deciding whether to undergo, 102
  types explained, 102, 195

Costs of specific medical procedures in local areas, 302–311

Council of Better Business Bureaus, 204

Council on Teaching Hospitals, 204

Countries of the World and Their Leaders, Yearbook, 135

CPR, how to administer, 62, 193

Cri Du Chat syndrome, 42, 183

Cri Du Chat Syndrome Society, 232

Cribs, safety standards and guidelines, 31

Crisis Centers, 88

Crohn's disease, 42, 184

Crutches, how to use, 82

Cryosurgery, latest research on, 193

Current Pediatric Therapy, 135

Cuts of beef, source of each cut, 66

Cystic fibrosis, 42, 184

Cystic Fibrosis Foundation, 233

D

Databases, health, major vendors, 165

Daycare centers
  a checklist for selecting, 18
  how to evaluate, 18
  safety, 18

Deafness, 42, 184, 278

Deafness Research Foundation, 233

D.E.B.R.A. (Dystrophic Epidermolysis Bullosa Research Association) of America, 250

Deciding on Surgery, 102

Delta Dental Insurance Plans, 11

Dental aesthetic problems, prevention, 36

Dental Appliances, Implants, Inlays, and Crowns, 33–34

Dental associations and organizations, 6, 179

Dental bite problems, treatments, 36

Dental care, hospitals specializing in, 76

Dental care for disabled persons, 193

Dental care guidelines for AIDS patients, 37, 154

Dental care for senior citizens, 37

Dental care and special medical problems, 35

Dental caries classified, 35

Dental cavities, research on prevention, 153–154, 278

Dental composite resin bonding, maintenance, 36

Dental diseases, disorders, and treatments explained, 35

Dental emergencies, what to do, 35

Dental examiners, state or regional boards of, 10

Dental fears, controlling, 35

Dental Features, 17–18

Dental fillings, inlays, and crowns explained, 34

Dental health directors, state and U.S. territorial, 12

Dental Hygiene, 34

Dental Implants: Are They For Me?, 111–112

Dental implants explained, 33–34

Dental injection sites for anesthetics, 35

Dental Instruments and Materials, 34

Dental insurance issues explained, 78

Dental problems, latest research on, 278

Dental restorations, methods to extend life of, 36
Dental specialists by specialty and city, 83
Dental specialties explained, 34
Dental specialty certifying boards, 9
Dental terms defined, 33
Dentist, how to find a, 86
Dentistry, continuing education requirements for
    relicensure, by state, 9
Dentists, 34
    how to evaluate, 34
    national directory, 83
Dentists: Listings and Specialties, 83–84
Dentures and bridges explained, 34
Depression
    causes, signs, and treatment, 89, 184
    latest research findings for treatment, 279
    treatment centers, directory, 91
Descriptions of Medicines, 54–56
Developmental disabilities treatment centers, direc-
    tory, 91
Developmental programs, infant and early childhood,
    listing, 91
Diabetes, 147
Diabetes
    in children, 22
    complications of, 279
    latest research findings on, 184
    newsletter, 28, 53
    supply sources for treating, 43
    symptoms and treatment, 42–43
Diabetes mellitus, questions to ask about, 28, 52
Diabetes Type II: Living a Long, Healthy Life Through Blood
    Sugar Normalization, 112
Diagnostic and Statistical Manual of Mental Disorders
    (DSM-111-R), 135
Diagnostic equipment, use in health care facilities, 159
Diagnostic Tests and Measurements, 18–20, 39–42
Diagnostics, 62, 88
Dictionary of Food Ingredients, 119
Diet plans, 157
Diet and the prevention and treatment of disease, 67,
    199
Dietary Guidelines for Age Groups, 63–64
Dietary guidelines for children, 30
Dietary guidelines for the elderly, 13
Dietary guidelines for infants, 29
Dietary supplements, calorie content, 64
Diets, fad, 283
Diets, Medicines, Tests (*re* the elderly), 13–14
Directories in Print, 108
Directory of Alzheimer's Disease Treatment Facilities and
    Home Health Care Programs, 123
Directory of Medical Rehabilitation Programs, 123
Directory of Medical Specialists, 123
Directory of Nursing Homes, 123–124
Directory of Pain Treatment Centers in the U.S. and Canada,
    124
Directory of Residential Facilities for Emotionally Handi-
    capped Children and Youth, 124
Directory of Special Libraries and Information Centers, 124–
    125
DIRLINE, 167
Disabilities
    articles on the functional evaluation of physical, 162
    current research on the treatment of, 162
    information sources regarding topics on, 87
Disability evaluations, physicians performing, 178
Disability types defined, 33
Disabled children

guidelines for involving them in sports and recre-
    ation, 39, 162
rights to special education services under the law, 39
Disabled persons
    independent living tips, 38
    organizations serving the needs of, 7
    organizations that provide information on the legal
    and civil rights of, 7
    patient education materials for, 154
    proper conduct when with, 38
    special nursing care for, 154
Disaster medical care, 198–199
Disciplinary records of physicians, by state, 10
Disciplining young children, 26
Diseases, diagnostic tests used with each disease, 18
Diseases and disorders (adult) explained, 42, 154, 155,
    197
Diseases of the brain and nervous system explained,
    47, 154
Diseases and disorders associated with aging, 13
Diseases and disorders (childhood), how each is
    treated, 20, 161
Diseases and disorders (childhood and adolescent) ex-
    plained, 20, 161
Diseases, Disorders, and Injuries (sports), 93–94
Diseases/medical disorders and the athlete, 22
Diseases and medical disorders, common, drugs used
    to treat each, 23, 49
Diseases and Disorders (mental), 88–90
Diseases that affect athletes, 93
Diseases, Disorders, and Their Therapies, 20–25, 35–
    37, 42–50
Disorders, medical, that affect athletes, 93
DNA fingerprints and paternity, 98
Doctors disciplined, 85
Dorland's Illustrated Medical Dictionary, 119
Down's syndrome, 42, 184
Drug, approval status of an experimental therapeutic,
    283
Drug Abuse, 72. *See also* substance abuse
Drug abuse
    educational materials for young children, 184–185
    organizations providing help for, 8
    prevention and education programs, directory, 56
    rehabilitation programs, 75, 279
    rehabilitation self-help organizations, directory, 57
    treatment trends, newsletter, 59
Drug Abuse and Treatment, 56–57
Drug Abuse Update, 148
Drug, Alcohol, and Other Addictions: A Directory of Treat-
    ment Centers and Prevention Programs Nationwide, 125
Drug and alcohol rehabilitation centers, evaluative pro-
    files, 75
Drug dosage levels for infants and children, 161
Drug dosage levels for the elderly, 156
Drug Evaluations Annual, 136
Drug (illicit) experimentation, warning signs, 24, 50
Drug Information Association, 267
Drug Interactions Guide Book, 136
Drug prevention programs and treatment centers, di-
    rectory with descriptive information, 74, 156–157
Drug problems in the workplace, educational materi-
    als for, 279
Drug Regulatory Authorities Abroad, 10
Drug-related terms defined, 32
Drug side effects and their impact on dental health
    and care, 35
Drug testing in the workplace, 159, 193
Drug testing program, U.S., 60

Drug (therapeutic) effects on food intake, 66
Drug (therapeutic) interactions with beverages, tobacco, foods, cocaine, and marijuana, 57, 157
Drug (therapeutic) interactions with specific foods, 66
Drug (therapeutic) interactions with the body's nutritional system, 57
Drug (therapeutic), toxicity of a, 54, 164
Drug treatment centers, guidelines for selecting, 74
Drug Treatment Programs, 74–75
Drug treatment programs, state listings, 56
Drug treatment protocol for cancer therapy, admission to, 156
Drugs
  adverse effects of specific medicinals, 156, 198
  adverse interaction with alcohol, 44
  and biological substances, descriptive monographs, 55
  FDA safety ratings for use during pregnancy, 60
  how they work in the body, 57
  and nutritional disorders, 44
  potential for abuse, 55
  and sexual function, 57
Drugs (prescription and non-prescription), descriptions and explanations, 54
Drugs (therapeutic)
  alcohol content, 55
  for the elderly
    general guidelines, 13
    precautions for use of specific medicines, 14
  use during pregnancy, 100, 156, 163
  used during breast-feeding, 60–61
Drugs affecting blood glucose level, 56
Drugs, Alcohol, and Your Children: How to Keep Your Family Substance-Free, 112
Drugs approved for therapeutic use by foreign authorities but not by the U.S., 55
Drugs arranged by categories of therapeutic use, 60
Drugs and Athletes, 94
Drugs Available Abroad: A Guide to Therapeutic Drugs Available and Approved Outside the U.S., 136
Drugs causing emotional disturbances, 89
Drugs causing visual impairments, 43
Drugs commonly used by athletes, effects of, 94
Drugs prescribed for treatment, questions to ask about, 60
Drugs that are often abused, 56
Drugs that induce emotional disturbances, 58
Drugs that sensitize skin to the sun, 21, 44
Drugs used to treat specific chronic medical disorders, 60
Drugs used to treat specific common diseases and medical disorders, 23, 49
Durable Power of Attorney, 79, 198
Dwarfism, latest treatment, 185
Dyslexia
  diagnosis of, 42, 185
  directory of special schools serving children with, 80

E

EAR Foundation, 243
Eating and Allergy, 112
Eating disorders, educational materials on the prevention of, 279
Economics of health care for the elderly, 158
Education of All Handicapped Act (P.L. 94–142), 72
Education of health care personnel, 85, 159
Effects of Drugs, 57–58

Elderly
  drug dosage levels for the, 156
  special nursing needs, 157
Electrocardiogram explained, 19, 41
Electronic Aids, 82
EMBASE, 167–168
Emergency
  pediatric, explained, 26
  when to call a doctor and what to say, 27
Emergency (medical) situation, how to assess, 61
Emergency Procedures and Actions, 62
Emotional disturbances, drugs that cause, 89
Emotional and intellectual development, 26
Emotionally disturbed children, residential treatment facilities
  directory, 82
  guidelines for finding and applying, 82
Emphysema/chronic bronchitis, questions to ask about, 52
ENCYCLOPEDIA OF ASSOCIATIONS, 168
Encyclopedia of Associations. Volume One. National Organizations of the U.S., 125
Encyclopedia of Medical Organizations and Agencies, 125
Endocrine glands explained, 17
Endocrine Society, 218
Endometriosis, 42, 185
Endometriosis Association, 236
Endoscopy, gastrointestinal diseases, 193, 282
Energy allowances, recommended daily, 63
Epilepsy
  drug therapy for, 279
  explained, 47, 154
  support groups, 185
  surgical treatment for, 194, 279
Epilepsy Foundation of America, 236
Epstein-Barr syndrome, 42, 185
Equipment and Devices, 38, 96
Essential Guide to Prescription Drugs, The, 136–137
Essential Principles of Chiropractic, 112
Estimated Safe and Adequate Daily Dietary Intake for vitamins and minerals, 69
Everybody's Guide to Chiropractic Health Care, 112
Exercise, 94–95, 96
Exercise physiology, articles on, 163
Exercises
  conditioning, how to perform, 94
  effectiveness of different methods for cardiovascular fitness, 45
  for relieving tension at work, 92
  for strengthening neck, back, and abdomen muscles, 15
Extra Pharmacopoeia (Martindale), The. See *Martindale, The Extra Pharmacopoeia*
Eye Bank Association of America, 229
Eye banks, directory, 81
Eye diseases, latest diagnostic methods and treatment for, 279
Eye disorders, latest research, 185
Eye examinations at home, 41
Eye surgeon, guidelines for selecting, 86

F

Familial polyposis, 42, 185
Familial Polyposis Registry, 236
Family Guide to Dental Health. See *The Mount Sinai Medical Center Family Guide to Dental Health*
Family planning service agencies, directory, 81

Family planning service agencies and organizations, 11

Family stress and caring for the elderly, 160

Fast foods, calorie content, 64

Fat, guidelines for lowering, 70

Fat content per serving, 65

Federation of the Handicapped, 271

Feeding guidelines for young children, 30

Feedings, infant, number of daily feedings and quantity per, 30

Feldenkrais work, source of names of practitioners, 84

Female disorders explained, 46–47

Fertility Research Foundation, 237

Fever, reducing a, 23

Fiber, recommended daily consumption, 69

Fiber and bulk, guidelines for diets high in, 71

Fiber content of foods, 65

Fibrocystic breast disease, 42, 185

Findex: The Directory of Market Research Reports, Studies, and Surveys, 108

First Aid Book. See *Johnson & Johnson First Aid Book*

First aid kit contents, 62

First Aid Preparation, 62

First aid procedures, 62

Florida Medical Association, 209

Fluorides as tooth protection explained, 37

Flying Wheels Travel, 271

Folk Name and Trade Diseases, 119

Folk names for occupational diseases, 33

Food Additives, 64

Food additives
  by type, purpose of each, 64
  guidelines for safe use, 64
  possible adverse effects, 64
  answers to questions about, 24, 48

Food Allergy, 112–113

Food contamination caused by pesticides, 157

Food and Drug Administration (FDA), 286

Food and Drug Interaction Guide, The, 137

Food and Drug Interactions, 66

Food and Nutrition Information Center, 286

Food Ingredients and Calories, 64–66

Food ingredients explained, 32

Food Poisoning, 66

Food poisoning explained, 66

Food sensitive diets, guidelines, 63

Food Sources, 66

Food Values of Portions Commonly Used, 137

Foods and their allergens, 63

Foods, irradiated, safety of, 283

Foods, non-carcinogenic, 35

Foods, vitamin and mineral content, 65

Foreign Travel and Immunization Guide, 137–138

Four basic food groups with recommended daily servings, 69

Fractured teeth repair, 36

Fractures, healing times, 22, 50

Fragile X Foundation, 237

Fragile X syndrome, 42, 185

Fraud in health care, 197

Friedreich's Ataxia, support group, 185

Friedreich's Ataxia Group in America, 237

G

Gaps between teeth, treatment, 36

Gastroplasty Support Group, 244

Gaucher disease, 42, 186

Gene structure, 98

Generic and Brand-Name Drugs, 58–59

Generic forms of individual drugs, description, 156

Generic-name drug glossary, purposes explained, 58

Generic-name drugs, brand names of, 59

Generic names of brand-name drugs, 58–59

Genetic diagnostic and counseling centers, directory, 81

Genetic disorders, 97–98

Genetic intervention, ethical considerations, 163

Genetics, 97–98

Geriatrics, hospitals and clinics specializing in, 76

Gerontological Society of America, 264

Gifted child development, 26

Gluten-restricted diet, 70

Government Departments and Agencies, 10–11

Great White Lie: How America's Hospitals Betray Our Trust and Endanger Our Lives, The, 113

Grief Education Institute, 268

Grieving, self-help groups, 198

Growth and Development, 25–26

Growth and development schedule, first year, 17

Guam Medical Society, 213

Guide Dog Foundation for the Blind Training Center, 229

Guide to Accredited Camps, 125–126

Guide to Prescription and Over-the-Counter Drugs, 138

Gynecological disorders and their symptoms, 46, 154

Gynecologist, guidelines for selecting, 86

H

Hair loss, latest research on, 186

Hair problems, answers to, 45

Hand surgery, latest research on, 194

Handicapped children, rights to special education services under the law, 39

Handicapped
  federal benefits for the, 283
  special nursing care for, 154

Hawaii Medical Association, 209

Hazardous substances, proper removal procedures, 161

Head injuries, latest treatment for, 186, 279

Headaches
  explained, 49, 186
  latest research on, 186
  newsletter, 54

Health and Healing, 113

Health and Healing: Understanding Conventional and Alternative Medicine, 113

Health associations, providers, programs, and services, directories of, 87

Health care associations, membership directories, 85

Health care products, manufacturers and providers, directories of, 83

Health Care Financing Administration, 287

Health Care U.S.A., 126

Health departments, state, 10–11, 321–330

HEALTH DEVICES ALERTS, 168

HEALTH DEVICES SOURCEBOOK, 168

Health foods, newsletter, 53

Health Hotlines: 800 Numbers from DIRLINE, 126

Health Industry Companies, 11–12

Health information centers and clearinghouses, national, addresses and telephone numbers, 7, 285–292

Health Information for Travelers, 51, 202

Health information sources, evaluative descriptions, 87

Health Insurance Association of America, 269

Health insurance companies, 11
Health insurance
  remedy for unfair insurance-claim rejection, 199
  reporting of a fraudulent claim, 199
Health Officials, 12
Health officials at all governmental levels—names, addresses, and telephone numbers, 12
HEALTH PERIODICALS DATABASE, 168
HEALTH PLANNING AND ADMINISTRATION, 168
Health promotion, educational materials on, 283
Health providers, quality control system, 85
HEALTH REFERENCE CENTER, 169
Health sciences journals, 87
Health Standards, 50–51
Healthcare Abroad, 274
Hearing disorders, 279
Heart disease
  newsletter, 29, 53
  prevention, 279
  rehabilitation programs for, 186
Heart diseases explained, 45, 154
Heart rate goal of exercise programs, 94
Heart rate, normal, by age, 17
Height and weight growth charts for children, 25
Height and weight standards for adults, 50
Helen Keller National Center for Deaf/Blind Youths and Adults, 229
Helpline telephone numbers, 77
Hemlock Society, 268
Hemochromatosis, 42, 186
Hemochromatosis Research Foundation, 239
Hemophilia, latest research on treatment of, 186
Hepatitis
  prevention of, 42, 186, 279
  questions to ask about, 52
Herbal Suppliers, 15
Herbs, toxic, 96
Herpes, latest treatment for, 279
Hiccups in babies, 22
High Blood Pressure Information Center, 287
High blood pressure, questions to ask about, 52
HIP (Help for Incontinent People), 254
HMOs accepting Medicare recipients, 283
HMOs
  addresses and telephone numbers, 7
  explained, 7
  guidelines for deciding whether to join, 77
  how to select, 77
HMOs: What They Are, How They Work, and Which One is Best for You, 113
Holistic medicine, source of names of practitioners, 84, 178
Home Health Care, 75
Home health care agencies, listing, 75
Home health care providers, accreditation of, 179
Home safety checklist, 30
Home safety for toddlers, tips, 31
Homeopathy as therapy for selected health conditions, 15
Homeopathy
  explained, 15, 196
  source of names of practitioners, 84
Hospice accreditation, 174
Hospice facilities
  for children, 80, 197
  evaluating for AIDS patients, 158
Hospice services, listing, 80
Hospital associations, state, 7
Hospitalization
  complaint guide for the inpatient, 76, 77, 174

  guidelines for checking out, 77
  how to prepare for, 76
  how to prepare a child for, 76, 197
  questions to ask a doctor before, 76
  reporting incorrect billing, 174
Hospitals, 75–77
  accreditation, 174
  affiliation with medical schools, 174
  behind the scene exposé of reprehensible conditions, 76
  descriptive profiles of some of the best, 75
  guidelines when selecting for childbirth, 76
  how they function, 75
  how to select, 75, 174
  local services available, 173
  state licensing agencies, 9
Hotline telephone numbers, 77
Hotlines and Helplines, 77
How to Defeat Alcoholism: Nutritional Guidelines for Getting Sober, 114
How to Talk to Your Doctor: The Questions to Ask, 114
Human Growth Foundation, 235
Huntington's disease explained, 47, 154, 186
Huntington's Disease Society of America, 239
Hyperbaric therapy, 194
Hypertension, 42, 186, 279
Hypoglycemia explained, 43, 154, 186

I

Idaho Medical Association, 209
Identification bracelets and cards, medical, how to obtain, 199
Ileitis and ulcerative colitis, newsletter, 53
Ileitis, latest treatment for, 186
Illinois State Medical Society, 209
Illness or injury of a child, what to do, 62
Illustrated Dictionary of Dentistry, 119–120
Immunization requirements, school, of each state, 321–330
Immunization schedule for childhood diseases, 20, 194
Immunizations needed for traveling, guidelines, 51
Impacted Wisdom Teeth in the Middle and Late Years, 114
Impotence, latest therapy for, 187
In vitro fertilization, success rates, 192
In vitro fertilization centers, directory, 80
Index Medicus, 106
Index to Dental Literature, 106
Indexes to dental articles, 87
Indexes to medical articles, 87
Indexing services, 87
Indiana State Medical Association, 209
Industrial chemicals and associated health risks, 92, 164, 198
Infant formulas, calorie content, 64
Infectious diseases, explanation of each, 42, 154, 155
Infertility, causes and treatment of, 99, 185, 194
Information materials for patients on chronic diseases and disorders, 155
Inhalation devices for asthmatic children, 24
Inherited traits, mechanism for, 98
Injection devices, identification of, 55
Injuries common to specific sports, 93
Injuries, sports
  causes and treatment of specific, 93, 163, 191, 195, 281
  how to prevent, 93
Instructions for Patients, 138
Instructions, medical, for patients with specific ailments, 21, 42

Insulin, mixing and injecting, 43
Insulin types described, 43
Insurance, 77–78, 199
Insurance companies, reporting complaints against, 293–302
Intellectual and emotional development, 26
International Association for Medical Assistance to Travelers (IAMAT), 6–7, 213
International Association for the Study of Pain, 245
International Childbirth Education Association, 272
International College of Surgeons, 222
International Directory of Corporate Affiliations, 126
International Hearing Dog Association, 233
International Ménière's Disease Research Institute, 243
Iowa Medical Society, 209
Iron overload disease, 187
Iron Overload Diseases Association, 240
Is Surgery Necessary?, 138

J

Johnson & Johnson First Aid Book, 138–139
Joint Commission on Accreditation of Health Care Organizations, 204
Journals that summarize state-of-the-art in medical specialties, 87, 154, 155
Juvenile Diabetes Foundation, 234

K

Kansas Medical Society, 210
Kentucky Medical Association, 210
Kidney dialysis, 42, 193
Kidney disease
 latest research on, 187
 questions to ask about, 28, 52
Kidney failure, information on financial issues associated with, 280
Kidney stones, prevention of, 280
Kidney transplantation, requirements for, 194

L

La Leche League International, 256
Learning disabilities, state associations for, 8
Legal-medical issues, a survey, 72
Legal Protections and Rights, 72
Legal responsibilities for drug and alcohol use by children, 72
Legislation and Judicial Cases, 92
Leprosy, 42, 187
Leukemia
 survival rates, 46, 187, 280
 treatment for, 280
Leukemia Society of America, 241
Libraries and Research Centers, 12
Libraries with services for the disabled, 12
Library collections in the health sciences, 12
Lion's Clubs International, 230
Lipid diseases, 42, 187
Liposuction, 194
Liquid diet for patients who cannot eat solid foods, 70
Lithotripsy for gall stones, 282
Lithotripsy for kidney stones, 42, 194, 282
Liver diseases, latest research on treatment of, 187
Living Bank, 273
Living Will, sample, 72, 198

Living With a Disability, 38–39
Living With Allergies, 148
Long-term illness, coping, 50
Look You Like: Medical Answers to 400 Questions on Skin and Hair Care, The, 114
Lou Gehrig's disease, 42, 187
Louisiana State Medical Society, 210
Lung diseases, 42, 187, 280
Lupus, 42, 187
Lupus Foundation of America, 242
Lyme Borreliosis Foundation, 242
Lyme disease, 23, 49, 187, 280

M

Macular diseases, 42, 187
MAGAZINE INDEX, 169
Maine Medical Association, 210
Male disorders explained, 47
Malpractice, physicians disciplined for, 85
Mammography, guidelines, 40, 195, 282
Managing the Side Effects of Chemotherapy and Radiation, 114–115
Manufacturers and Suppliers, 67
March of Dimes Birth Defects Foundation, 229
Marfan syndrome, 42, 187
Marijuana, adverse effects, 185
Market research reports on health care industry companies, 12
Martindale, The Extra Pharmacopoeia, 139
Massachusetts Medical Society, 210
Maternity care provider, guidelines for selecting, 101
Maxillofacial and oral surgery explained, 37
Medic Alert Foundation, 268
Medic Alert Organ Donor Program Foundation, 273
Medicaid explained, 77
Medicaid programs, information about individual state operations, 302–311
Medical Acronyms and Abbreviations, 120
Medical acronyms, abbreviations, and contractions explained, 32
Medical assistance information centers abroad, 79
Medical Association of Georgia, 209
Medical Association of the State of Alabama, 208
Medical Care, 26–28, 51–52
Medical & Chirurgical Faculty of the State of Maryland, 210
Medical consulting specialist, questions to ask a, 26, 52
Medical Device Register, 127
Medical Device Register: International Volume, 127–128
Medical devices, safety records, 283
Medical equipment, problems with or recall of, 158
Medical equipment and supplies, market research reports on, 82
Medical examinations (adults), schedule for, 39
Medical examinations (pediatric), schedule for, 19
Medical and Health Care Books and Serials in Print, 108–109
Medical and Health Information Directory. Vol. 1. Organizations, Agencies, and Institutions, 126
Medical and Health Information Directory. Vol. 2. Publications, Libraries, and Other Information Services, 127
Medical and Health Information Directory. Vol. 3. Health Services, 127
Medical herbalism explained, 15
Medical herbalism as therapy for selected health conditions, 15
Medical illustrators, listing, 179
Medical malpractice, newsletters, 73

Medical Malpractice Litigation Reporter, 148

Medical Malpractice: Verdicts, Settlements, and Experts, 148

Medical organizations for health professionals, 6, 152, 159, 205–224

Medical passport, 202

Medical Passport Foundation, 275

Medical products suppliers, directory, 83, 158, 159

Medical Questions, 27–28, 52

Medical record, procedure for obtaining, 199

Medical record, retrieving in the event of physician's death or retirement, 199

Medical record form, 27

Medical records administrator, educational requirements, 179

Medical schools, addresses and telephone numbers, 174

Medical Sign Language: Easily Understood Definitions of Commonly Used Medical, Dental and First Aid Terms, 120

Medical Society of Delaware, 209

Medical Society of the District of Columbia, 209

Medical Society of New Jersey, 211

Medical Society of the State of New York, 211

Medical Society of Virginia, 212

Medical specialist for a child, how to find a, 26

Medical specialists at selected hospitals, 84

Medical specialists by specialty, national directory, 84, 174–176

Medical specialties

explained, 85

meaning of board certification in. *See* Board certification, meaning of, in

state-of-the-art in, 87, 154, 155

Medical specialty certifying boards, 9

Medical (state) licensing boards, 8, 312–321

Medical terms and phrases explained, 32, 153

Medical tests

answers to questions about, 40

effects of exercise on, 04

Medical Tests and Diagnostic Procedures: A Patient's Guide to Just What the Doctor Ordered, 139

Medical trade shows, 12

Medical writers, identification of, 179

Medicare, filing complaint about a health care provider, 77

Medicare explained, 77

Medication Instruction Sheets, 198

Medicine and the Law, 115

Medicines

calorie content, 64

for the elderly

general guidelines, 13

precautions for use of specific drugs, 14

use of specific drugs during pregnancy, 100, 156, 163

MEDLINE, 169

Meeting the Needs of People With Disabilities: A Guide for Librarians, Educators, and Other Service Personnel, 139–140

Melanoma Letter, The, 148

Melloni's Illustrated Medical Dictionary, 120

Membership lists of professional health associations, 6

Menière's disease, 42, 187

Mental Development, 90

Mental disorders, diagnostic descriptions, 88

MENTAL HEALTH ABSTRACTS, 169

Mental health agencies and institutions, 81, 280

Mental Health Services: Directory, 90

Mental illness, drug treatment case studies, 161

Mental Retardation, 90–91

Mental retardation

explained, 90–91

medical services for children with, 81

research centers, 91

social programs for, 160

treatment centers, directory, 80

Merck Index: An Encyclopedia of Chemicals, Drugs, and Biologicals, The, 140

Merck Manual of Diagnosis and Therapy, The, 140

Michigan Medical Society, 210

Midwifery, the practice of, 179

Milk-restricted diet, 70

Mineral content of foods, 65

Mineral and vitamin supplements for children, nutrient contents, 29

Minerals and vitamins—explanations, sources, daily requirements, and treatment for deficiency, 65

Minnesota Medical Association, 210

Misalignment of vertebrae and discs explained, 16, 17

Mississippi State Medical Association, 210

Missouri State Medical Association, 210

Mobility International, 272

Modern Nutrition in Health and Disease, 140

Montana Medical Association, 211

Mount Sinai Medical Center Family Guide to Dental Health, The, 140–141

MRI explained, 40–41

Multiple births

parents with, self-help groups, 201

statistics on, 201

Multiple sclerosis, latest research on, 188

Muscular dystrophy

diagnosis and treatment, 280

support group, 188

Muscular Dystrophy Association, 243

Muscular sclerosis, current treatment for, 280

Musculoskeletal disorders, 280

Myasthenia gravis, 42, 188

Myasthenia Gravis Foundation, 243

N

Narcolepsy, 188

Narcolepsy and Cataplexy Foundation of America, 244

Narcotics Anonymous, 235

Narcotics Educational Foundation of America, 235

National Aids Information Clearinghouse, 287

National Alliance for the Mentally Ill, 248

National Alliance of Blind Students, 230

National Alliance of Breast Cancer Organizations, 230

National Alopecia Areata Foundation, 238

National Arthritis and Musculoskeletal and Skin Diseases Information Clearinghouse, 287

National Association to Aid Fat Americans, 244

National Association of Disability Examiners, 218

National Association of Insurance Commissioners, 269

National Association for Sickle Cell Disease, 249

National Asthma Center, 228

National Brain Research Association, 230

National Brain Tumor Foundation, 230

National Cancer Institute Cancer Information Service, 288

National Captioning Institute, 233

National Center and Caucus on Black Aged (NCBA), 264

National Center for Education in Maternal and Child Health, 266

National Center for Health Education, 267

National Center for Homecare Education and Research, 225

National Center for Homeopathy, 265

National Child Safety Council, 266
National Cholesterol Education Program NCEP Information Center, 288
National Chronic Pain Outreach Association, 8, 245
  directory of chapters, 82
National Clearinghouse for Alcohol and Drug Information, 288
National Coalition Against the Misuse of Pesticides, 267
National Commission for the Certification for Acupuncture, 255
National Committee for Prevention of Child Abuse, 265
National Continuing Care Directory: Retirement Communities With Nursing Care, 128
National Council Against Health Fraud, 266
National Council on the Aging, 264
National Council on Alcoholism, 226
National Council for International Health, 207
National Council on Patient Information and Education, 267
National Council of Senior Citizens, 264
National Council on Stuttering, 251
National Depressive and Manic Depressive Association, 234
National Diabetes Information Clearinghouse, 288
National Digestive Diseases Information Clearinghouse, 289
National Down's Syndrome Society, 235
National Easter Seal Society, 229
National Eye Institute Information Center, 289
National Eye Research Foundation, 236
National Federation of Parents for Drug-Free Youth, 235
National Fitness Foundation, 269
National Foundation of Dentistry for the Handicapped, 257
National Foundation for Ectodermal Dysplasia, 250
National Foundation for Ileitis and Colitis, 8, 232
National Foundation for Ileitis and Colitis—Foundation Focus, 148
National Foundation for Infectious Diseases, 239
National Gaucher Foundation, 237
National Head Injury Foundation, 238
National Headache Foundation, 238
National Headache Foundation—Newsletter, 148–149
National Health Council, 205
National Health Directory, 128
National Health Information Center, 289
National Healthcare Anti-Fraud Association, 269
National Hearing Aid Society, 233
National Heart, Lung, and Blood Institute Information Center, 289–290
National Hemophilia Foundation, 239
National Hypoglycemia Association, 240
National Indian Council on Aging, 264
National Information Center for Orphan Drugs and Rare Diseases, 247
National Institute on Aging Information Center, 290
National Institute of Allergy and Infectious Diseases, 290
National Institute of Child Health and Human Development Information Center, 290
National Institute on Deafness and Other Communication Disorders Clearinghouse, 290–291
National Institute of Dental Research Information Center, 291
National Institute of Mental Health Public Inquiries Branch, 291
National Institute of Neurological Disorders and Stroke, 291

National Institutes of Health, how to get treatment from, 80
National Insurance Consumer Organization, 270
National Kidney Foundation, 240
National Kidney and Urologic Diseases Information Clearinghouse, 291
National League of Nursing, 207
National Leukemia Association, 241
National Lipid Diseases Foundation, 241
National Lupus Erythematosus Foundation, 242
National Marfan Foundation, 243
National Multiple Sclerosis Society, 243
National Neurofibromatosis Foundation, 244
National Odd Shoe Exchange, 255
National Organization of Mothers of Twins Clubs, 272
National Organization for Rare Disorders, 247
National Osteoporosis Foundation, 245
National Pacific/Asian Resource Center on Aging, 264
National Parent-Teachers Association, 225
National Parkinson Association, 246
National Rehabilitation Association, 271
National Retinitis Pigmentosa Foundation, 247
National Reye's Syndrome Foundation, 247
National Safe Workplace Institute, 273
National Scoliosis Foundation, 248
National Second Surgical Opinion Program, 292
National Self-Help Clearinghouse, 267
National Sickle Cell Disease Program, 292
National Society for Children and Adults with Autism, 228
National Society to Prevent Blindness, 230
National Spinal Cord Injury Association, 251
National Stroke Association, 252
National Sudden Infant Death Syndrome Foundation, 252
National Tay Sach's and Allied Diseases Association, 253
National Tuberous Sclerosis Association, 254
National Vitiligo Foundation, 254
National Wheelchair Athletic Association, 271
National Wheelchair Basketball Association, 271
Natural Health, Natural Medicine: A Comprehensive Manual for Wellness and Self-Care, 115
Natural Medicine, 15–16
Natural Medicine Practitioners, 84
Natural medicine treatment programs for specific ailments, 48
Naturopathic medicine
  explained, 196
  source of names of practitioners, 84, 196
Nebraska Medical Association, 211
Neck, chiropractic recommendations for exercising muscles in the, 94
Neonatal intensive care units, 76
Neurofibromatosis, genetic testing for, 188
Neurological and neuromuscular disorders in children, 23
Nevada State Medical Association, 211
New Family Medical Guide, 141
New Hampshire Medical Society, 211
New Mexico Medical Society, 211
Newborn baby, items needed for, 31
Newborn infants
  normal physical characteristics, 17
  potential health problems, 22
Newsletters
  medical, bibliography with publishers, 87, 145
  on natural health care, 16
  re the elderly, 14
Newsletters in Print, 109

9479 Questionable Doctors: Disciplined by States or the Federal Government, 120–121
Non-toxic substances, 95
North American Riding for the Handicapped Association, 271
North Carolina Medical Society, 211
North Dakota Medical Association, 211
NURSING AND ALLIED HEALTH, 169
Nursing care for an individual disease or disorder, 155
Nursing education, 180
Nursing home administrator examining boards, by state, 10
Nursing homes, 78
  accreditation, 174
  checklist of selection considerations, 78
  classified by type of sponsor, 78
  corporate, headquarters' addresses and telephone numbers, 78
  directory with descriptive profiles, 78
Nursing profession, 179
Nutrient deficiency and the immune system, 46
Nutrients, food sources, 66
Nutrients and Dietary Guidelines, 29–30
Nutrition Almanac, 141
Nutrition, daily, ways to improve, 200
Nutrition: Disorders and Diseases, 67–68
Nutrition guidelines for athletes, 69
Nutrition and individual diseases, 69
Nutritional and health food products used to prevent or treat diseases, newsletter, 67
Nutritional, proper, practices during pregnancy, 69–70
Nutritional disorders explained, 67
Nutritional requirements for supporting different disease and medical disorder therapies, 157
Nutritional Standards, 68–69

O

Obesity
  health risks, 280
  support groups, 188
  surgical treatment for, 195
Obsessive compulsive neurosis, 42, 188
Obstetrician, guidelines for selecting, 86
Occupational health and safety, newsletter, 73
Occupational medicine, physicians specializing in, 178
OCCUPATIONAL SAFETY AND HEALTH, 169–170
Occupational safety and health, legal issues in the workplace, 160
Occupational Safety and Health Reporter, 149
Occupational Stress, 149
Occupational stress, newsletter, 91
Occupational stress and legal recourse, newsletter, 92
Occupations, health hazards of selected, 283
OCD Foundation, The, 245
Office on Smoking and Health Technical Information Center, 292
Ohio State Medical Association, 211
Oklahoma State Medical Association, 212
Old Enough to Feel Better: A Medical Guide For Seniors, 115
Older Women's League, 265
Once A Month: The Original Premenstrual Syndrome Handbook, 115–116
Ophthalmologist, guidelines for selecting, 86
Optical supply houses and manufacturers, directory, 83
Optometric associations (state), addresses and telephone numbers, 7
Optometric boards of examiners, by state, 10
Optometrists

education and training of, 180
  national directory, 84
Optometrists: Listings, 84
Oral and maxillofacial surgery explained, 37
Oral Features, 37–38
Oral tumors, how to detect, 36
Oregon Medical Association, 212
Organ and tissue transplantation donation, newsletter, 29, 54
Organ donations, procedure for making, 201
Organ transplantation
  ethical issues, 164
  latest research on, 201
  survival statistics, 282
Organizations for diseases and disorders, addresses and telephone numbers, 5–6, 152, 224–254
Organizations and government agencies that protect or advocate consumer health rights, 7, 197, 199
Organizations specializing in information about prenatal care and health care for children, 5, 197
Orphan drugs, availability, 198
Orthodontic appliances explained, 33
Orthodontic treatment for adults, 154
Orton Dyslexia Society, 235
OSHA, summary of major federal cases, 92
OSHA's safety and health standards, 73
Osteogenesis imperfecta, 42, 188
Osteogenesis Imperfecta Foundation, 245
Osteopathic hospitals
  addresses and telephone numbers, 76
  U.S. listing with addresses and telephone numbers, 16
Osteopathic Medicine, 16
Osteopathic physicians
  education and training of, 180
  national directory, 85
  state licensing boards for, 9
Osteopathic specialty certifying boards, 9
Osteopathy as therapy for selected health conditions, 15
Osteopathy
  explained, 15
  source of names of practitioners, 84
Osteoporosis explained, 44, 154, 188, 280
Osteoporosis: The Silent Thief, 116
Ostomies, support group, 195
Outpatient facility, guidelines for selecting, 75
Overcoming Bladder Disorders, 116
Overuse sports injuries explained, 93
Oxbridge Directory of Newsletters, 109

P

Pacifiers, use of, 31
Paget's disease, 42, 188
Paget's Disease Foundation, 245
Pain, recent research findings on, 188
Pain control, dental, 35
Pain treatment centers, directory, 82
Pancreatic transplants, 195, 282
Parkinson Support Group of America, 246
Parkinson's disease, newsletter, 54
Parkinson's disease explained, 47, 154, 189, 281
Parkinson's Disease Foundation—Newsletter, 149
PASS Group (Panic Attack Sufferers' Support Group), 225
Paternity and DNA fingerprints, 98
Patient's Guide to Medical Tests, The, 141
Patients' rights, 72, 160, 198
PDQ: PATIENT INFORMATION FILE, 170

PDQ PROTOCOL FILE, 170
Peak flow meter, how to use, 19
Peak flow rates for asthmatic children, 20
Pediatric brain disorders, support groups, 182
Pediatric emergency calls, prior information to assemble, 27
Pediatric emergency explained, 26
Pediatric illnesses, hospitals and clinics specializing in severe, 76
Pediatric surgical procedures explained, 102–103, 195
Pediatrician, guidelines for selecting a, 26
Pennsylvania Medical Society, 212
People's Book of Medical Tests, The, 141–142
Periodontal disease explained, 36
PET explained, 40–41
Pharmaceutical manufacturers abroad, 11
Pharmaceuticals, calorie content, 55
Pharmacists, education of, 180
Phobia Society of America—Newsletter, 149
Phobias, types of, 89
Phobic disorders, newsletter, 91
Physical fitness of adolescents, articles about, 162
Physical fitness of children, measurements, of, 162, 199
Physical fitness programs for the elderly, 162, 199
Physical medicine and rehabilitation, physicians practicing in, 178
Physical rehabilitation centers (inpatient), listing, 97
Physical therapists, education and training of, 180
Physical therapy for the disabled, 154
Physician, personal, questions to ask when interviewing a, 86
Physician disciplinary records, by state, 10
Physician information centers worldwide, 85, 178, 179
Physician Licensure and Certification, 174–177, 312–321
Physician Rights and Responsibilities, 84
Physician training, 85
Physicians
  biographical information, 84, 174
  Canadian, addresses and training of, 178
  disciplined, 85
  English, addresses and training of, 178
  English-speaking, in specified foreign countries, 85, 178
  filing complaints against, 176, 312–321
  in Foreign Countries, 178–179
  how to check qualifications, 85
  Mexican, addresses and training of, 178
  national directory, 84, 174
  in Specific Practices, 178
  U.S., temporarily located in foreign countries, addresses, 84, 179
  U.S., volunteering to practice in foreign countries, 179
  when and how to change, 86
Physicians' Desk Reference (PDR), 142
Physicians' Desk Reference for Nonprescription Drugs, 142
Physicians and Surgeons: Listings and Specialties, 84–85
Planned Parenthood Federation of America, 206
Plastic surgery. *See* Cosmetic surgery
Plastic surgery clinics, accreditation, 174
Playground safety checklist, 31
PMS: A Positive Program to Gain Control, 116
Podiatrists, education and training of, 180
Poison Control Centers, 78
Poisoning of children, types and treatment, 24
Poisons
  common poisonings of children with symptoms and treatment, 95

symptoms and physician response to specific, 96
Polio Survivors Association, 246
Pollen calendar by state, 24, 48
Pollen and spores in different U.S. cities, 24, 48
Porphyria, 42, 189
Post-Polio League for Information, 246
Post-polio symptoms, 189
Potassium, foods high in, 65
Potsmokers Anonymous, 235
PPOs
  addresses and telephone numbers, 7
  explained, 7
Pregnancy
  childbirth explained, 101
  distinguishing between true and false labor, 101
  exercising during, 101, 189
  factors that may cause a high risk, 101
  FDA safety ratings for use of specific drugs during, 100
  fetal developmental phases, 99
  how to reduce sickness during, 101
  level of alcohol consumption and risk to fetus, 100
  medical tests administered, 99
  methods for preventing, 99
  physical and emotional changes, 99
  potential complications, 100
  proper nutritional practices, 69–70
  recommended dietary allowances, 100
  risks from video display terminals, 201
  signs of, 98
  test products, descriptions, 98
  tests, how to perform and interpret at home, 98
  use of specific medicines during, 100, 156, 163
  warning signs justifying physician's attention, 101
  weight gain, 99–100
  what to do during emergency childbirth, 101
Premenstrual syndrome
  clinics and support groups, by state, 8, 189
  coping with and controlling emotional effects, 89
  dietary guidelines for, 67
  explained, 49, 154
  as a legal defense, 72
  self-diagnostic questionnaire, 41
  and sexuality, 102
Premenstrual Syndrome Action, 246
Prenatal visit, information checklist in preparation for, 99
Prescriptions, 59
  abbreviations and terms explained, 31–32
Presidents Council on Physical Fitness and Sports, 269
Principal International Businesses, 128
Professional Training, 85
Prostate enlargement, treatment for, 281
Prostheses
  evaluation of, 82, 158
  explanation of new, 159
Protein
  high, diet guidelines for, 71
  low, diet with, 71
Protein content per serving, 65
Psychiatrists, education and training, of, 178
Psychoanalysts, education and training of, 178
Psychological problems of youth, 89
Psychological therapies and their ethical considerations, 160
Psychologists, addresses and telephone numbers, 180
Psychoses, types explained, 88
Psychosomatic medicine, physicians practicing, 178
PSYCINFO, 170
Public Citizen Health Research Group, 267

Public health laws of the individual states, 321–330
Public Voice for Food and Health Policy, 270
Publications, health fact-sheets and pamphlets, 153
Publications in-print in the health sciences, 86
Puerto Rico Medical Association, 213
Pulse rate, measuring and interpreting, 19, 41

Q

Quality Control, 85
Questions, medical inquiries that will elicit information needed, 52
Questions to ask a pediatrician, 27

R

Rachel Carson Council, 267
Radiation (external) therapy, side effects, 25, 46
Radiologic tests, safety of, 282
Radiological Society of North America, 221
Radiology, therapeutic, current research on, 195
Ragweed density by state, 24, 48
Raising the young child, guidelines, 30
Rare diseases, current therapies for, 189
Rare skin disorders, 190
Readers' Guide to Periodical Literature, 106–107
Rearing the Child, 30
Recipes emphasizing natural ingredients, 70
Recommended Dietary Allowances, 116
Recommended Dietary Allowances (RDAs), daily, 68
Recommended Dietary Allowances (RDAs) during pregnancy, 68
Recommended Dietary Allowances for minerals and vitamins, 29
Rectal temperatures (child), interpretation, 62
Regurgitation by babies, 22
REHAB: A Comprehensive Guide to Recommended Drug-Alcohol Treatment Centers in the United States, 128
Rehab Developments, 97
REHABDATA, 170
Rehabilitation
   changes in the field of, 97
   exercises, how to perform, 96
   federal laws, 72
   programs and facilities, 81, 200, 279
   robotics used in, 82
Rehabilitation engineering centers for technological developments, 83
Rehabilitation International, 271
Reproduction, 98–101
Reproductive technology, ethical considerations, 163
Research Centers Directory, 128–129
Research centers in the medical and health sciences, 12, 158
Resolve, 237
Respiratory diseases, 42, 189, 281
Retinal disorders, laser surgery, 194, 282
Retinitis pigmentosa, support group, 189
Retirement, economic and psychological adjustment to, 157
Reye's syndrome, 42, 189
Rheumatism, 42, 189
Rhode Island Medical Society, 212
Right to die, 198
Root canal therapy explained, 35
Royal College of Physicians, 214
Royal College of Surgeons, 214

S

Safety Guidelines, 30–31
Safety issues, 197–198
Safety Standards, 73
Salicylate content of foods, 65
Salt, low, diet guidelines, 70
Sarcoidosis Family Aid and Research Foundation, 248
Sarcoidosis, support group, 189
Schizophrenia
   new drug therapies, 189–190
   treatment programs for, 90, 281
Schools for blind and visually-impaired children, 39
Schools for deaf and hearing-impaired children, 39
Schools
   health services and health education programs, 197
   Organizations, and Services (for the disabled), 39
SCIENTIFIC AMERICAN MEDICINE, 170–171
Scleroderma, 42, 190
Scoliosis, recent research findings on, 190
Scoliosis Association, The, 248
Second medical opinion
   assistance locating a surgeon for a, 282
   when to consider, 50
Seizures described, 23
Selecting A Health Professional, 85–86
Selecting Professional Care (pregnancy), 101
Self-diagnostic medical tests explained, 41
Self-help organizations and support groups, addresses and telephone numbers, 79, 181, 182, 183, 185, 188, 189, 190, 191, 192, 195, 198, 201
Self-Help Organizations, 79
Self-Help for Premenstrual Syndrome, 117
Sexual dysfunction clinics, listing, 101
Sexual dysfunction, research studies on treatment of, 163
Sexuality, 101–102
Sexuality and premenstrual syndrome, 102
Sexually transmitted diseases, 42, 190, 192, 281
SHHH (Self Help for Hard of Hearing People), 233
Sibling rivalry, guidelines for managing, 30
Sick building syndrome, 201
Sickle cell disease, latest research on treatment of, 190, 281
SIDS
   explained, 22, 154
   support group, 191
SIECUS (Sex Information and Education Council of the US), 225
Sign Language for medical and dental terms, 33
Simon Foundation, 254
Sinusitis, 42, 190, 195
Sjögren's syndrome, support group, 190
Sjögren's Syndrome Foundation, 249
Skin aging, 13
Skin Cancer Foundation, 250
Skin problems
   answers for, 21, 44
   psychosocial factors, 281
   sports related, 94
Sleep disorders explained, 49, 190
Sleeping pattern, baby, 26
Smoke, second-hand, adverse effects on children, 162
Smoking and disease, court cases, 160
SMOKING AND HEALTH, 171
Smoking
   how to stop, 45, 283
   hypnosis therapy, 194
   related health problems, 156
Snakes, poisonous, worldwide, 96

Society for the Advancement of Travel for the Handicapped, 272
Society for Investigative Dermatology, 218
Society of Thoracic Surgeons, 224
Society for Vascular Surgery, 204
Soft diet, suggestions for, 71
South Carolina Medical Association, 212
South Dakota State Medical Association, 212
Special Diets and Controls, 69–71, 199
Specialists, medical, national directory, 84, 174–176
Speech disorders, therapy for, 281
Speech-language pathology, rehabilitation programs, 81, 191
Sperm banks, directory, 80, 201
Spina bifida, support group, 191
Spina Bifida Association of America, 251
Spinal cord injuries
    drug therapy for, 191
    latest treatment for, 281
    newsletter, 54
Spinal Cord Injury Life, 149
Spinal Cord Society, 251
SPORT, 171
Sports
    children's participation in, 93, 163
    for children, organized, guidance for adults involved with, 93
    for the disabled, articles on, 154
    and the disabled child, 39, 162
    diseases/medical disorders and the athlete, 22
    health issues regarding participation of girls and women, 95
    how to involve disabled children in, 93, 154, 200
    injuries
        causes and treatment of specific, 93, 163, 191, 195, 281
        common to specific, 93
        and fitness, organizations providing services regarding, 8
        how to prevent, 93
        newsletter, 95
    medical conditions that may prevent participation, 93
    medicine, hospitals and clinics specializing in, 76
    organizations for disabled persons, 8, 200
    overuse injuries, prevention, control, and treatment, 93
    stress and psychological injuries, 94
    team, how to modify for disabled children, 93
Sports Health: The Complete Book of Athletic Injuries, 142
Sports Medicine Digest, 149
Sports-related diseases and medical disorders explained, 48
Sportswise: An Essential Guide for Young Adult Athletes, Parents, and Coaches, 117
Stained teeth, treatments, 36
Standards for health care facilities, 158
State Administrative Officials Classified by Function, 129
State Executive Directory Annual, 129
State Medical Society of Wisconsin, 213
Stedman's Medical Dictionary, 120
Steroids, negative side effects, 58
Story of Impacted Wisdom Teeth, The, 117
Stress, test for, 88
Stress reduction, 281
Stroke
    prevention of, 42, 191, 281
    questions to ask about, 52
Stroke Foundation, The, 252
Strollers, how to use, 31
Stuttering Resource Foundation, 251

Substance Abuse and Kids: A Directory of Education, Information, Prevention, and Early Intervention Programs, 129
Substance abuse by children, parent's guidebook, 25
Substance abuse prevention and education programs, directory, 56
Substance abuse prevention programs for children, directory, 75
Substance Abuse Residential Treatment Centers for Teens, 129–130
Substance abuse treatment programs, directory, 74, 75
Sudden Infant Death Syndrome Clearinghouse, 253
Sugar content of foods, 65
Suicide prevention centers, 88
Suicide, teenage statistics, 198
Summer Camps, 79
Suppliers, 83
    of equipment and devices for persons with disabilities, 38
    of organic produce and herbal products, sources of, 67
Surgery: A Layman's Guide to Common Operations, 142
Surgery
    citations to articles on specific procedures, 164
    different operating procedures explained, 102–103, 163–164, 192, 193, 194, 195, 196
    guidance on deciding whether to undergo, 102
    heart, latest procedures, 194
    questions to ask before undergoing, 52, 102
Surgery On File: Eye, Ear, Nose and Throat Surgery, 143–144
Surgery On File: General Surgery, 144
Surgery On File: Obstetrics and Gynecology, 144
Surgery On File: Orthopedics and Trauma Surgery, 144–145
Surgery On File: Pediatrics, 145
Surgery: Yes or No?, 142
Surgical Procedures, 102–103
Surgical procedures to treat cancer, newest techniques, 164
Surgical versus non-surgical approaches to specific disorders, 102
Surgicenters, accreditation, 174
Surrogate Parent Foundation, 273
Surrogate parenthood, legal aspects, 201
Surviving With AIDS: A Comprehensive Program of Nutritional Co-Therapy, 117
Sutures, surgical, different types illustrated, 103
Symptoms
    illness or medical disorder that is indicated, 20, 42
    in infants for which a doctor should be called, 21
    their causes and what to do about them, 42

T

Tablets, identification of, 55
Take This Book to the Hospital With You, 117–118
Tattoo removal, 45
Tay Sach's disease, 42, 191
Teeth
    crowded and crooked, treatment, 36
    development schedule, 38
    how to clean, 34
    primary and secondary, depiction, 38
Temperature, measuring and interpreting, 19, 41
Temporomandibular disorders explained, 37, 191
Tennessee Medical Association, 212
Tension Relief, 92
Terms and Phrases, 32–33
Tests, diagnostic
    abnormal results explained, 19, 40